MORPHOGENESIS AND PATTERN FORMATION

Morphogenesis and Pattern Formation

Editors

Thomas G. Connelly
Department of Anatomy and
Center for Human Growth
and Development
University of Michigan Medical School
Ann Arbor, Michigan

Linda L. Brinkley
Department of Anatomy
University of Michigan Medical School
Ann Arbor, Michigan

Bruce M. Carlson
Departments of Anatomy
and Biological Sciences
University of Michigan Medical School
Ann Arbor, Michigan

Raven Press ■ New York

Raven Press, 1140 Avenue of the Americas, New York New York 10036

Made in the United States of America

International Standard Book Number 0-89004-635-2
Library of Congress Catalog Number 80-5538

Great care has been taken to maintain the accuracy of the information contained in the volume. However, Raven Press cannot be held responsible for errors or for any consequences arising from the use of the information contained herein.

Materials appearing in this book prepared by individuals as part of their official duties as U.S. Government employees are not covered by the above-mentioned copyright.

Library of Congress Cataloging in Publication Data
Main entry under title:

Morphogenesis and pattern formation.

Proceedings of a Symposium on Morphogenesis and Pattern Formation, held in Ann Arbor, Mich., Apr. 11-13, 1980, which was organized through the Center for Human Growth and Development, University of Michigan.
Includes bibliographies and index.
1. Morphogenesis–Congresses. I. Connelly, Thomas G. II. Brinkley, Linda L. III. Carlson, Bruce M. IV. Symposium on Morphogenesis and Pattern Formation (1980: Ann Arbor, Mich.) V. University of Michigan. Center for Human Growth and Development. **VI.** Title.
QH491.M67   611'.013   80-5538
ISBN 0-89004-635-2   AACR2

PREFACE

Morphogenesis, although an old field, has experienced a revival and a resurgence of research activity during the past decade. This is due to both new ways of looking at old problems and the availability of new methods of examining morphogenetic systems. In some areas of morphogenesis the development of hypothetical model systems has been a dominant approach whereas in others the experimental approach has been widely used. Commonly, the production and interpretation of abnormal form has been a valuable tool in clarifying morphogenetic mechanisms.

This volume reports the proceedings of the Symposium on Morphogenesis and Pattern Formation, which was organized through the Center for Human Growth and Development at the University of Michigan. One of the Center's major objectives is to stimulate new directions in research or outlook by bringing together people from different disciplines who are working on similar problems, but from different points of view. One of the goals of this symposium was to provide for the interaction of people who conduct laboratory or theoretical research on normal morphogenesis and those who must deal with the consequences of abnormal morphogenesis in the clinical setting. This was accomplished not only by the formal presentations but also by discussion periods. Much of the discussion material has been recorded in this volume. We hope that the inclusion of the discussion sessions will help to convey the spirit of excitement which prevailed during the entire meeting and added much to the element of dynamism associated with the study of emerging form in developing systems.

Thomas G. Connelly
Linda L. Brinkley
Bruce M. Carlson

ACKNOWLEDGMENTS

The editors thank the University of Michigan Center for Human Growth and Development and its director, Dr. Robert E. Moyers, for continuing support in both organizing the symposium and preparing the subsequent proceedings. In order to achieve its objectives, the symposium was organized as a continuing education course in collaboration with the Department of Postgraduate Medicine at the University of Michigan. We are indebted to the Department for making available the excellent facilities of the Towsley Center for Continuing Medical Education and to Dr. Robert Means and his staff for their capable help in planning and executing the meeting.

The organizers and attendees were disappointed that Dr. Jan Langman was unable to address the group due to illness. We hope that the three rousing cheers to his health led by Dr. David Smith helped speed him on the road to recovery. We were grateful to Dr. Eugene Perrin for filling in for Dr. Langman on short notice.

We must express appreciation to Ms. Kathy Ribbens, Ms. Hattie Robertson, and Ms. Barbara Nesbitt for their help in preparing the final manuscripts of the symposium talks and discussion, and to Ms. Rachel Must for transcribing the taped discussions. We thank Mr. Ken Guire for his help in dealing with the computer-assisted text processing system of the University of Michigan and Wayne State University Computer Systems, and Mr. John Beckerman and Mr. William Brudon for their help with the artwork associated with the proceedings.

Contents

vii

IV: Dysmorphogenesis

V: Modeling of Morphogenesis

Contributors

Merton R. Bernfield
Department of Pediatrics
Stanford University School of Medicine
Stanford, California 94305

Fred L. Bookstein
Center for Human Growth and
*   Development*
University of Michigan
Ann Arbor, Michigan 48109

Bruce M. Carlson
Department of Anatomy & Division of
*   Biological Sciences*
University of Michigan
Ann Arbor, Michigan 48109

Verne S. Caviness, Jr.
Department of Neurology
Eunice Kennedy Shriver Center
Waltham, Massachusetts 02154

Philippe Evrard
Department of Neurology
Eunice Kennedy Shriver Center
Waltham, Massachusetts 02154

John F. Fallon
Department of Anatomy
University of Wisconsin
School of Medicine
Madison, Wisconsin 53706

H. L. Frisch
Departments of Chemistry & Physics
State University of New York at Albany
Albany, New York 12222

Salome Gluecksohn-Waelsch
Department of Genetics
Albert Einstein College of Medicine
Bronx, New York 10461

Antone G. Jacobson
Department of Zoology
University of Texas at Austin
Austin, Texas 78712

Marketta Karkinen-Jaaskelainen
Department of Pathology
University of Helsinki
Helsinki, Finland

Robert O. Kelley
Department of Anatomy
University of New Mexico
School of Medicine
Albuquerque, New Mexico 87131

Edward J. Kollar
Department of Dental Medicine
University of Connecticut Health Center
Farmington, Connecticut 06032

Stuart A. Newman
Department of Anatomy
New York Medical College
Valhalla, New York 10595

Mary Ann Perle
Genetics Division
Department of Pediatrics
Children's Hospital Medical Center
Boston, Massachusetts 02115

M. Cecilia Pinto-Lord
Department of Neurology
Eunice Kennedy Shriver Center
Waltham, Massachusetts 02154

Lauri Saxén
Department of Pathology
University of Helsinki
Helsinki, Finland

David W. Smith
Dysmorphology Unit
Department of Pediatrics
Child Development & Mental
*   Retardation Center and the*
Center for Inherited Diseases
University of Washington
School of Medicine
Seattle, Washington 98195

Malcolm S. Steinberg
Department of Biology
Princeton University
Princeton, New Jersey 08544

James J. Tomasek
Department of Anatomy
Harvard Medical School
Boston, Massachusetts 02115

L. Wolpert
Department of Biology as Applied to
  Medicine
Middlesex Hospital Medical School
London W1P 6DB, United Kingdom

Morphogenesis and Pattern Formation,
edited by T. G. Connelly et al.,
Raven Press, New York © 1981.

Introduction

Bruce M. Carlson

Department of Anatomy and Division of Biological Sciences, University of Michigan, Ann Arbor, Michigan 48109

Most living beings start out their life as a tiny sphere -- the fertilized egg. From such a geometrically simple, single cell the developing organism must create a vast array of complex structures. The genesis of form is accomplished in a variety of ways, many of which will be dealt with in considerable detail by the participants in this symposium. As a brief introduction, I would like to review certain aspects of early embryogenesis in vertebrates, with particular emphasis on processes and properties that are particularly relevant to pattern formation and morphogenesis.

At the time of fertilization, the genetic material contained in the two haploid gametes is combined to permit the expression of a certain degree of genetic diversity within the overall constraints of species specificity and the traits that characterize strains or races within the species. While permitting diversity, the same diploid genetic constitution protects the embryo from the untoward effects of most deleterious genes. Somewhere, within the fertilized ovum is essentially all of the information that is required to construct an adult individual. The extent to which the information contained within the DNA of the zygote interacts with other components of the system to produce specific form is little understood and remains one of the central problems of morphogenesis.

One of the earliest, and most critical events of early embryogenesis is the establishment of polarity. In a number of vertebrate groups, particularly those whose eggs contain significant amounts of yolk, polarity, at least along one axis, is inherent in the unfertilized egg. Other axes (traditionally viewed in the Cartesian coordinate system) may be established on

1

the basis of the site of sperm penetration, or possibly even factors extrinsic to the egg or embryo. There is evidence that polarity in mammalian embryos is not fixed until late in the cleavage period. Whenever it occurs and whatever the coordinate system, the existence of an overall reference system (axes) has been an intrinsic feature of a number of general theories of morphogenesis and pattern formation.

The period of cleavage, sometimes viewed in the past as a relatively uninteresting period in vertebrate embryogenesis, is assuming greater significance, particularly with respect to cellular interactions and molecular biological aspects of development. In addition to these features, cleavage results in a striking increase in the number of cells and the amount of genetic material. The latter is required for differential gene expression at a given time, and a minimum or critical number of cells is required for many morphogenetic phenomena.

In mammalian embryos cleavage leads to the blastocyst stage, at which time an inner mass of largely embryo-forming cells has become distinguished from an outer shell of extraembryonic trophoblastic cells. According to the "inside-outside" hypothesis of Tarkowski and Wroblewska (1) cells of the morula which have no contact with the exterior are destined by virtue of their position within the embryo to form the inner cell mass, whereas those in contact with the exterior will become trophoblast. This is but one example of a positional effect in development. Positional effects, or positional information (3) are often currently viewed as the ability of a cell or group of cells in a morphogenetic field to read their relative positions in that field and then differentiate accordingly.

Regulation is an important property of entire early embryos and of certain developing structures in later embryos. In some respects, regeneration can be looked upon as a post-embryonic manifestation of regulation. Regulation in the early embryo can be looked upon as the ability of the entire embryo to compensate for altered numbers and arrangements of cells. The ability of an experimentally bisected embryo to form two complete individuals has a natural counterpart in identical twinning. The production of single tetraparental (allophenic) embryos by combining the dissociated cells of two embryos is a classical example of a regulative process integrating duplicate information into developmental unity.

It is becoming increasingly apparent that at a given stage of early development small numbers of cells act as clonal sources for major populations of cells seen later in development. How these sources are selected and what happens to the cells that do not serve as clonal sources are major problems of contemporary interest and of considerable relevance to pattern formation and morphogenesis. The small number of cells (as few as three) from the inner cell mass of mammalian embryos that apparently give rise to the tissues of the embryo proper is one example of this phenomenon.

As the embryo approaches the period of gastrulation, profound changes in the cells lead to the formation of distinctly different populations of cells which begin to move, either singly or in aggregates, into different locations relative to one another. Many of the differences among the various kinds of cells in the embryo during gastrulation are reflected in different properties of the cell surface, which in turn are often translated into cell movement (2). The net result of the morphogenetic movements that take place during gastrulation is the forming of the three germ layers of the embryo. The germ layers form the material basis for further embryonic development.

The morphogenetic movements of gastrulation lead to the apposition of groups or sheets of cells with markedly different properties. Some of these groups of cells interact in a way such that the action of one tissue changes the developmental course of another tissue with which it is closely associated. This type of action and reaction constitutes an embryonic induction; a process that initiates the formation of many structures within the embryo. The action of the chordamesoderm (notochord) upon the overlying ectoderm, resulting in formation of the neural plate, is called primary induction, and it is one of the central events in organizing subsequent embryonic development.

Shortly after primary induction and formation of the neural plate, one of the most obvious manifestations of pattern formation appears, namely the sequential formation of pairs of somites alongside the nascent nervous system. There have been many attempts to explain the basis for somite formation, and this phenonomenon remains an important one in our quest for understanding morphogenetic mechanisms.

The subsequent formation of organs and structures highlights other factors controlling morphogenesis. The internal glandular organs form as the result of continuous inductive interactions between an epithelial and a mesenchymal component, but there is much evidence that the interactions are mediated by the extracellular matrix interposed between the cellular components of the system. The relative roles of direct cellular interactions and matrix-mediated interactions in morphogenesis will be a major theme of this symposium.

Another, more specialized system that depends upon epithelio-mesenchymal interactions in its development is the limb bud. In contrast to most glandular organs, highly specific morphology must result from this interaction or the limb will not develop into a functionally useful structure. There is now little doubt that the mesenchymal component of the limb bud is pre-eminent in specifying form, but how this is accomplished is subject to widely varying interpretations. A number of these viewpoints are represented in the presentations of participants in this symposium.

A final process that is critical in this introductory glossary of morphogenetic terms and concepts is growth. Growth, represented by an increase in either cell numbers and/or cell size, is a little explored and often neglected aspect of morphogenesis and development.   A burst of cell proliferation commonly follows an inductive stimulus; thereafter, local variations in growth can have a profound influence upon the ultimate shape of an organ, as well as its size.   A critical element in morphogenesis is how early morphogenetic events are translated into different patterns of growth among groups of cells within the same tissue type.   During most phases of development, growth is profoundly affected by extrinsic factors, and extreme variation in these factors can lead to abnormal development.

The field of morphogenesis is so vast that a single meeting can cover only a small portion of the morphogenetic phenomena that have received significant attention.   This symposium was designed to expose both the speakers and the audience to a selection of well-investigated morphogenetic phenomena and systems with the hope that not only common threads or clear-cut differences among the systems and approaches might be obvious, but some clues toward the genesis of abnormal form might become apparent as well.

REFERFNCES

1.   Tarkowski, A. K. and J. Wroblewska (1967):   J. Embryol. Exp. Morph., 18: 155-180.

2.   Townes, P. L. and J. Holtfreter (1955); J. Exp. Zool., 128: 53-120.

3.   Wolpert, L. (1969):   J. Theoret. Biol. 25: 1-47.

Morphogenesis and Pattern Formation,
edited by T. G. Connelly et al.,
Raven Press, New York © 1981

Positional Information, Pattern Formation, and Morphogenesis

L. Wolpert

Department of Biology as Applied to Medicine, Middlesex Hospital Medical School, London
W1P 6DB, United Kingdom

"Their lives were simple and well regulated and they usually followed in their parents' footsteps. They made few decisions, but when they decided to do something different, this was because of their social position, and childhood experiences. Strangely, they talked little and their language was dull and monotonous, comprising one or two phrases repeated again and again. But they had good memories, and having decided at an early age to change careers, they stuck to it, and were able to carry out a long programme of work. What they knew best, and cared most about, was their inborn potential, their position in society, and their childhood experiences." --N. Kaim

There is an important distinction between pattern formation and morphogenesis, which in its more limited meaning, refers to changes in form. Pattern formation is the process whereby the spatial organization of cellular differentiation is specified, whereas, changes in form involve a process whereby cell sheets change shape or cells move to new positions. In general, pattern formation precedes changes in form since it is by this process that cells are specified so that they will generate the forces that bring about the cellular movements. Thus, in sea urchin gastrulation, the secondary mesenchyme cells provide the force for gastrulation, and these cells are specified earlier by a patterning process (9). In the formation of the neural tube, the specification of the neural cells includes the specification of the generation of forces that will cause the tube to fold (see Jacobson, this volume). Both pattern formation and changes in form are different from cellular differentiation, which is the process by which specialized cells, such as muscle and cartilage, develop, and here the key question is how the synthesis of appropriate luxury molecules are controlled. These distinctions can be illustrated by the arm and leg which contain the same differentiated cell types, yet have substantially different patterns and forms. The differences in skeleto-muscular morphology between vertebrates do not reflect differences in cell differentiation, but in pattern formation. In general, I would suggest that cellular differentiation and changes in form can be considered as the result of cells carrying out a programme of activity that has been specified by the process of pattern formation.

Positional Information

A mechanism for pattern formation is that based upon positional information (45-46, 50). This suggests that the cell states required for pattern formation are specified in a manner analogous to assigning position in a coordinate system. The positional values thus assigned may determine the later behavior of the cell. The cells may interpret the positional information by a particular program of cellular differentiation, or growth, or cell movement, and this will depend on the cell's genetic constitution and developmental history. Positional value, which is a record of the cell's position, is the key parameter in pattern formation, and it underlies the concept of non-equivalence.

Pattern formation using positional information is a two-step process. The cells are assigned a positional value in the positional field and the cells then interpret this. This mechanism has several important implications. Firstly, the observed pattern arises from the interpretation of the gradient in positional values, and the smooth gradient in positional values can give rise to patterns with discontinuities in cell types and behaviors. There need be no obvious correspondence between the observed pattern and the underlying set of positional values. Secondly, and this follows from the previous point, the same positional field can give rise to quite different patterns, since only the interpretation need be altered. It follows that the mechanism for specifying and recording position may be the same in different systems, and universal mechanisms may be involved. Thirdly, the only cell-to-cell interactions required may be those required to specify position. After position is specified, much of the cell's behavior may be autonomous.

Non-equivalence

The principle of non-equivalence says that cells of the same differentiation class may have intrinsically different internal states (such as different positional values) and they will, as a rule, be non-equivalent, if the cells give rise to structures differing in shape or pattern (17). This means that cells are to be characterized, not merely by their histological type, but by other characteristics such as their positional value which can affect, for example, their surface properties or growth. The mesenchyme of the leg and wing buds are non-equivalent since leg tissue grafted into the wing maintains its character, and can form a toe if placed distally (28). In amphibian limb regeneration, the structures that regenerate depend on the level of the cut yet the same classes of cells are present at all the levels.

Non-equivalence means that there are more cell states than is generally recognized. For example, discussion of development in terms of binary choices (12) is almost always couched in terms of overt terminal states, such as muscle and cartilage and neglects positional values. While at any stage of development the number of options open to a cell is restricted, it is not necessarily two, and the specification of a new positional value must be taken into account (48, 52).

Cell Lineage and Cytoplasmic Localization

In insects, segregated cytoplasmic factors can play an important role in specifying germ cells. In the vertebrates such cytoplasmic localization does not seem to play a major role in pattern formation. An exception may be exemplified by amphibian development in which cytoplasmic differences in the egg may be important in defining the major body axes and setting up the boundaries of the coordinates for positional information. In the case of mammals, no differences have been detected between blastomeres up to the 8-cell stage, and the earliest example of pattern formation -- the specification of trophectoderm and inner cell mass -- appears to be position dependent: the cells on the outside form trophectoderm (26). Pattern formation in vertebrates in general seems to arise from position dependent cell-to-cell interactions (4).

Much attention has been given to the importance of cell lineages in development. However, I would argue that cytoplasmic localization apart, where two daughter cells differ from one another, this is invariably due to position dependent cell interactions (48). This in no way excludes the importance of change of state associated with cell lineages, or the importance of cell divisions for such changes as in, for example, quantal mitoses (12). The particular maturation lineage a cell may undergo is part of the program a cell possesses by virtue of its past history and external signals.

The Setting Up of Positional Information

A simple monotonic gradient can provide positional information. For example, if a source is present which releases a diffusible molecule, and if this is broken down at a rate proportional to its concentration, then an exponential concentration gradient will be set up. The concentration at any point effectively provides a measure of distance, and thus acts as a positional signal. The source, in turn, which is kept at a constant concentration can be regarded as the boundary or reference region of the coordinate system. It is not necessary to have the source specified as a discrete unique region. Meinhardt and Gierer (23) have shown how such a gradient can be self-organizing, making use of plausible biochemical reactions. It can comprise two diffusible molecules, an activator which is slowly diffusible and an inhibitor which diffuses more rapidly. The synthesis of the activator includes a positive feedback loop, and its synthesis is inhibited by the inhibitor. The synthesis of the inhibitor is dependent on the concentration of the activator. Such a system will autonomously set up a gradient and the inhibitor concentration could provide the positional signal.

This positional signal must be distinguished from the positional value which can be regarded as the memory or more permanent record of position. Positional signals may be transitory whereas positional values may persist over very long periods.

All the available evidence suggests that when a positional field is being set up the time required is of the order of hours and the distances over which interactions take place small, less than 50 cell diameters (43). This is one of the reasons why Crick (3) suggested that diffusion would be a satisfactory way of setting up a positional field.

There are other ways of setting up positional fields. One class of mechanism makes use of time. The basic idea is that cells can measure time and that under appropriate conditions this can specify their positional values. Thus, in the progress zone model, for the proximo-distal axis of the chick limb we have suggested that cells measure the time they spend in a zone near the tip (36). Since all the cells in this zone are dividing, cells continually leave the zone: those that come out last, and thus farthest away from the body wall, have been in longest. In this way, a gradient in positional values is generated.

Another possible mechanism involves the direct transfer of positional value from one cell to another. For example, it seems that the positional field in the neural plate in amphibia is specified by direct transfer of positional values from the underlying mesodermal tissue. In general, directive or instructive embryonic induction, may be thought of as the direct transfer of positional values from the inducing tissue to the responding one. This usually involves epidermal cells acquiring the positional values of underlying mesoderm.

Positional Information and Chick Limb Development
====

The development of the chick wing can be used to illustrate some of the above concepts (reviewed 43). Here I will briefly consider only two axes, the anteroposterior and the proximodistal, which define a two-dimensional Cartesian positional field (Fig. 1).

Position appears to be specified in a zone at the tip of the limb, we have called the progress zone (36, 53) and we have assumed that this zone, about 350 microns wide, is specified by the apical ectodermal ridge. All the cells in the progress zone are dividing and it is only when the cells have left the progress zone that overt cytodifferentiation can be seen, and development is largely autonomous.

Position along the anteroposterior axis may be specified by a graded signal from the polarizing region (38, 39, 42) which was discovered by Saunders and Gasseling (29). This region is at the posterior margin of the limb bud, and in our model it is the source of a diffusible morphogen whose concentration specifies

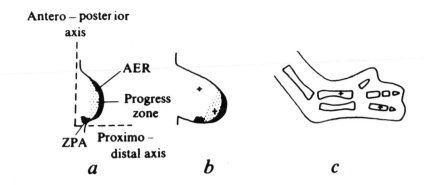

Antero – posterior axis

AER

Progress zone

ZPA   Proximo – distal axis

a   *b*   *c*

FIG. 1. The skeleto-muscular system is laid down in the mesenchyme in a proximo-distal sequence as the bud grows out. It is suggested that cells are assigned positional information in the progress zone, which is beneath the apical ectodermal ridge (AER). Position along that antero-posterior axis appears to be specified by a signal from the polarizing region (ZPA). In (b) two points are marked (+). The one outside the progress zone has already had its positional information specified. The one inside the progress zone is in the process of being specified. At a later stage (c) the cells at these points have interpreted the positional information forming part of the radius and digit 4, respectively (after Tickle et al., (42).

****

position along the anteroposterior axis (Fig. 2). The different digits form at different thresholds. When the polarizing region is grafted to the anterior margin of an early limb bud, it causes the limb to have mirror-image symmetry along the anteroposterior axis. Instead of the normal pattern of digits 2 3 4, the pattern is now 4 3 2 2 3 4. More proximally, there will often be two ulnas side by side, and the pattern of muscles and tendons is also reduplicated (31). Our suggestion is that the signal from the polarizing region has specified new positional values in the anterior region of the limb bud to which it was grafted. If the signal from the polarizing region is a diffusible morphogen, then the concentration at any point will vary with distance from the polarizing region, and in general, we have found this to be the case. Following a graft of a polarizing region to the anterior margin, the limb widens by 50% in 36 hours, and effectively increases the distance between the grafted and host polarizing regions (34). This has the effect of lowering the maximum concentration of morphogen between them. If this widening is prevented by low doses of X-rays then the typical pattern of

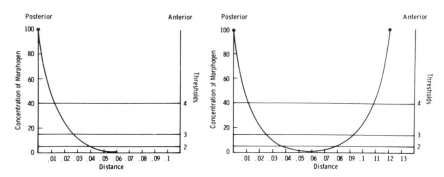

FIG. 2. The concentration of morphogen across the antero-posterior axis of the limb. The polarizing region is represented as a point source at the posterior margin, and the concentration is kept at 100 units. An exponential gradient is set up since the morphogen is assumed to be broken down (left panel). The digits are specified at different thresholds. If an additional polarizing region is grafted at the anterior margin, and the limb widens by a factor of 1.5 then this will result in a pattern of digits 4 3 2 2 3 4 (right panel).

****

digits is 4 3 4. Not only does a new digit 2 not develop, but the host digit 2 is suppressed. We interpret this as a rise in morphogen concentration that results from the widening being suppressed.

Further evidence for a graded signal comes from the following experiments. (1) If the polarizing region is placed so far anterior in the. limb bud that only occasionally an additional digit is specified, this digit is always digit 2, which has the lowest threshold. As the graft is placed in a somewhat more posterior position, digits 3 2 are specified, and eventually 4 3 2 (42). (2) The signal from the polarizing region can be attenuated in several ways. If quail polarizing region is treated with gamma-irradiation and it is then grafted to the anterior margin, the most anterior new digit formed falls from 4 through 3 to 2 (33). Similarly, Tickle (40) has shown that by diluting the number of polarizing region cells with anterior margin cells, similar results can be obtained. She has demonstrated this directly by grafting a monolayer of polarizing region cells beneath the apical ectoderm. About 120 cells were required for digit 4 and only 20 for digit 2.

For the proximo-distal axis the mechanism we have suggested for specifying position is one based on the cells measuring the time they spend in the progress zone (36). Since all the cells in the progress zone are dividing, cells are continually leaving the progress zone and thus those that leave last, have been in the longest and have the most distal positional values. It is possible that the cells measure time by counting cell divisions -- there are about 7 cycles during the laying down of the limb. In this model, the main interaction is between the apical ridge and the underlying mesoderm. If the ridge is removed the progress zone is abolished and depending on the stage, distal positional values cannot be specified, and this leads to the limb being truncated (27).

This mechanism for specifying position along the proximo-distal axis makes predictions as to the effect of killing off cells in the progress zone. In Fig. 3, this is illustrated diagramatically, and shows that if the killing is done at an early stage, proximal structures will be most affected, since, as the progress zone becomes repopulated with successive cell cycles, distal structures will be the most normal. Our experiments involving X-irradiation of early limb buds with doses up to 2,000 rads, on the whole, give the expected results (54) and phocomelic limbs develop. Any treatment which kills off a large number of cells in the early limb bud should result in phocomelia. Application of cytosine arabinoside to mouse embryos at an early stage of limb development has just that effect (16). It may be that thalidomide exerts its effect in this way, possibly by causing haematomas (Poswillo, personal communication).

Universality of Positional Fields

The coordinate system involved in setting up a positional field is analogous to the classical field concept (45). In terms of positional information, a field may be defined as that group of cells whose position is specified with respect to the same set of boundary values. That is they belong to the same coordinate system. There is quite good reason to believe that the basic system for setting up and recording positional values is the same in many different systems and may, in fact, be universal. The difference between different fields would lie in how cells interpret positional information and this of course depends upon the cell's genome and developmental history. The best evidence for this comes from studies on insects where the positional fields of imaginal discs appear to be the same. This can be shown by making genetic mosaics using the technique whereby somatic crossing over is induced. The classical example is the homeotic mutant, aristapaedia. With this mutant, a leg forms in place of the antenna. In mosaics that comprise patches of wild type cells adjacent to cells with the aristapaedia genotype, the cells behave according to their position and their genome (24). This suggests that the positional values, along with the antenna and leg, are the same, but the cells interpret the positional values in leg and antenna differently because they have different developmental histories. For antenna to form, the wild type aristapaedia gene must apparently be activated, presumably because of its position in an earlier positional field. Further evidence comes from

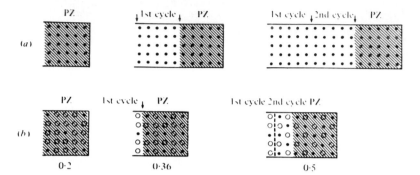

FIG. 3.   A simplified model to show the effect of x-irradiation on
the progress zone. Two discrete cell cycles in the outgrowth of
an idealized limb are shown. In the control (a) 25 cells leave
the progress zone PZ at each cell cycle and these are assumed to
form   a   limb   rudiment such as a humerus, or radius and ulna. In
the irradiated case (b) the open circles represent cells no longer
capable of dividing and the fraction of dividing cells is 0.2.
That is 80% of the cells have been inactivated. At the first cell
cycle only 5 cells come out of the progress zone and only 1 of
these is normal. However, at the next cell cycle, 10 cells will
emerge, of which 5 are normal. Note that the fraction of normal
cells in the progress zone is now 0.5.

****

Bryant (1) who studied intercalary regeneration in imaginal discs
and found that different discs would interact one with the other,
just as if the positional field in each was the same.
    Evidence for identity of positional fields also comes from
studies on the chick limb. Saunders et al., (28) showed that if
proximal tissue from the early leg bud was grafted to the tip of
the developing wing bud, it developed into a toe. This shows that
the grafted tissue could respond to the mechanism in the wing bud
that specifies position along the proximo-distal axis, but it is
interpreted according to its own developmental program. Again,
the polarizing region from wing and leg in the chick are
equivalent.
Moreover, the signal from an homologous region of mouse, man and
turtle appear to give similar signals and can all specify
additional digits in the chick limb (6, 4). We have also just
found that Hensen's node which is equivalent to the dorsal lip of
the blastopore and can signal the mesoderm to form additional
somites (13), can also signal in the chick limb.

Interpretation of Positional Information and Thresholds

In terms of positional information, the process of interpretation is the key step in the development of the pattern, since it is this process that can make the pattern overt. If positional values are specified as a continuous function, the problem is how this is converted into the observed pattern. It seems very likely that any mechanism must involve thresholds: the cells behave in one way if the concentration of some substance is above a particular value, and in another if below it. Given a gradient in a morphogen over say 50 cells, how could thresholds specify the cell states. Our model (18) assumes that the gene can be turned on by a signal provided by a morphogen S and provided the gene product feeds back on itself, then when S increases to a critical threshold concentration, the system suddenly 'jumps' to a new stable state in which the gene remains on even when S is removed. The crucial factor which determines precision of the threshold response is how well the cells can specify their own threshold: that is how well they can control their own concentration of macromolecules. The presence of gap junctions could even out differences in the concentration of a small molecule.

In our model an increasing morphogen concentration will activate additional genes, those activated at lower concentrations remaining turned on. Meinhardt (22) has put forward and analyzed a more complex model in which specific genes are activated at different concentrations of the morphogen. In order to activate just one out of a set of genes at a particular morphogen concentration, it is necessary to introduce a repressor which acts on other genes in the set. In addition, it is also necessary to assume that genes have an overlap and the product of gene g_i, can not only activate gene g_i, but g_{i+1} and g_{i-1}. Then, if there is a hierarchy in the positive feedback loops (autocatalysis) such that gene g_{i+1} is more stimulated by its product, than gene g_i, a stepwise activation of genes will occur with an increase in morphogen concentration. This is an important model as it provides a detailed analysis of how a morphogen can specify genes and may be the first step in recording positional value.

A rather different model for interpretation has been put forward by MacWilliams and Papageorgious (21) and it is capable of generating patterns based on ellipses of varying shape.

Directive Embryonic Inductions and the Direct Transfer of Positional Value

Embryonic induction is classically defined as the interaction between two different tissues such that the behavior of the one is altered. The paradigm is the induction of the nervous system by the underlying mesoderm in amphibian gastrulation. Saxén (30) usefully distinguishes between directive and permissive inductions. In directive inductions, cells are committed to a new pathway of differentiation, whereas with a permissive induction, the cell is already committed but still requires a stimulus to express its new phenotype, as in the induction of kidney tubules.

I wish to suggest that all directive inductions are similar and involve the direct transfer of positional values from the one tissue to the other, and that the responding tissue can then interpret these positional values. It seems that this is the way ectoderm acquires positional values. It differs from the usual way of setting up a field and is a direct transfer from one that is already set up. In these terms embryonic induction is a means of positional signalling. It is a convenient coordinating mechanism for making sure that positional values in adjacent, but different, tissues is the same. If this interpretation is correct then the specificity of the inductive signal bears no relation to the structure induced, and it is possible that the same principles and even molecules may underly all inductions.

The idea of transfer of positional values specifying positional values in primary embryonic induction can be illustrated by two experiments (11). In the first, small pieces of gastrula ectoderm are placed at different positions along the axis of the endomesoderm of an exogastrula. The cephalic end induces brain structures, and the trunk portion a tail. The second experiment relates to homoiogenetic induction. The crucial point is that induction of specific structures can be brought about by the tissues that have already been induced. These tissues can induce structures similar to themselves in adjacent tissues. Thus, after the neural plate has acquired its positional values from the underlying mesoderm it can induce similar structures in competent ectoderm. The neural plate retains up to the stage of the free swimming larva, the power of inducing structures of its own type when grafted to competent embryos.

These ideas may be related to the gradient concepts of induction of the nervous system (44) which is based on gradients of neuralising and mesodermalising factors in the mesoderm. It may be that these gradients represent gradients in positional value. The beautiful experiment of Toivonen and Saxen (44) in which they combined presumptive forebrain with posterior mesoderm and obtained more caudal neural structures might be interpreted as averaging of positional values.

Xenoplastic inductions provide very good evidence for transfer of positional values from the mesoderm to overlying ectoderm (11). The larvae of urodeles and anurans differ in various order-specific structures. The urodeles have a pair of balancers on the ventro-lateral side of the head whereas the anurans have a pair of suckers in a more ventral position. The urodele larva has both whereas the anuran tadpole only horny denticles. When belly ectoderm of an anuran gastrula is transplanted to the prospective head region of a urodele gastrula, it forms suckers and horny denticles in a ventral position. Clearly, it is position that is being specified followed by order-specific interpretation. This is also a nice example of universality of positional fields.

One of the most dramatic demonstrations of position dependent differentiation relates to melanoblasts. Rawles (25) has shown that irrespective of the immediate source of the melanoblasts, if they are introduced into foreign feather germs, the results consistently give a specific colour and pattern in homologous feathers which are characteristic of the donor melanoblasts. Thus, Pheasant melanophores into White Leghorn give the Pheasant pattern. Even when there are sex-linked differences the pattern is consistent with the donor. The obvious interpretation is that the melanophores can acquire the local positional values by template transfer from the ectoderm and are programmed to differentiate in a particular way according to their positional value.

The Program of Growth

It is proposed that the varying patterns of growth in development can be viewed as an aspect of pattern formation, and the different growth programs are specified at an early stage (49). Once the program of growth is specified, it is largely autonomous. It is possible that the program of growth is specified in a manner similar to other aspects of pattern formation. That is the cells interpret their positional values by a particular growth program. For example, in the chick limb, the length of the cartilaginous elements is determined by their initial length and later growth. Since the initial sizes of the elements are more or less the same when they are laid down, differences in size reflect differences in growth. This, in turn, reflects how much the cells divide and enlarge, and how much matrix they secrete. This is well illustrated by a comparison between the wrist elements and the adjacent radius and ulna (35). While the radius and ulna show substantial increase in length, the wrist hardly grows at all which probably is due to the cells in the wrist not increasing in size. This is a good example of the non-equivalence of cartilage. It is even possible that the time of ossification of the growth plates is also specified at this early stage.

There is also considerable evidence for the autonomy of such growth programs. For example, by grafting in the chick limb bud a young progress zone in place of an older one, limbs develop in which elements are repeated in tandem, such as humerus, radius and ulna, humerus, radius and ulna, wrist, digits. In such limbs, the length of the elements always corresponds with the donor embryo, and are unaffected by the host (37). This is similar to the observation of Harrison (10) on chimaeras from salamanders. For example, Ambystoma tigrinum has limbs that develop somewhat later but are ultimately much larger than those of Ambystoma punctatum. Reciprocal transplantation showed that their growth is almost entirely autonomous. If an A. tigrinum limb is grafted to an A. punctatum embryo, its development initially lags behind, but eventually grows to its normal size, resulting in a larva with an absurdly large limb.

While the examples above have emphasized autonomy and lack of interactions there are situations where growth of one element is coordinated with another. Thus, while the pattern of muscles and tendons is specified early in limb development (31) their subsequent growth is coordinated with that of the cartilage and is dependent on it (20). Their growth is dependent on their being stretched by the growing cartilage. If the growth of the cartilage is inhibited (19) or the tendon cut (8) the muscles are shorter.

Pattern Regulation and Regeneration

There is a classical distinction between morphallaxis and epimorphosis. In morphallaxis the missing parts are formed by remodeling what remains in order to form a normal, though smaller system, whereas in epimorphosis the new structures are generated locally by growth. Both may be treated within the context of positional information, since both regulation and regeneration can be viewed as generating new positional values. In morphallaxis positional values may change without cell division as in Hydra (51) whereas in epimorphosis new positional values are generated in association with localized growth, as in amphibian limb regeneration. As Cooke (5) has pointed out the distinction is not absolute and both may be involved in a particular system. Thus, we should concentrate rather on the different processes involved in the generation of the new positional values. Are new boundary regions specified? Over what distance does interaction occur? Is cell division required? Are any positional values lost?

A powerful model for epimorphic regulation has been put forward by French, Bryant and Bryant (7). The model is based on positional values being specified in terms of polar coordinates. For the amphibian limb, for example, the radial axis corresponds to the proximo-distal axis, and the angular coordinate corresponds to a set of values around the circumference of the limb when viewed in transverse section. Two main rules have been proposed (1) when cells are placed next to each other such that positional values, that are normally non-adjacent, are now adjacent, positional values are intercalated by the shortest route, to produce a sequence of positional values such that all discontinuities are removed. (2) More distal positional values are generated during regeneration only when there is a complete set of circumferential positional values: the degree of distal-transformation is related to how complete a set of circular values is present. The rules have been shown to account for a wide range of phenomena in cockroach legs, insect imaginal discs and amphibian limb regeneration, and some surprising predictions have been made. For example, if amphibian limbs are constructed which are symmetrical about the anteroposterior axis, that is they are made of two posterior halves, then there is an incomplete set of circumferential positional values. Such limbs only undergo partial regeneration if amputated after several weeks of healing (2). While there are several aspects of the model particularly in relation to distal transformation which are controversial (32), it has generated a whole new set of experimental and theoretical studies.

An important question is how such a polar coordinate system is set up. My own intuition is that the coordinate system is initially set up as a Cartesian system, but for reasons not yet clearly understood, the system behaves as if it were a polar coordinate system. However, it could be that the initial specification of positional values involves intercalation and a polar coordinate sytem, and Iten and Murphy (15) have suggested that the results of the grafts of the polarizing region discussed above are best understood in this way.

Towards a Molecular Basis

We know nothing about the molecular basis of pattern formation in general, and positional information in particular. Even where there is good evidence for positional signalling involving a diffusible morphogen, direct evidence is lacking, and other possibilities remain. We do not even know the pathway for such signals, or, for example, whether or not gap junctions are involved (47). Thus far it has not been possible to design a suitable assay for isolating a morphogen and our failure is in the grand tradition of the failures to understand the molecular basis of the action of the primary organiser. We can, at this stage, exclude neither ions, such as calcium, nor macromolecules - RNA - as a morphogen. Worse still, we are only beginning to think about the nature of positional value, and how it can program cell behavior. This is the central problem, and it is about how the genome is organized so that the cell responds to simple signals in the appropriate manner in pattern formation. That is, of course, only true if the conceptual framework is correct. If it is, then we are in a position similar to Mendelian genetics at the beginning of the century. We have models that can account for a wide variety of phenomena, but the physical basis is quite unknown. What we need now is a great deal of hard work and not a little luck.

This work is supported by the Medical Research Council.

REFERENCES

1.   Bryant, P. J. (1979): In: Determinants of Spatial Organization, edited by S. Subtelny and I. R. Konigsberg, pp. 295-316, Academic Press, New York.

2. Bryant, S. (1978): In: The Clonal Basis of Development, edited by S. Subtelny and I. M. Sussex, pp. 63-82, Academic Press, New York.
3. Crick, F. H. C. (1970): Nature, 225-420-422.
4. Cooke, J. (1975): Ann. Rev. Biophys. Bioeng., 4:185-217.
5. Cooke, J. (1979): J. Embryol. Exp. Morphol., 51:165-182.
6. Fallon, J. F. and Crosby, G. M. (1977): In: Vertebrate Limb and Somite Morphogenesis, edited by D. A. Ede, J. R. Hinchliffe and M. Balls, pp. 55-71, Cambridge University Press, Cambridge.
7. French, V., Bryant, P. J., and Bryant, S. V. (1976): Science, 193:969-981.
8. Goldspink, G. (1974): In: Differentiation and Growth of Cells in Vertebrate Tissues, edited by G. Goldspink, pp. 69-100, Chapman Hall, London.
9. Gustafson, T. and Wolpert, L. (1967): Biol. Rev., 42:442-498.
10. Harrison, R. F. (1969): Organization and Development of the Embryo, edited by S. Wilens, Yale University Press, New Haven.
11. Holtfreter, J. and Hamburger, V. (1955): In: Analysis of Development, edited by B. N. Willier, P. A. Weiss and V. Hamburger, pp. 230-296, Saunders, Philadelphia.
12. Holtzer, H. (1978): In: Stem Cells and Tissue Homeostasis, edited by B. L. Lord, C. S. Potten and R. J. Cole, pp. 1-28, Cambridge University Press, Cambridge.
13. Hornbruch, A., Summerbell, D., and Wolpert, L. (1979): J. Embryol. Exp. Morphol., 51:51-62.
14. Illmensee, K. (1976): In: Insect Development, edited by P. A. Lawrence, pp. 76-96, Blackwells, Oxford.
15. Iten, L. E. and Murphy, D. J. (1980): Devel. Biol., 75:373-385.
16. Kochhar, D. M. and Agnish, N. D. (1977): Devel. Biol., 61:388-395.
17. Lewis, J. H. and Wolpert, L. (1976): J. Theoret. Biol., 62:479-490.
18. Lewis, T., Slack, J. M. W. and Wolpert, L. (1977): J. Theoret. Biol., 65:579-590.
19. McLachlan, J. (1980): J. Embryol. Exp. Morphol., 55:307-318.
20. McLachlan, J. and Wolpert, L. (1980): In: The Development and Specialization of Muscle, edited by D. F. Goldspink, Cambridge University press, Cambridge (in press).
21. MacWilliams, H. K. and Papageorgiou, S. (1978): J. Theoret. Biol., 72:385-411.
22. Meinhardt, H. (1978): J. Theoret. Biol., 74:307-321.
23. Meinhardt, H. and Gierer, A. (1974): J. Cell Sci., 15:321-346.
24. Postlethwait, J. H. and Schneiderman, H. A. (1974): Ann. Rev. Genet., 7:381-433.
25. Rawles, M. E. (1948): Physiol. Rev., 28:383-408.
26. Rossant, J. (1977): In: Development in Mammals, Vol. 2, edited by M. H. Johnson, pp. 119-150, Elsevier, North Holland

Biomedical Press, Amsterdam.
27. Saunders, J. W. (1948): J. Exp. Zool., 108:363.
28. Saunders, J. W., M. T. Gasseling and J. M. Cairns (1959): Develop. Biol., 1:281.
29. Saunders, J. W. and M. T. Gasseling (1968): In: Epithelial-mesenchymal Interactions, edited by R. Fleischmajer and R. E. Billingham, pp. 78-97, Williams and Wilkins, Baltimore.
30. Saxén, L. (1977): In: Cell and Tissue Interactions, edited by J. W. Lash and M. M. Burger, pp. 1-9, Raven Press, New York.
31. Shellswell, G. B. and L. Wolpert (1977): In: Vertebrate Limb and Somite Morphogenesis, edited by D. A. Ede, J. R. Hinchliffe and M. Balls, pp. 71-87, Cambridge University Press, Cambridge.
32. Slack, J. M. W. (1980): J. Theoret. Biol., 82:105-140.
33. Smith, J. C., C. Tickle, and L. Wolpert (1978): Nature, Lond., 272:612.
34. Smith, J. C. and L. Wolpert (1980): In preparation.
35. Summerbell, D. (1976): Embryol. Exp. Morphol., 35:241.
36. Summerbell, D., J. H. Lewis, and L. Wolpert (1973): Nature, Lond., 244:492.
37. Summerbell, D. and J. H. Lewis (1975): J. Embryol. Exp. Morphol., 33:621.
38. Summerbell, D. and C. Tickle (1977): In: Vertebrate Limb and Somite Morphogenesis, edited by D. A. Ede, J. R. Hinchliffe and M. Balls, pp. 41-55, Cambridge University Press, Cambridge.
39. Tickle, C. (1980): In: Development in Mammals, Vol. 4, edited by M. H. Johnson, Elsevier, Amsterdam.
40. Tickle, C. (1980): In preparation.
41. Tickle, C., G. Shellswell, A. Crawley and L. Wolpert (1976): Nature, Lond., 259:396.
42. Tickle, C., D. Summerbell, and L. Wolpert (1975): Nature, Lond., 254:199.
43. Tickle, C. and L. Wolpert (1980): In: Scientific Foundations of Paediatrics, Second Edition, edited by J. Dobbing and J. Davis, Heinemann, London (in press).
44. Toivonen, S. and L. Saxén (1968): Science (US), 159:539-546.
45. Wolpert, L. (1969): J. Theoret. Biol., 25:1-47.
46. Wolpert, L. (1971): Current Top. Devel. Biol., 6:183.
47. Wolpert, L. (1977): In: Intercellular Junctions and Synapses in Development, edited by J. D. Feldman, N. B. Gilula and J. D. Pitts, pp. 83-96, Chapman and Hall, London.
48. Wolpert, I. (1978): In: Stem Cells and Tissue Homeostasis, edited by B. I. Lord, C. S. Potten and R. J. Cole, pp. 29-48, Cambridge University Press, Cambridge.
49. Wolpert, L. (1978): In: Paediatrics and Growth. Report of the 5th Unigate Paediatric Workship, edited by D. Barltrop, pp. 15-24, Blackwells, Oxford.
50. Wolpert, L. (1978): Sci. Amer., 239:154-164.
51. Wolpert, L., A. Hornbruch, and M. R. B. Clarke (1974):

    Amer. Zool., 14:647-663.

52.   Wolpert, L. and J. H. Lewis (1975): Fed. Proc., 34:14-20.
53.   Wolpert, L., J. H. Lewis, and D. Summerbell (1975): In: Cell Patterning, Ciba Foundation Symposium, 29, edited by R. Porter and J. Rivers, pp. 95-130, Elsevier, Amsterdam.
54.   Wolpert, L., Tickle. C., and Sampford, M. (1979): J. Embryol. Exp. Morphol., 50:175.

Morphogenesis and Pattern Formation,
edited by T. G. Connelly et al.,
Raven Press, New York © 1981.

Biology and Pathology of Embryonic Induction

Lauri Saxén and Marketta Karkinen-Jaaskelainen

Department of Pathology, University of Helsinki, Helsinki, Finland

Differentiation of cells during embryogenesis is reflected in the appearance of new phenotypic characteristics and the restriction of developmental options. At the tissue level, this is followed by morphogenesis, the organization of cells into organ anlagen composed of several types of cells which are spatially strictly arranged to ensure a functional entity. The selection of certain phenotypes from the genetically homogenous cell population and the organization of them into organs and tissues is under constant guidance of various epigenetic control systems. Along with organismal factors like hormones, growth factors and the unknown forces operative in "positional information" (Wolpert, this volume), the micromilieu of the differentiating cells is of decisive importance. The micromilieu is composed of cells intimately associated with the target, and it is known to "induce" both cytodifferentiation and morphogenesis.

The Epigenetic Landscape

Waddington (105) has illustrated cytodifferentiation and the forces that guide it by his "epigenetic landscape (Fig. 1). The undifferentiated totipotent zygote starts its development from the top of the landscape, running downhill through branching valleys which force it to certain pathways. Each cell finds a series of channels, reaching ultimately a plateau or stationary state as a fully differentiated, phenotypically specific unit of a complex organism. We shall employ this model for the illustration of morphogenetic cell interactions (induction) and the various biological characteristics of this guiding system. The branching valleys and the downhill movement of the cells illustrate the sequential nature of induction, the ultimate state of a cell being determined by a series of interactive processes. The model also

21

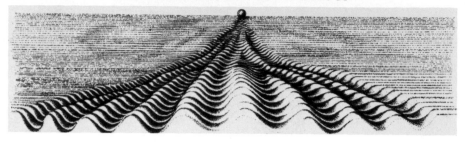

FIG. 1. The "epigenetic landscape" illustrating cytodifferentiation and its control (after 105).

****

illustrates the two basically different stages of the sequential event: as soon as the cell reaches a branching point, a decision will be made between two or more alternative pathways. At the same time some of the developmental options will be lost. After this the cell can only follow that direction in the valley which provides favorably permissive conditions for the expression of previously acquired options. During the permissive stages developmental options are not restricted. We shall refer to these two distinct types of epigenetic control as "directive" and "permissive" interactions.

What is not shown in the scheme is the reciprocity of the interactions. While becoming exposed to the guiding forces of the inductor, the target cell exerts a reciprocal action on it; while travelling in the epigenetic landscape, the cell leaves a trace on the landscape and may alter its profile.

In the following, we shall give examples illustrating the main features of morphogenetic cell and tissue interactions, and finally give a few examples of experimentally or hereditarily disrupted inductions and their consequences.

Interactions in Early Mammalian Development

When a mammalian zygote cleaves, the two daughter cells are identical having the same genome and phenotype, and both retain the ability of forming an entire conceptus if isolated and allowed to develop separately. Each cell of a mouse eight-cell embryo evidently retains this totipotency. Shortly thereafter, however, the cells are restricted as to their developmental options, presumably in response to positional clues (45). The geometry of cleavage has been thoroughly analyzed, but no clear concept has yet emerged of how two cell populations derive from a homogenous population of the blastomeres.

At about the 16-cell stage, one or some of the blastomeres become encircled by other cells, continue to divide rapidly and show little sign of overt differentiation. Differentiation can be brought about experimentally, and within approximately 8h, determination may be irreversible. The cells of the inner cell mass and those of the outer cell sheet, the trophectodermal cells, are no longer interconvertible (35, 39). If the inner cells are isolated, they fail to implant or to provide a decidual response in the endometrium, as the trophoblastic cells do; if grown alone in vitro, they are unable to form a blastocyst. The trophectodermal cells are capable of all this, and also, even if devoid of the inner cells, they hatch (shed off the zona pellucida). DNA synthesis goes on and progesterone synthesis is initiated (91). The different behavior of the two cell populations has been studied and tested by developing methods for the separation of the two. The inner cells are readily destroyed by chemicals toxic to rapidly dividing cells (1, 91). The trophoblast layer of the blastocyst can also be selectively killed by immunosurgery, a two-step procedure involving incubation with antiserum, followed by an exposure to complement, resulting in lysis of cells with the attached antibody. Tight junctions between the trophectodermal cells seal off the inner cells from the antibody, and they can be obtained in great numbers and cultured free of trophectodermal cells (93).

Several interesting findings have been reported in the two populations grown separately. An empty trophoblast vesicle implanting and differentiating soon ceases to grow if devoid of the inner cells. It needs the inductive stimulus of the latter for continuous cell proliferation and formation of the ectoplacental cone. Otherwise, only giant cells are formed, and the vesicle survives for only 10 days. If, however, an inner cell mass is microsurgically introduced to such an empty trophoblastic vesicle, an area of proliferating cells appears in the region of the trophectoderm overlying the inner cell mass, and normal development ensues (28-32, 35).

If the inner masses are grown alone, they soon differentiate and eventually resemble the normal conceptus. Not only does the embryonic moiety develop with a beating heart, blood islands and other embryonic organs, but it also clusters, and sheets of trophectoderm-like cells with desmosomes and interdigitating membranes and polyploid giant cells, typical of the trophectoderm, are found (40, 41). Electron microscope findings confirm these cells to be trophoblast yet they derive from inner cells. Similar findings were reported by Johnson (45), who speculated on the timing and underlying technique of transcriptional mechanisms. It can be concluded that the inner cells do not seem to be irreversibly determined, as suggested earlier, or that they, at least, possess some totipotent cells, possibly the stem cells of the germinal cell line (46). The inner cells exert a degree of plasticity even after new protein synthesis has started (57). Apparently, the initiation of new gene activity does not necessarily involve the switching off of previously active genes (45).

Could it thus be that the very early cells, exposed to the exterior, are triggered to differentiate towards trophoblasts while those inside escape the influence and remain totipotent, and not vice versa as previously thought?

Another recent finding of considerable interest, from the inductive point of view, is the report by Dziadek who (21) describes an "inhibitory induction." This can occur in an embryo with two germ layers. The cells of the inner cell mass adjacent to the blastocoel cavity form a primitive endoderm which can be divided into embryonic and extraembryonic parts, according to the structure it overlies (Fig. 2). There is a striking difference in vivo between the two: the embryonic endoderm synthesizes serum alphaglobulin, while the extraembryonic part does not (22). However, if grown alone in vitro the two of them synthesize it equally with equal efficiency. But if the extraembryonic ectoderm is combined with the endoderm in culture, it is capable of inhibiting the synthesis entirely (21).

Alphafetoprotein has proved to be a useful marker in other respects as well. When an isolated inner cell is grown in culture, the surface exposed to the exterior becomes covered with endodermal cells which do not synthesize alphafetoprotein. If this "primary" endoderm is removed by immunosurgery, a new endoderm is formed, and this layer synthesizes alphafetoprotein (22). It can be concluded that the "primary" endodermal cells are those of the future parietal endoderm, while those in the second layer are the ones of the visceral ectoderm. In other words, they do not have a common stem cell, but are formed from the inner cell mass in a consecutive manner. The first exposure of the inner cell mass to the exterior induces the formation of parietal endoderm which possibly induces the next layer to form visceral endoderm. This in turn may induce the next layer to form mesoderm and definitive endoderm.

Another point of interest is the finding that embryonic cells of common origin carry some marker on or within them, known to the members of the same clan. Gardner and Rossant (33) injected two different cell types into the blastocoel cavity and noticed that the primitive endodermal cells always found their way into the endoderm of the visceral yolk sac, while primitive ectodermal cells were regularly found in the embryonic mesoderm or in the mesodermal structures of the yolk sac. The mechanism by which this is controlled is unknown, but it shows that the cells behave in a biologically meaningful way, confirming earlier findings that primitive ectoderm forms the entire embryo plus the extraembryonic mesoderm.

Sequential Interactions

As already suggested by the model of the epigenetic landscape and the description of the early interactive events in the embryo, organogenesis involves a chain of consecutive interactive events as illustrated in the scheme of Rutter and his collaborators (72) (Fig. 3). Two examples of sequential inductive interactions of this kind will be given.

Primary induction. Primary induction, starting with the formation of the mesoderm and ending in the regional segregation of the neural plate, is a typical multistep process. As pointed out by Nieuwkoop (66), an interaction can take place during embryogenesis as soon as two tissue components have developed. In amphibian embryos this occurs at the blastula stage, when a distinct ectodermal half (animal pole) and an endodermal half (vegetal pole) are recognized. By isolation and recombination experiments with different zones of the blastula, Nieuwkoop (66) has shown that neither the animal half nor the vegetal endoderm (zones I and IV in Fig. 4) give rise to mesodermal derivatives if cultured in isolation. If cultured after recombination, mesoderm is frequently formed. Xenoplastic recombinations have shown that this mesoderm is exclusively of ectodermal origin (68). Thus, the endoderm acts as the inductor for mesodermalization of the ectoderm.

When mesoderm has been formed, a second step is taken in the sequential "primary" induction: the invaginating axial mesoderm induces the overlying ectoderm, giving rise to neural plate (reviews: 80, 95). But this is still a multistep process: first the ectoderm becomes uniformly neuralized, and only later is its regional differentiation determined by axial mesoderm. This is shown in the following experiment (Fig. 5). Competent gastrula ectoderm is exposed either to a purely "neuralizing" heterotypic inductor, or to a "spinocaudal" type of inductor, which normally causes formation of the spinal cord and mesodermal derivatives as well. If the inductor is removed after 24 h when induction is complete, and the ectodermal cells are disaggregated, reaggregated and subcultivated two distinct spectra of structures are created. In the first experiment the neuralized cells form exclusively cranial neural structures (forebrain), whereas in the second experiment, caudal structures of the CNS (spinal cord) are formed. If, however, the two "predetermined", disaggregated cell populations are combined and cultured as a mixed reaggregate, a "new" type of induction is created in which neural structures of the hindbrain region are the most common (81). Therefore, one can conclude that regionalization of the predetermined neural plate is determined during the second inductive step, an interaction between the neuralized and the caudalized cells. The same result is obtained when fragments of normal neurulae are similarly combined: cells from the anterior neural plate mixed with mesodermal cells change their prospective fate and transform into cells of the more caudal CNS regions (104).

Development of the cutaneous appendages. Another example of a multistep inductive process is the development of the cutaneous appendages. It is well established that in this both the dermis and the epidermis play a decisive role, and that their interaction is precisely timed. Much has been learned about the biological nature of induction by experimentally combining dermis and epidermis from regions of the embryo which normally produce different structures, either homo- or heterospecifically (review:

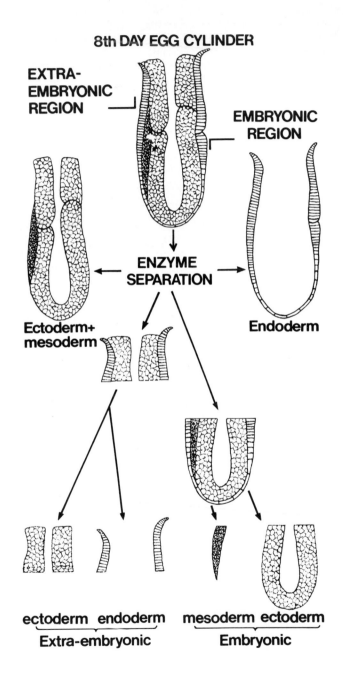

8th DAY EGG CYLINDER

EXTRA-EMBRYONIC REGION

EMBRYONIC REGION

ENZYME SEPARATION

Ectoderm+ mesoderm

Endoderm

ectoderm   endoderm

Extra-embryonic

mesoderm ectoderm

Embryonic

FIG. 2. A schematic figure of an early embryo showing the experimental separation of the embryonic and extraembryonic endoderms which both synthesize alphafetoprotein when grown in vitro. The extraembryonic ectoderm is, however, able to inhibit the synthesis if grown in combination with the endoderm. The mesoderm at this stage is hardly detectable but able to accumulate alphafetoprotein like the ectoderm, yet neither is capable of synthesizing it.

****

84, 85). The most studied species have been the chick and the duck, but a striking similarity has been noted also in reptilian and mammalian embryos.

It has been shown that two inductive waves are needed to complete development of the cutaneous adnexa. Epidermis possesses the intrinsic information needed for the determination of the type of the appendages (scales for reptilians, feathers for birds and hair for mammalian skin), but the dermis determines the size and distribution of the appendages. The first step is rather non-specific. During this induction the distribution pattern characteristic of the region from which the dermis is derived is established. Even in interclass combinations, in which the appendages remain rudimentary, the overall pattern is faithfully copied according to the dermal counterpart. In other words, region-specific characteristics are signalled and received (14, 16, 51, 52, 90). The appendages remain rudimentary in interclass recombinations, but in intraclass recombinations full development ensues. If the ectoderm from a feather-bearing region of chick embryo dorsal skin is combined with dermal mesenchyme from a tarsometatarsal region where the normal appendages are scales, the epidermis fails to produce feathers but produces scales instead (71, 83). Indeed, even epidermis from glabrous regions responds to this induction. However, even if this induction is received and the overall distribution of the appendages is laid down, another inductive stimulus is needed for full development of the appendages, and that is a class-specific one (15, 16, 18, 19). Chick and duck epidermal-mesodermal interactants can be exchanged, and their signal is transmitted and interpreted correctly. This is not possible in lizard-chick-mouse-type recombinations in which the adnexes remain rudimentary. When the chick ectoderm is combined with the mouse dermal mesoderm, rudimentary appendages are formed, they follow the distribution pattern of the mouse skin, but no further development takes place. If, however, chick dermal cells are added to the dermal part, full development of the feather ensues (87) (Fig. 6). Thus at least two inductive steps are needed for development of the cutaneous appendages. The first, unspecific by the regional dermis guiding the distribution and the size of the appendages, and another, class-specific, for the full development of the cutaneous appendages.

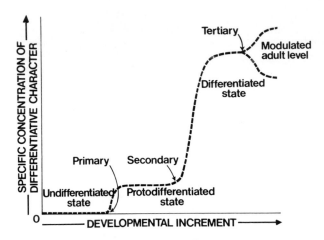

FIG. 3. A scheme of sequential inductions and different levels of differentiation (after 72).

****

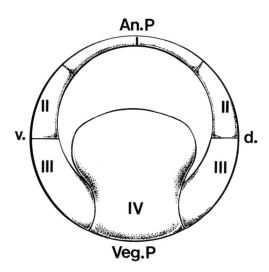

FIG. 4. Subdivision of the Ambystoma blastula into four animal-vegetal zones (after 66).

****

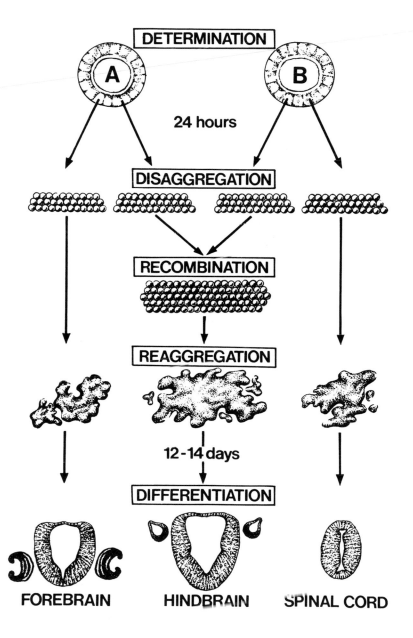

FIG. 5. A scheme of the experiment demonstrating the two-step induction of the CNS (after 91).

****

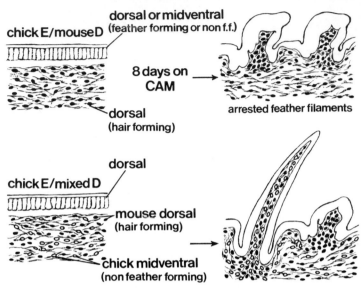

FIG. 6. A scheme demonstrating the two-step process of feather formation. Step 1 (upper): The mouse dermis initiates the formation and determines the overall patterning of cutaneous appendages which, however, remain rudimentary. Step 2 (lower): If chick dermal cells are added to the mouse dermis, this chimeric dermis allows full differentiation of the feather (after 87).

****

Directive and Permissive Inductions

The sequential processes described in the previous paragraph include two basically different types of steps (Fig. 7) also illustrated in the epigenetic landscape: the <u>directive</u> one where the cell actually becomes committed to a new pathway of development, and the other, often prolonged period, during which the cell expresses its new phenotype characteristics in <u>permissive</u> conditions. The directive step results in a restriction of the developmental options, which does not take place during the permissive phase. Some examples will be given of such interactive steps, alternating in the course of normal development.

<u>Induction of the lens</u>. Induction of the lens, a morphogenetic interaction between the presumptive lens ectoderm and the optic cup, was first detected and experimentally demonstrated by Spemann (94). Originally the optic cup was considered the only specific inductor determining the lens, but subsequent experiments on amphibian embryos showed that a variety of heterotypic tissues had this capacity (43, 80). Based on such observations and experiments on amphibian embryos, Jacobson (44) presented his

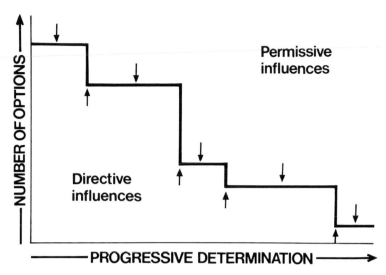

FIG. 7. A scheme of directive and permissive inductions and the gradual restriction of developmental options during embryogenesis (after 77).

****

hypothesis on sequential induction of the lens. The first inductor brought in contact with the head ectoderm during embryogenesis was, accordingly, pharyngeal endoderm. A second inductive stimulus was produced by the precardiac mesoderm, and the inductive chain was completed by an interaction with the optic cup. A two-step process was also proposed for avian embryos by Mizuno (64), who made in vitro combinations between the cephalic epi-hypoblast and various heterotypic mesenchymes (Fig. 8). The epiblast and the hypoblast combined with dermal and certain other heterotypic mesenchymes formed lenses, whereas an isolated epiblast without hypoblast failed to do so. The author suggested that at the first step the hypoblast acts upon the epiblast and subsequently, this "determined" target tissue can be triggered by several tissues, other than the optic cup, to become transformed into lens.

Such instructive and permissive types of induction in lens development were recently demonstrated also by Karkinen-Jaaskelainen (47). The permissive influence of heterotypic tissues and even cell-free materials was shown when the presumptive lens ectoderm was dissected long before it had made contact with the optic cup and then cultured in various conditions. Combined with various mesenchymes (head, metanephric, salivary) and cultured in protein-rich medium, both the mouse and the chick ectoderm formed lentoid bodies. Expression of the genes

LENS DIFFERENTIATION IN VITRO

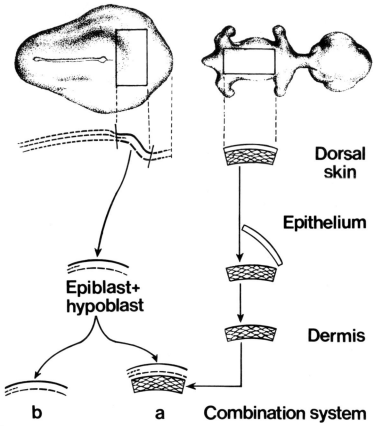

FIG. 8. An experiment suggesting a two-step process in lens induction: First the hypoblast acts upon the undetermined epiblast, whereafter lens formation can be triggered with heterotypic inductors such as the dorsal dermis (after 64).

****

for crystallins in these lentoids could be demonstrated by immunofluorescence.

A definite directive effect of the optic cup became evident when this inductor was experimentally combined with trunk ectoderm of 4- and 14-somite chick embryos. Morphologically detectable lentoids, expressing crystallin were regularly formed by heterotypic target tissue. The ectodermal origin of these lenses could be confirmed in heterospecific combinations between chick and quail tissues since the latter carried a nuclear marker (43).

Development of the tooth. Tooth development involves a series of interactive events, beginning during migration of the preodontoblastic neural crest cell (82). During the bell stage, final determination of the odontoblasts and the epithelial ameloblasts is completed. By then the odontoblasts need only a permissive epithelial influence for expression of their phenotype. Apparently their developmental options have become restricted at this stage, but they can still express some alternative pathways; e.g., when the mesenchymal cells of a 17-day mouse tooth rudiment were combined with avian limb epithelium, cartilage was formed, and collagen type II could be demonstrated in the mesenchyme. Obviously this represents a true induction of de novo synthesis of a protein normally not produced by teeth (38).

Odontoblasts have also developed a directive signalling system. When combined with various heterotypic epithelia, they can induce the differentiation of ameloblasts, resulting in the formation of a complete tooth (53). A most striking example of this directive influence was recently reported (54). The epithelium was separated from the pharyngeal arches of a 5-day chick embryo combined with the dental mesenchyme of 16- to 18-day mouse embryos and subsequently cultured in the anterior eye chamber of adult nude mice. In many cases, good odontoblast differentiation was seen in the mesenchyme, and in some cases well developed teeth were found with ameloblasts secreting enamel proteins. The authors concluded that the evolutionary loss of teeth in birds did not result from a loss of the gene for enamel production, but rather from an altered epigenetic control mechanism.

Induction of integumental derivatives. The embryonic ectoderm and the basal layer of an adult ectoderm possess pluripotential cells with many options for a developmental course. Some of these are triggered by permissive environmental conditions such as suitable substrata, nutrients and growth factors (108, review: 109). For instance, a fully differentiated, keratinizing epidermis has been obtained from a 12-day chicken embryonic epidermis (which normally consists of only two undifferentiated cell layers) by cultivating it on collagen or on frozen-killed dermis devoid of living cells (see 109). Cutaneous appendages have also been obtained by "permissive" conditions. With agar, aluminum, paraffin and various tissue fragments, Sengel and Kieny (88, 89) obtained ectopic feathers from 2-day chicken embryonic midventrum which normally never forms this kind of appendage. The underlying mechanism presumably involved a regional increase in the number of cells in the subectodermal mesenchyme.

In vivo development of the epidermis and its appendages is strictly controlled by the underlying dermis, while the basal epidermal layer is proliferating and the outer-most layer is worn off. Billingham and Silvers (3) made reciprocal combinations of adult guinea pig skin by recombining tissues from the sole of the foot, trunk and ear. They followed the development of the recombinants for more than 100 days, allowing several renewals of the epidermis. In each case, the epidermis was directed by the

MESODERM

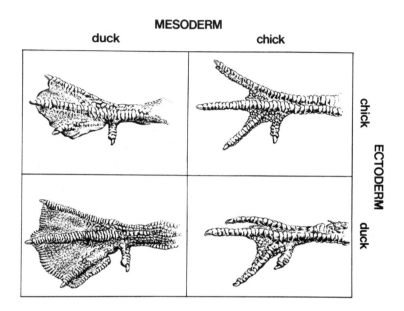

FIG. 9. If the dermal component of the duck and chick are interchanged, the inductive stimulus is received and fully interpreted within one class of the amniotes: the duck forms a foot indistinguishable from the chick and the chick foot webs like that of the duck (after 84).

****

underlying dermis to assume the characteristics of the particular dermal region. Thus, the ear epidermis remained pigmented, but it showed the histological features of the sole epidermis when combined with the unpigmented dermis of the sole.

Even fairly advanced, differentiated epidermal structures can be diverted from their developmental pathway. If chick embryonic corneal epithelium which is already depositing a collagenous matrix at 5 days is combined with heterotypic mesenchyme of trunk dermis of a mouse, corneal differentiation stops and skin appendages form.

The directive inductive influence on epidermal differentiation within one class of amniotes is exemplified by interchanging the dermal component of duck and chick embryonic feet. The chicken epidermis develops webbing and the duck feet are indistinguishable from ordinary chick feet (90) (Fig. 9). Dhouailly and her collaborators demonstrated recently that the strong dermal influence "not only induces the formation of cutaneous appendages in conformity with its regional origin, but also triggers off in the epidermis the biosynthesis of either of the two different keratin types, in accordance with the regional type (feather, scale or pad) (17). They showed that chick embryonic feather-forming epidermis can be made to form scales and scale-type keratin when combined with dermis from the metatarsal region, and vice versa. The type of keratin, however, remained unchanged from the original species, in interspecies combinations. In interclass combinations they used mouse plantar dermis and chick dorsal feather-forming epidermis, and obtained foot pads in a typical mouse plantar pattern, but a synthesis of mouse plantar scale keratin (17).

Differentiation of ganglioblasts. The adrenergic and cholinergic ganglia of the autonomic nervous system are neural crest-derived, and find their ultimate location after migration. LeDouarin and her collaborators (60, 61) followed this migration in interspecies transplantations between quail and chick with the quail cells identifiable by their nuclear marker. She made recombinations of the progenitor cells with various heterotypic tissues. When presumptive adrenergic ganglioblasts were cultured in contact with limb bud mesenchyme, they developed into neurons, but were devoid of catecholamines. If the cells were brought into contact with the notochord or the adjacent mesenchyme, catecholamine synthesis was initiated. Finally, when these ganglioblasts from the "adrenomedullary" level were transplanted into the "vagal" level of another embryo, they migrated into the gut, developing there into functional cholinergic neurons. These experiments led LeDouarin (59) to conclude that the ganglioblasts are uncommitted prior to their migration, and thus possess the option of developing into adrenergic or cholinergic elements. Their fate is determined by environmental influence along the process of migration.

Reciprocal Interaction

The structural and functional maturation of an organ requires exact spatial organization of its various cell types. This takes place at the level of cells, of their complementary surfaces and reactive peripheries, extracellular products and synchronized function. For the sake of adjustment to this procedure, a two-way interaction must exist. Several well-documented examples of this interdependence have, indeed, been reported.

Primary induction. Discussing the various steps of primary induction, we ended with the stage of segregation of the neural plate. There is evidence that this stage offers an example of reciprocal inductive interaction. Neural tissue affects the differentiation of its inductor, the chordamesoderm (65, 97, 103). Recently two independent investigations confirmed these observations using a rather similar experimental approach.

Kurrat (58) made recombinations of the neural ectoderm and the chordamesoderm of different developmental stages, from early gastrula to late neurula. Such recombinations qualitatively and quantitatively stimulated differentiation of the mesoderm, in comparison with cultures of isolated chordamesoderm.

Nieuwkoop and Weijer (67) compared the stimulatory effect of competent and non-competent ectoderm on invaginating gastrula mesoderm - when competent ectoderm was used, massive neural structures were induced. These in turn, stimulated the growth and development of the notochord, whereas the non-competent ectoderm with only small and occasional neural structures did not.

Differentiation of the metanephric kidney. The metanephric kidney develops from two tissue components, the epithelial ureter and the mesenchymal blastema into which the epithelial bud intrudes. The secretory part of the nephron is derived from the mesenchyme, and it joins the collecting branches of the epithelial component. This precise, temporally and spatially synchronized development suggesting an interdependence between the two components, was experimentally demonstrated by Grobstein (36). When the two components were separated and cultured in isolation, they failed to complete morphogenesis. No tubules were formed in the mesenchyme, and the epithelium, instead of branching, rounded up into a solid mass. The induction of the tubules in the isolated mesenchyme was obtained by recombining it with the ureter with various heterotypic tissues, whereas the branching of the ureter seemed to require a specific stimulus from the metanephric mesenchyme. None of the other mesenchymal tissues tested supported normal branching (36). The induction of the tubules is less specific, apparently permissive in nature, as the tubule inductors have no effect on other embryonic mesenchymes. This suggests that the kidney mesenchyme is "predetermined" (74). We have also considered this induction "terminal", because a relatively short induction pulse is followed by the differentiation of all three segments of the nephron, the distal tubules, the proximal tubules and the glomeruli (24, 27).

Differentiation of the odontoblasts and ameloblasts. The interactions during tooth development, involving both permissive and directive stages, are also reciprocal. The predetermined odontoblasts are induced by epithelial ameloblasts, probably by their basement membrane components (12, 50, 102). The induction is followed by polarization of the odontoblasts and the onset of predentin secretion into the mesenchymal-epithelial interspace. Subsequently, differentiation of the ameloblasts is seen, accompanied by the secretion of their unique product, enamel. It is not exactly known how and when the odontoblasts (or their products) induce differentiation of the ameloblasts, but if this interaction is blocked by physical barriers or with antimetabolites, ameloblast differentiation is prevented (42, 101, 102).

Differentiation of cutaneous appendages. The induction of cutaneous appendages offers a good example of the reciprocal nature of morphogenetic interactions. During normal development

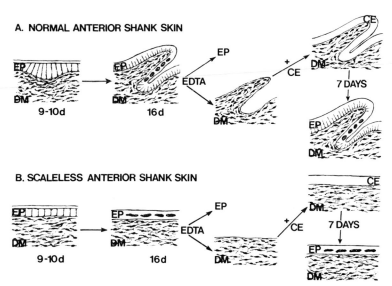

A. NORMAL ANTERIOR SHANK SKIN

B. SCALELESS ANTERIOR SHANK SKIN

FIG. 10. Diagram of the epidermal (EP) and the dermal (DM) components of the normal and the scaleless mutant skin in reciprocal inductive interactions. Normal epidermis conditions the underlying dermis to induce feather formation in the chorionic epithelium (CE). The mutant epidermis fails to do so and, subsequently, the mutant dermis is incapable of inducing feather formation in the CE (after 73).

****

of the avian embryo, feather formation is initiated by an epidermal thickening, followed by condensation of dermal cells within 3-6h. The time is too short to be explained by local cell proliferation, and Stuart and Moscona (96) showed that the condensates were indeed formed from migrating cells which followed a birefrigent lattice within the dermis. There is a scaleless mutant lacking scutellate scales, feathers, spurs and footpads. Dermal-epidermal combinations between normal and mutant tissues suggested that the mutant ectoderm was the defective component (34, 86). When mutant dermis was combined with normal epidermis, normal differentiation took place and feathers were formed, while the reciprocal combination failed to produce feathers. The mutant epidermis does not induce formation of the birefrigent lattice in normal dermis, epidermal thickening does not take place, and further development is defective. If, however, chick chorionic epithelium is used instead of normal skin ectoderm, a new feature becomes apparent: mutant dermis is unable to induce feather formation in chorionic epithelium (Fig. 10). The interesting thing is that normal dermis is fully capable of inducing feather formation in a similar combination. The chick chorionic epithelium is a "neutral target", widely used in experimental work, and it readily responds to external stimuli (48, 49). Here results with mutant dermis clearly show that the induction of feather formation is a multistep, reciprocal process. The epidermis first induces the dermis, which, in turn, induces feather formation. If the initial step is defective, the dermis is not conditioned for the next step. The normal epidermis can compensate for the missing signal to the mutant dermis, but when chorionic epithelium is used, the defect surfaces (73).

PATHOLOGY OF INDUCTION

As the significance of inductive tissue interactions for normal cytodifferentiation and morphogenesis has been demonstrated, one would expect to find impaired interactions as the pathogenetic mechanism behind abnormal differentiation and development. Two apparent consequences of an abnormal or defective interaction could be speculated upon: abnormal embryonic development (dysmorphogenesis) and uncontrolled cell differentiation and proliferation (neoplasia). Examples of these have been presented, although left partially open for criticism as far as the actual defective mechanism is concerned (reviews: 75, 76, 99, 100).

Dysmorphogenesis

Inductive tissue interactions can be thought to be disrupted or inhibited in three ways: the production and release of the "signal substances" of the inductor tissue might be affected, the responsiveness, "competence" of the target could be defective or, finally, the actual transmission of signals might be blocked by physical or chemical means. Examples of such inhibited inductions can be found from both aberrant mutant strains and from experimental work.

Defective inductor. There are only a few mutant strains known in which the abnormalities of the embryo can be conclusively traced to a defective inductor, devoid of its normal morphogenetic function. The classic example derives from the experiments of Zwilling (summarized:110) on a mutant, wingless chick strain. Reciprocal combinations of the normally interacting apical ectodermal ridge (AER) and limb bud mesenchyme were made between the mutant strain and wild-type chick embryos. Normally, the mesenchyme produces a "maintenance factor" (MF), responsible for the maintenance of the AER, and the latter, in turn, induces the sequential differentiation of the mesenchymal counterpart. When mesenchyme from the mutant strain is combined with the AER from the wild-type embryo, the latter soon regresses and fails to induce the differentiation of the mesenchyme. In the reverse combination of the mutant AER and wild-type mesenchyme, the latter will respond normally to the inducing AER, suggesting that the primary defect is to be sought in the lack of or insufficient production of the MF.

Another type of defect in the inductor tissue has recently been thoroughly explored in the androgen-insensitive mutant mouse Tfm

IN VIVO DEVELOPMENT OF MAMMARY RUDIMENTS

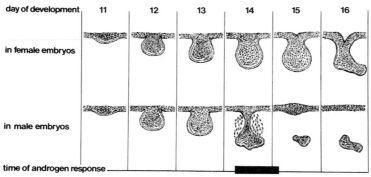

FIG. 11. A scheme of the in vivo development of the mammary gland rudiment in female and male embryos. On day 14 mesenchymal cells become condensed around the epithelial rudiment and the anlagen develops an androgen-sensitivity, leading to the regression of the bud in male embryos (after 57).

****

(testicular feminization syndrome). The males of this particular mutant have a very low level of functional androgen receptor proteins and express a female phenotype, devoid of male sex glands (review: 8). The development of the mammary gland is not controlled only by an epithelio-mesenchymal interaction, but also by "morphogenetic" hormones. After an initially similar development of the mammary epithelia, the anlagen of the female and the male diverge after 14 days (Fig. 11). In the male, the mesenchymal cells become condensed around the epithelial bud which regresses soon thereafter. As shown by Kratochwil (55, 56), this regression is induced by the mesenchyme but requires stimulation by androgenic hormones. To clarify this dual control system, Kratochwil and Schwartz (57) made reciprocal epithelio-mesenchymal combinations between the Tfm-strain mice and the normal wild-type embryos, exposing them to androgen steroids. The epithelium of the androgen-insensitive strain combined with the wild type mesenchyme regressed normally after androgen stimulation, whereas the reverse combination (wild-type epithelium + Tfm mesenchyme) did not respond. Hence, the authors conclude that the genetic defect lies in the mesenchyme which is incapable of becoming activated by the androgen steroids to exert its action upon the epithelium.

Mammalian urogenital epithelia differentiate under a similar stroma-mediated hormonal action (5-7). For example, the female urogenital sinus epithelium, in association with the mesenchymal stroma, can be converted into prostatic glands by androgenic hormones. The above mentioned Tfm mice with a female phenotype were used by Cunha and Lung (8) in reciprocal combination experiments. The combination of the wild-type mesenchyme and the

urogenital epithelium of the Tfm embryos formed prostatic acini
when exposed to androgens, whereas in the reverse combination with
the mutant mesenchyme, the wild-type epithelium was converted into
vaginal-type cells. Thus the results are in good agreement with
those of Kratochwil and Schwartz (57) and show that "the
expression of morphogenetic inductive activities in urogenital
sinus mesenchyme requires the presence of the wild-type allele of
the Tfm locus in the mesenchymal component." (8).

Lack of responsiveness. Several mutant strains have been
described where dysmorphogenesis can be traced back to the
unresponsiveness of the target tissue to an inductive action. The
scaleless mutant, already described, is one of them, and two
others will be discussed here.

One of the mutants of the T-locus in the mouse is characterized
by severe developmental disturbances in the vertebral column.
Since it is well established that the chondrogenesis of the
somites, leading to the formation of the vertebrae, is under the
inductive action of the spinal cord, Dunn and Bennett (20) used
the reciprocal combination technique to examine this induction in
the mutant embryos. The mutant spinal cord proved to be an
effective inductor when combined with the somitic mesenchyme of
the wild-type embryo, but no cartilage was formed when the mutant
mesenchyme was combined with an active, wild-type spinal cord.

Another example of the action of a mutant gene on tissue
responsiveness is provided by the "eyeless" mutant of the axolotl.
The sterile, abnormally pigmented e/e homozygote animal develops
no optic vesicles and, hence, Van Deusen (106) undertook a series
of experiments to explore the mechanism of the eyelessness. The
presumptive forebrain area of the ectoderm and the inducing
mesoderm from late blastula stages of the mutant embryos were
transplanted into the mutant and the wild-type embryos of the same
stage (Fig. 12). Reciprocal transplantations were also performed.
The wild-type forebrain ectoderm, transplanted into the normal or
mutant blastulae, invariably developed normal eyes, whereas the
presumptive forebrain ectoderm of the e/e embryos failed to do so
when transplanted into the wild-type blastulae. Hence, it is
justified to conclude that the primary action of the e-gene is
exerted on the presumptive forebrain ectoderm not responding to a
normal inductor.

Experimental interference with induction. Normal inductive
interactions can be affected in vivo by a microsurgical removal or
displacement of one of the interactants. This has been done
repeatedly in amphibian embryos, easily accessible for such
interventions, and the consequences are detectable as
corresponding defects in one or both of the interacting tissue
components (reviews: 62, 80). In higher vertebrates such delicate
experiments are technically difficult and, hence, in vitro
techniques have been employed. In such model systems of
induction, the process can be interrupted by both physical and
chemical means. Physically, the interactants can be separated by
various materials, e.g., by filters of varying pore sizes. Such
experiments show that certain inductive interactions require a

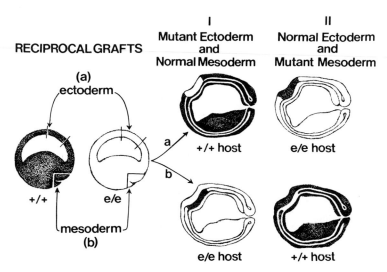

FIG.   12.   The   experimental   design   to   demonstrate   the
unresponsiveness   of   the   presumptive   eye   ectoderm   of   the   eyeless
(e) mutant (after 106).

****

close   apposition   of   the   interacting   cells,   and   if   that   is
prevented   by   certain   filter   types,   induction   is   blocked.   The
induction   of   the   kidney   tubules   is   one   of   these   contact-dependent
inductions   (79, 107).   Only   a   restricted   period   in   the   development
of   the   tubules   is   sensitive   to   the   physical   separation   of   the   two
components.   After   a   contact   time   of   20   to   24   h,   long   before   any
morphogenetic   response   is   detectable   in   the   mesenchyme,   the
interactants   can   be   separated   and,   subsequently,   the   tubules   will
develop   into   an   advanced   stage,   expressing   all   the   major   segments
of   the   nephron.   Two   further   observations   might   be   of   interest   in
this   respect.   Firstly,   it   has   been   shown   that   the   metanephric
mesenchyme   is   responsive,   "competent"   to   the   inductor   only   for   a
restricted   period   of   time   (69)   and,   secondly,   that   that   the
induction   of   the   tubules   is   not   an   all-or-none   phenomenon   but   a
function   of   the   time   and   extent   of   the   contacts   between   the
inductor   and   the   responding   mesenchyme   (78).

    It   is   difficult   to   judge   to   which   extent   such   physical
obstacles   or   disrupted   contacts   are   involved   in   dysmorphogenesis.
The   ultrastructural   observations   by   Ede   and   his   collaborators   (23)
suggest   altered   intercellular   relations   as   the   causal   mechanism
for   the   severe   limb   malformations   in   the   talpid[3]   mutant   chick.   In
the   normal   embryos,   the   AER   and   the   limb-bud   mesenchyme   are
interconnected   with   abundant,   thin   cytoplasmic   processes,
extending   from   the   mesenchymal   cells   to   the   basal   lamina   of   the
AER.   In   the   talpid[3]   embryos,   the   number   of   these   processes   is
reduced;   the   contact   area   between   them   and   the   basal   lamina   is

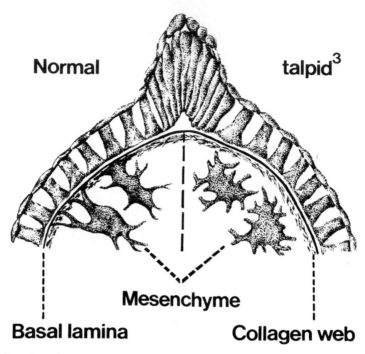

FIG. 13. A scheme of the epithelial-mesenchymal relationships in the limb bud of a wild-type chick embryo and of an embryo from the talpid[3]-mutant strain (after 23).

****

restricted (Fig. 13). It is feasible to postulate that this decreased contact between the interacting components affects their mutual communication and leads to abnormal limb development. As long as the actual molecular mechanisms of inductive tissue interactions remain unknown, a specific chemical interference of these processes or a search for teratogens, acting specifically upon them, must wait. However, some *in vitro* experiments could be described in which inductive interactions have been blocked during a certain "critical" period without actual toxic, irreversible effects.

Based on the hypothesis of a contact-mediated process in kidney induction and on some suggestive evidence for the significance of the surface-associated glycoconjugates mediating this induction, two compounds known to interfere with the molecules or the synthesis of these molecules were tested. Diazo-6-oxonorleucine (DON), a glutamine analogue and tunicamycin, an antibiotic inhibiting protein glycosylation, were tested during and after the critical induction period. A dose-dependent inhibitory action was demonstrated and shown to be restricted to the actual induction period. It also proved to be reversible, since after the withdrawal of the drug, morphogenesis was triggered and proceeded normally (25, 26).

It has been repeatedly suggested that the glycosaminoglycans of the basement membrane are involved in certain epithelio-mesenchymal interactions (2). Hence, an experiment was made to inhibit their synthesis during the induction of the odontoblasts. Both DON and tunicamycin interfered with their synthesis and with the morphological development of the basement membrane. This inhibition clearly correlated with the impaired differentiation of the odontoblasts. Both temporal and spatial correlation as well as the dose-dependence suggested a causal relationship (42, 101).

Induction and Neoplasia

An attempt to bring together two poorly understood phenomena, induction and carcinogenesis, can not yet lead to any general conclusions. The idea of disrupted inductive interaction being involved in malignant transformation is by no means new, but it still lacks direct experimental evidence. Three main lines of approaching this problem can be thought of: direct morphological and biochemical observations on the early changes in the inter-relationship of neoplastic and normal cells, the analysis of the significance of inductive interactions in the production of experimental cancer and, finally, reciprocal combination experiments on normal and neoplastic cells.

Early changes in the dermo-epidermal junction in the mouse after carcinogenic treatment have been described (98). At the ultrastructural level, the first detectable change is the detachment of the basal epidermal cells from the basal lamina which subsequently shows degenerative changes. The epidermal cells thus come into direct contact with the stroma where a patchy dissolution is seen. Simultaneously, an increased collagenase activity is demonstrable, and the collagen content of the dermal stroma decreases (63). These events preceed overt malignant transformation of the epidermis, and it has been repeatedly suggested that the primary target of the skin carcinogen is the stroma (reviews: 70, 100). Morphogenesis of the rodent salivary gland has been shown to be guided by an epithelio-mesenchymal interaction. This interaction is also required for tumor formation in the gland. Infection is also required for tumor formation in the gland. The infection of young salivary glands with polyoma virus results in transplantable epithelial tumors (11). If, instead of infecting the intact rudiment, its epithelial and mesenchymal components are enzymatically separated, then infected and cultivated separately, neither component gives rise to tumors. Recombination of the infected components, however, results in tumor formation. Apparently, normal interaction of the tissue components is required for tumorigenesis, since the infected epithelium combined with various heterotypic non-inducing mesenchymes fails to produce tumors (9, 10).

Several investigators have combined neoplastic cells with non-neoplastic ones to see whether the latter could "induce" changes in the neoplastic tissue. The experiments of De Cosse and his collaborators may serve as an example (12, 13). The mouse mammary adenocarcinoma BW10232 is an anaplastic epithelial tumor which only very rarely shows any tubular differentiation (0.7%). When this tumor was cultured transfilter to the normal mammary mesenchymes taken from 12-day embryos, tubular structures developed frequently (57%) and a reduction of DNA synthesis was noted in the cancer cells. A similar, though weaker effect was obtained with two heterotypic mesenchymes, salivary and limb.

SUMMARY

Cytodifferentiation and morphogenesis during embryonic development and tissue renewal are guided by heterotypic interactions between cells and tissues. These interactive events are sequential and reciprocal, and they vary from true instructive influences to merely permissive actions. Defective interactions are apparently involved in both dysmorphogenesis and malignant transformation.

REFERENCES

1. Ansell, J. D. (1975): In: The Early Development of Mammals, edited by M. Balls and A. E. Wild, pp. 133-144. Cambridge University Press, Cambridge.
2. Bernfield, M. R. (1978): In: Birth Defects, edited by J. W. Littlefield, J. de Grouchy, and F. J. G. Ebling, pp. 111-125. Excerpta Medica, Amsterdam-Oxford.
3. Billingham, R. E. and W. K. Silvers (1968): In: Epithelial-Mesenchymal Interactions, edited by R. Fleishmajer and R. E. Billingham, pp. 252-266. Williams and Wilkins, Baltimore.
4. Coulombre, A. J. and J. L. Coulombre (1971): In: The Structure of the Eye, edited by G. K. Smelser, pp. 405-420. Academic Press, New York.
5. Cunha, R. (1972): Anat. Rec., 172:179-195.
6. Cunha, R. (1975): Endocrinology, 97:665-673.
7. Cunha, R. (1976): Int. Rev. Cytol., 47:137-194.
8. Cunha, R. and B. Lung (1979): In Vitro, 15:50-71.
9. Dawe, C. J. (1972): In: Tissue Interactions in Carcinogenesis, edited by D. Tarin, pp. 305-358. Academic Press, London.
10. Dawe, C. J., W. D. Morgan, and M. S. Slatick (1966): Int. J. Cancer, 1:419-450.
11. Dawe, C. J., J. Whang-Peng, W. D. Morgan, E. C. Hearson, and T. Knutsen (1971): Science N.Y., 171:394-397.
12. DeCosse, J. J., C. L. Gossens, and J. F. Kuzma (1973): Science N.Y., 181:1057-1058.

13. DeCosse, J. J., C. L. Gossens, J. F. Kuzma and B. R. Unsworth (1975): *J. Nat. Cancer Inst.*, 54:913-922.
14. Dhouailly, D. (1970): *J. Embryol. Exp. Morphol.*, 24:73-94.
15. Dhouailly, D. (1975): *Wilhelm Roux's Arch.*, 177:323-340.
16. Dhouailly, D. (1977): *Wilhelm Roux's Arch.*, 181:3-10.
17. Dhouailly, D., G. E. Rogers, and P. Sengel (1978): *Dev. Biol.*, 65:58-68.
18. Dhouailly, D. and P. Sengel (1972): *C. R. Acad. Sci.*, 275:479-482.
19. Dhouailly, D. and P. Sengel (1973): *C. R. Acad. Sci.*, 275:1221-1224.
20. Dunn, L. C. and D. Bennet (1964): *Science N.Y.*, 144:260-267.
21. Dziadek, M. (1978): *J. Embryol. Exp. Morphol.*, 46:135-146.
22. Dziadek, M. (1979): *J. Embryol. Exp. Morphol.*, 53:367-379.
23. Ede, D. A., R. Bellairs, and M. Bancroft (1974): *J. Embryol. Exp. Morphol.*, 31:761-785.
24. Ekblom, P. (1980): In preparation.
25. Ekblom, P., S. Nordling, L. Saxén, M.-L. Rasilo, and O. Renkonen (1979): *Cell Differ.*, 8:347-352.
26. Ekblom, P., J. W. Lash, E. Lehtonen, S. Nordling, and L. Saxén (1979): *Exp. Cell Res.*, 121:121-126.
27. Ekblom, P., A. Miettinen, and L. Saxén (1980): *Dev. Biol.*, 74:263-274.
28. Gardner, R. L. (1974): In: *Birth Defects and Fetal Development, Endocrine and Metabolic Factors*, edited by K. S. Moghissi, pp. 212-233. Charles C. Thomas, Springfield, Illinois.
29. Gardner, R. L. (1974): In: *The Immunobiology of Trophoblast*, edited by R. G. Edwards, C. W. S. Howe, and M. H. Jonson, pp. 45-65. Cambridge University Press, Cambridge.
30. Gardner, R. L. and V. E. Papaioannou (1975): In: *Early Development of Mammals*, edited by M. Balls and A. E. Wild, pp. 107-132. Cambridge University Press, Cambridge.
31. Gardner, R. L., V. E. Papaioannou, and S. Barton (1973): *J. Embryol. Exp. Morphol.*, 30:561-572.
32. Gardner, R. L. and J. Rossant (1976): In: *Embryogenesis in Mammals*, pp. 5-18. North-Holland, Amsterdam.
33. Gardner, R. L. and J. Rossant (1979): *J. Embryol. Exp. Morphol.*, 52:141-152.
34. Goetinck, P. F. and U. K. Abbott (1963): *J. Exp. Zool.*, 154:7-19.
35. Graham, C. F. (1971): In: *Control Mechanisms of Growth and Differentiation*, edited by D. D. Davies and M. Balls, pp. 371-378. Cambridge University Press, Cambridge.
36. Grobstein, C. (1955): *J. Exp. Zool.*, 130:319-340.
37. Haundyside, A. H. (1978): *J. Embryol. Exp. Morphol.*, 45:37-53.
38. Hata, R. and H. C. Slavkin (1978): *Proc. Natl. Acad. Sci. USA*, 75:2790-2794.

39. Hillman, N., M. I. Sherman, and C. Graham (1972): J. Embryol. Exp. Morphol., 28:263-278.
40. Hogan, B. and R. Tilly (1978): J. Embryol. Exp. Morphol., 45:93-105.
41. Hogan, B. and R. Tilly (1978): J. Embryol. Exp. Morphol., 45:107-121.
42. Hurmerinta, K., I. Thesleff, and L. Saxen (1979): J. Embryol. Exp. Morphol., 50:99-109.
43. Jacobson, A. G. (1958): J. Exp. Zool., 139:525-558.
44. Jacobson, A. G. (1966): Science, 152:25-34.
45. Johnson, M. H. (1979): J. Embryol. Exp. Morphol., 53:335-344.
46. Johnson, M. H., A. H. Handyside, and B. R. Braude (1977): In: Development in Mammals 2, edited by M. H. Johnson, pp. 67-95. North-Holland, Amsterdam.
47. Karkinen-Jaaskelainen, M. (1978): J. Embryol. Exp. Morphol., 44:167-179.
48. Kato, Y. (1969): J. Exp. Zool., 170:229-252.
49. Kato, Y. and Y. Hayashi (1963): Exp. Cell Res., 31:599-602.
50. Koch, W. E. (1967): J. Exp. Zool., 165:155-170.
51. Kollar, E. J. (1966): J. Invest. Derm., 46:254-262.
52. Kollar, E. J. (1970): J. Invest. Derm., 55:374-378.
53. Kollar, E. J. and G. R. Baird (1970): J. Embryol. Exp. Morphol., 24:173-186.
54. Kollar, E. J. and C. Fisher (1980): Science, (in press).
55. Kratochwil, K. (1971): J. Embryol. Exp. Morphol., 25:141-153.
56. Kratochwil, K. (1977): Dev. Biol., 61:358-365.
57. Kratochwil, K. and P. Schwartz (1976): Proc. Natl. Acad. Sci. USA, 73:4041-4044.,
58. Kurrat, H. J. (1977): Biol. Zbl., 96:79-93.
59. Le Douarin, N. (1977): In: Cell Interactions in Differentiation, edited by M. Karkinen-Jaaskelainen, L. Saxén, and L. Weiss, pp. 171-190. Academic Press, London.
60. Le Douarin, N. and M.-A. Teillet (1974): Dev. Biol., 41:162-184.
61. Le Lievre, C. and N. Le Douarin (1975): J. Embryol. Exp. Morphol., 34:124-154.
62. Mangold, O. (1961): Acta Genet. Med. Gemellol., 10:1-49.
63. Mazzucco, K. (1972): In: Tissue Interactions in Carcinogenesis, edited by D. Tarin, pp. 377-398. Academic Press, London.
64. Mizuno, T. (1972): J. Embryol. Exp. Morphol., 28:117-132.
65. Muchmore, W. B. (1958): J. Exp. Zool., 139:181-188.
66. Nieuwkoop, P. D. (1969): Wilhelm Roux's Archiv, 162:341-373.
67. Nieuwkoop, P. D. and C. J. Weijer (1978): Med. Biol., 56:366-371.
68. Nieuwkoop, P. D. and G. A. Ubbels (1972): Wilhelm Roux's Archiv, 169:185-199.
69. Nordling, S., H. Miettinen, J. Wartiovaara, and L. Saxén (1971): J. Embryol. Exp. Morphol., 26:231-252

70. Orr, J. W. and W. K. Spencer (1972): In: Tissue Interactions in Carcinogenesis, edited by D. Tarin, pp. 291-303. Academic Press, London.

71. Rawles, M. E. (1963): J. Embryol. Exp. Morphol., 11:765-789.

72. Rutter, W. J., W. R. Clark, J. D. Kemp, W. W. Bradshaw, T. G. Sanders, and W. D. Ball (1968): In: Epithelial-Mesenchymal Interactions, edited by R. Fleischmajer and R. E. Billingham, pp. 113-131. The Williams and Wilkins Company, Baltimore.

73. Sawyer, R. H. (1979): Dev. Biol., 68:1-15.

74. Saxén, L. (1970): Dev. Biol., 23:511-523.

75. Saxén, L. (1973): In: Pathobiology of Development, edited by E. V. D. Perrin and M. Finegold, pp. 31-51. Williams and Wilkins, Baltimore.

76. Saxén, L. (1977): In: Handbook of Teratology, edited by J. Wilson and C. Frazer, pp. 171-197. Plenum Press, New York.

77. Saxén, L. (1977b): In: Cell Interactions in Differentiation, edited by M. Karkinen-Jaaskelainen, L. Saxén, and L. Weiss, pp. 145-151. Academic Press, London.

78. Saxen, L. and E. Lehtonen (1978): J. Embryol. Exp. Morphol., 47:97-109.

79. Saxén, L., E. Lehtonen, M. Karkinen-Jaaskelainen, S. Nordling, and J. Wartiovaara (1976): Nature, 259:662-663.

80. Saxén, L. and S. Toivonen (1962): Primary Embryonic Induction. Academic Press, London.

81. Saxén, L., S. Toivonen and T. Vainio (1964): J. Embryol. Exp. Morphol., 12:333-338.

82. Sellman, S. (1946): Odont. T., 54:1-128.

83. Sengel, P. (1958): Annee Biol., 34:29-52.

84. Sengel, P. (1975): In: Ciba Foundation Symposium 29 (new series), pp. 51-70. North-Holland, Amsterdam.

85. Sengel, P. (1976): In: Morphogenesis of Skin. Cambridge University Press, Cambridge.

86. Sengel, P. and U. K. Abbott (1963): J. Hered., 54:254-262.

87. Sengel, P. and D. Dhouailly (1977): In: Cell Interactions in Differentiation, edited by M. Karkinen-Jaaskelainen, L. Saxén, and L.Weiss, pp. 153-169. Academic Press, London.

88. Sengel, P. and M. Kieny (1967a): Arch. Anat. Microsc. Morphol. Exp., 56:11-30.

89. Sengel, P. and M. Kieny (1967b): Dev. Biol., 16:532-563.

90. Sengel, P. and M. P. Pautou (1969): Nature, 222:693-694.

91. Sherman, M. I. (1975): In: The Early Development of Mammals, edited by M. Balls and A. E. Wild, pp. 145-165. Cambridge University Press, Cambridge.

92. Slavkin, H. C. (1974): In: Oral Sciences Reviews., edited by A. H. Melcher and G. A. Zarb, pp. 1-136. Munksgaard, Copenhagen.

93. Solter, D. and B. B. Knowles (1975): Proc. Natl. Acad. Sci. USA, 72:5099-5102.

94. Spemann, H. (1901): Verh. Anat. Res., 61-79.
95. Spemann, H. (1938): Embryonic Development and Induction. Yale University Press, New Haven, Connecticut.
96. Stuart, E. S. and A. Moscona (1967): Science, 157:947-948.
97. Suzuki, A. (1968): Kumamoto J. Sci., 1:1-8.
98. Tarin, D. (1967): Int. J. Cancer, 2:195-211.
99. Tarin, D., editor (1972): Tissue Interactions in Carcinogenesis. Academic Press, London.
100. Tarin, D. (1976): In: Fundamental Aspects of Metastasis, edited by L. Weiss, pp. 151-187. North-Holland Publishing Company, Amsterdam.
101. Thesleff, I. and R. M. Pratt: J. Embryol. Exp. Morphol., (in press).
102. Thesleff, I., E. Lehtonen, J. Wartiovaara, and L. Saxén (1977): Dev. Biol., 58:197-203.
103. Toivonen, S. and L. Saxén (1966): Ann. Med. Exp. Biol. Fenn., 44:128-130.
104. Toivonen, S. and L. Saxén (1968): Science N.Y., 159:539-540.
105. Waddington, C. H. (1956): Principles in Embryology. Allen and Unwin, London.
106. Van Deusen, E. (1973): Dev. Biol., 34:135-158.
107. Wartiovaara, J., S. Nordling, E. Lehtonen, and L. Saxén (1974): J. Embryol. Exp. Morphol., 31:667-686.
108. Wessells, N. K. (1964): Proc. Natl. Acad. Sci. USA, 52:252-259.
109. Wessells, N. K. (1977): Tissue Interactions and Development. W. A. Benjamin, Inc., Menlo Park.
110. Zwilling, E. (1956): Cold Spring Harbor Symp. Quant. Biol., 21:349-354.

Morphogenesis and Pattern Formation,
edited by T. G. Connelly et al.,
Raven Press, New York © 1981.

The Developing Limb: An Analysis of Interacting Cells and Tissues in a Model Morphogenetic System

Robert O. Kelley and *John F. Fallon

*Department of Anatomy, University of New Mexico, School of Medicine, Albuquerque, New Mexico 87131; *Department of Anatomy, University of Wisconsin, School of Medicine, Madison, Wisconsin 53706*

Problems of morphogenesis, the development of form, are central to contemporary developmental biology. Several experimental systems exist which permit the investigator to probe fundamental questions of induction, tissue interactions and pattern formation and their causal and regulatory mechanisms. The developing limbs of amniote embryos comprise such a model system and are receiving considerable theoretical and experimental attention from investigators attempting to define the nature of morphogenetic interactions which lead to the development of definitive structure.

To briefly state the features of this experimental model, limb buds of reptiles (62), birds (98) and mammals (55, 56) are capped apically by a thickened epithelium termed the apical ectodermal ridge (a developmental sequence for mammals is illustrated in Figs. 1-4). Saunders (65) and Zwilling (98) demonstrated the vital role of the apical ridge during normal development of avian limbs. When the apical ectoderm is removed, further development ceases and only those proximal limb parts established prior to ridge removal will form. As illustrated in Figure 5, the earlier the ridge is removed, the fewer distal parts will develop (see also 81). In essence then, the apical ectodermal ridge may be considered an inducer of limb development.

In addition, it has been demonstrated by Kieny (43, 44) and Saunders and Reuss (68) that an earlier, necessary relationship exists between limb mesoderm and overlying ectoderm. The initial aggregate of mesodermal cells induces the adjacent ectoderm to become active; i.e., to take on the properties of the apical ectodermal ridge. Subsequently, the underlying mesoderm serves to maintain the ridge in its active, thickened form (101). Other embryonic mesoderm (e.g., somite) fails to support the apical

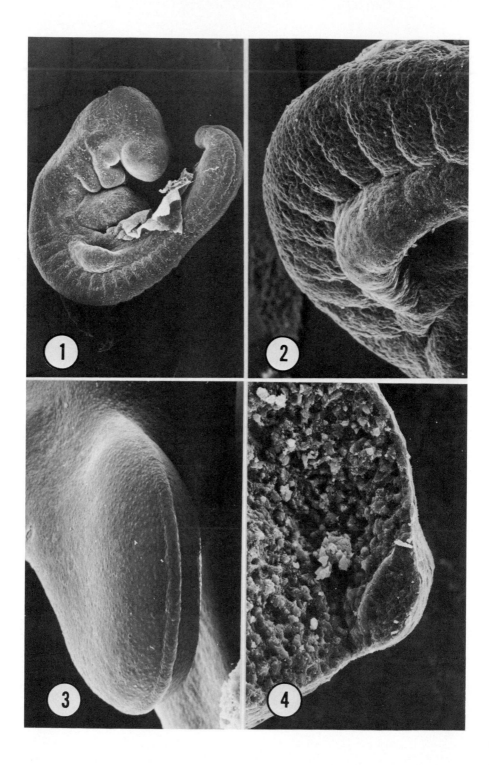

Figure 1. Scanning electron micrograph of a hamster embryo revealing early development of a limb bud on the right flank. X 100.

Figure 2. Higher magnification of bud illustrated in Figure 1. Early limb bud develops immediately ventrolateral to segmentally arranged somites and forms in a cranio-caudal direction along the body of the embryo. X 300.

Figure 3. As development proceeds, a prominent thickening of apical ectoderm, the "apical ectodermal ridge", forms along the anteroposterior axis of the bud. X 300.

Figure 4. By breaking the specimen open, the thickened apical ectoderm is clearly contrasted to the thinner dorsal and ventral ectoderm. In addition, subjacent mesoderm and investing extracellular matrix is revealed for examination. X 300.

****

thickening and the ridge flattens to a thin, cuboidal epithelium (72, 100). These observations have been synthesized into the Saunders-Zwilling hypothesis of limb development (67, 99).

It should be noted that because of technical difficulty, there have been relatively few experimental studies of limb development in mammals. Most of our present knowledge of limb morphogenesis has been gleaned from experiments on the chick embryo. However, the evidence that is available (e.g., 57), together with morphological observations (34, 36) and studies of developmental mutants (28) are essentially in agreement with the Saunders-Zwilling hypothesis.

In this report, we shall limit our attention to an examination of the central question posed by the organizers of this symposium; viz., to what extent do specific structures employ common or unique forms of morphogenetic control. However, to proceed, it will be necessary to review briefly (1) the origin and morphogenetic properties of limb mesoderm; and (2) the inductive role of the apical ectodermal ridge. We will then investigate the structural features of the matrix in which mesodermal cells reside and, finally, examine ultrastructural specializations which may facilitate and regulate the transfer of developmental information throughout the interacting tissues of developing limbs.

Since it is not our intention to provide a comprehensive, exhaustive review of literature relating to the broader aspects of limb development (e.g., pattern formation, regeneration, etc.), the reader is referred to several review articles which provide experimental and theoretical details as well as historical perspectives (3, 16, 24, 56, 67, 85, 96, 99; also see Wolpert, this volume). In addition, the British Society for Developmental Biology recently chose "Vertebrate Limb and Somite Morphogenesis" as the topic of its third annual Symposium (15). The book of collected papers presented at that meeting provides a compendium of research on limb morphogenesis through 1976 and serves as an excellent resource to the reader in stating the multiple problems facing the investigator of developing vertebrate limbs.

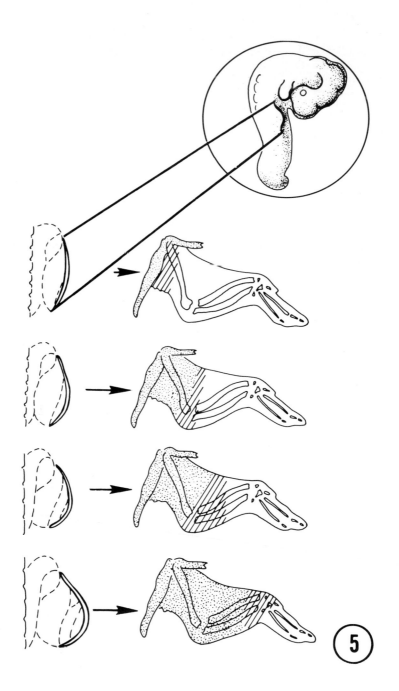

⑤

Figure 5. A schematic tabulation of the results following removal of the entire apical ridge from chick wing buds in progressive stages of development. Stippled outlines in the left column show the approximate boundaries of future wing areas in the stages used for the operation. In the right hand column, stippled areas illustrate the wing parts always formed after excision of the apical ridge whereas lined areas reveal the range of terminal development of wing parts. The inset illustrates a chick embryo at approximately 72 hours of incubation revealing the position and stage of development of the early wing bud used in the first step of the experiment (diagram redrawn from reference 65).

****

Origin and Morphogenetic Properties of Limb Mesoderm

The exact origin of cells which form the limb mesoderm has been the object of study by Dr. Madelein Kieny's group in Grenoble for several years (10, 14, 43). Studying chick embryos, they have shown that limb buds emerge as thickenings of the somatopleure and, in particular, of the somatopleural mesoderm at somite levels 15-20 (for the wing) and levels 26-32 (for the leg). In addition, the somatopleural mesoderm at early stages (up to the 13 somite stage for the wing and the 19 somite stage for the leg) requires the presence, and stimulation, of the adjacent unsegmented somitic mesoderm to be morphogenetically active (44, 45). This early somite-somatopleure relationship which exists prior to the emergence of the limb does not seem to depend on a cellular contribution of the segmental plate to the limb-forming somatopleure. For similar evidence in mammals, refer to the work of Agnish and Kochhar (1).

In marked contrast to the apparent structural homogeneity of the early limb mesoderm (see Fig. 6 for reference), it has recently been demonstrated that the developmental potential of limb mesenchymal cells to differentiate into cartilage and muscle reflects a clear dual origin of mesodermal components within the limb (2, 10). Muscle tissue appears to be of somitic origin, whereas tendons and chondrogenic tissues are of somatopleural origin. In addition, precursor cells remain as distinct cell types and do not appear to mix to any great extent in the developing limb mesoderm (proximo-distal; anteroposterior; and dorsal-ventral) within the limb (32). The experiments of Saunders and his co-investigators (50, 52, 67) have demonstrated the presence of at least one specialized region of mesodermal cells at the posterior border of the chick wing (see Fig. 7 for orientation) which, when grafted to the apex of another limb bud, causes additional (i.e., supernumerary) parts to develop from anterior tissues (Figs. 8-10). It is important to realize that the supernumerary digits which form as a result of these experiments always exhibit a sequence in which the most postaxial digit formed is nearest to the implanted graft (Fig. 10). Because

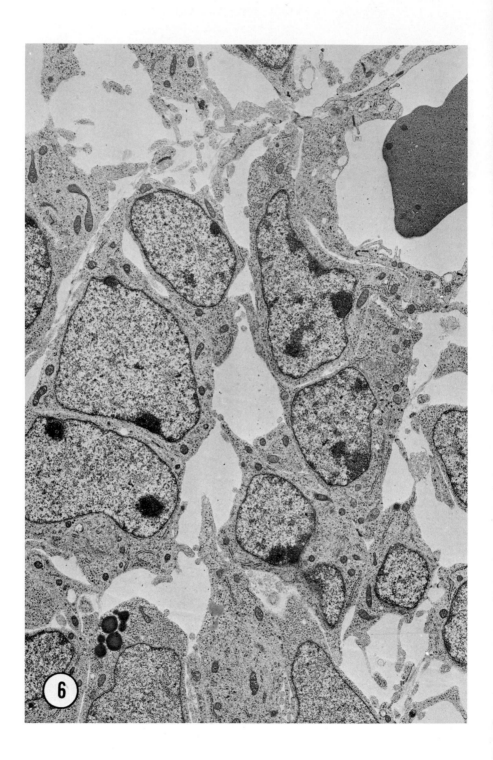

Figure 6. Transmission electron micrograph of mesenchymal cells in an early mammalian limb bud. Note structural homogeneity. However, cells are of dual origin in the embryo: those derived from somitic mesoderm will contribute to limb musculature whereas those cells which migrate from the somatopleure into the limb bud will form cartilage, tendon and bony components of the limb. X 10,000.

****

the graft appears to determine the anteroposterior polarity of the additional limb parts formed by the experiment, the postaxial limb region has been called the zone of polarizing activity (5).

Considerable research has centered on the several morphogenetic properties of the polarizing zone and readers are referred to the text edited by Ede, Hinchliffe and Balls (15) for a thorough review. However, it is germane to our present discussion to note that the the zone appears to be the source of at least two groups of apparently diffusible materials. One is capable of influencing subridge mesoderm to evoke the maintenance of a thickened apical ridge in vitro (51). In addition, the zone also serves as a center for intercellular signalling which dictates "positional information" within the mesoderm (86, 95) for the specification of the digits within the chick wing.

However, despite the clear morphogenetic effects of the zone of polarizing activity in grafts and in vitro tests, Saunders' group (50, 52) and Fallon and co-investigators (12, 17, 18, 19) have seriously questioned whether this region of mesoderm actually performs a "polarizing" role during limb bud stages of development. Most notable of these experiments is the observation that removal from an early limb bud of the mesodermal region with the highest potential for polarizing activity results in the development of a normal limb. The zone of polarizing activity does not regenerate after removal. As noted by Fallon and Crosby (18), cells of the polarizing zone, in their normal environment, may be inactive in producing an inductive (i.e., "polarizing") substance or, if produced, the substance is not required for normal development during limb bud stages. For another point of view, see Summerbell (83).

It is interesting to note that the developing limbs of all tetrapods tested have a zone of polarizing activity. In the case of urodeles (73, 74) and anurans (9), this has been demonstrated by duplications after tissue grafting similar to that described for the chick. Technical problems with such procedures for mammalian embryos have already been mentioned, and similar problems are encountered with reptiles. Therefore, the polarizing zone was demonstrated in amniotes other than birds by grafting pieces of limb bud mesoderm of reptiles and mammals to the anterior border of the chick wing bud. Duplications did develop, but only in cases where the posterior border pieces of mesoderm were grafted. The graft did not contribute to the outgrowth, and mammalian or reptilian toes did not develop. In these experiments posterior border limb bud mesoderm from as widely divergent

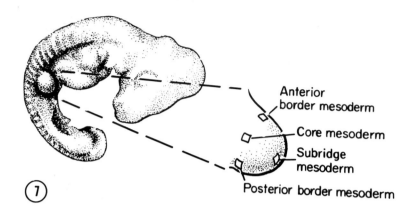

Figure 7. Schematic illustrating the regions of limb mesoderm which have been extensively studied for morphogenetic activity. The subridge mesoderm is a growth center whereas a portion of the posterior border is often called the "zone of polarizing activity." Core mesoderm is essentially prechondrogenic. In addition, limb axes (proximodistal; anteroposterior; dorsoventral) can be determined from the illustration (reproduced from reference 41).

****

amniotes as possible (viz. human and snapping turtle) caused the chick wing to duplicate. Clearly there has been conservation of the position and informational content of the zone of polarizing activity through evolutionary time. However, as noted, no function has been unequivocally demonstrated for these cells.

The polarizing zone does induce new and polarized outgrowths under experimental conditions. However, this induction takes only 12-15 hours, after which time the grafted zone can be removed and a duplication will still develop (21, 66, 77). It is possible that this action is similar to the polarizing zone's function in normal limb development. It is clear in the chick that the mitotic rate in prospective limb and non-limb regions of the body wall are the same before stage 17. After this time the original rate is maintained in the prospective limb regions and drops in the flank (71). In later stages the mitotic rate falls in the limb bud, but never to the level of the flank. It is reasonable to propose that the polarizing zone is required for maintenance of the mitotic rate in the limb bud regions of the body wall, and that this occurs before the limb bud actually forms. Further, the source or high point of this morphogenetic activity proscribes the posterior border of the subsequent outgrowth (19). In formal terms, the zone would be responsible for the induction of outgrowth and the polarization of the limb field in all tetrapods. After this is accomplished the zone of polarizing activity is simply residual in amniote limb buds and lost altogether in adult amniote limbs.

We think it is useful to point out the possibility that descendants of polarizing zone cells must be present in <u>anamniotes</u> that do regenerate their limbs. The initial dedifferentiation after limb amputation in these animals may reactivate the polarizing zone cells. Thus the earliest events during regeneration including the <u>initial proliferation</u>, and the ultimate polarization of the urodele regeneration blastema as well, may be under the direction of the reactivated zone of polarizing activity. In contrast, the proliferation of the polarizing zone cells along the posterior limb bud border of <u>amniotes</u> that cannot regenerate may reflect only the long standing requirement for their continued existence in common ancestors that could regenerate. In this context we note that animals that normally do not regenerate limbs, but are stimulated to form an outgrowth by various means, do not form a polarized outgrowth.

One other morphogenetic region of mesoderm deserves mention in this review, a region which maintains an elevated mitotic index and which may contribute to the outgrowth of the limb bud. Termed the "progress zone", Summerbell, Lewis and Wolpert (84) have proposed that the mesoderm at the distal tip of the the limb bud is maintained in a state of developmental lability by the apical ectodermal ridge. The <u>in vitro</u> experiments of Kosher, Savage and Chan (46) may provide support for this suggestion in that cells maintained in culture within .4-.5 mm of a fragment of apical ridge retain proliferative and structural characteristics of nonspecialized mesenchymal cells, whereas those explants cultured in the absence of apical ectoderm (or those cells cultured).5 mm from a ridge explant) initiate chondrogenic differentiation during the first day of culture. Removal of the apical ridge causes a reduction in the rate of bud outgrowth (33) and, more specifically, a short term increase in cell density and cell death. Thus, Summerbell (82) has hypothesized that mesenchymal cells <u>in vivo</u> are relieved of increased cell density in the region immediately beneath the apical ridge, a condition facilitated by the ridge, which permits subsequent proliferation and ultimate distal growth as daughter cells come to be positioned more proximal to the progress zone.

Role of the Apical Ectodermal Ridge

As we have seen in the previous discussion, the apical ectodermal ridge (Figs. 3 and 4) exhibits profound effects on normal limb development. In essence, the ridge provides the conditions under which axial elongation of the limb can occur and is required for the progressive definition of mesodermal limb parts (65). In addition, it also affects the events of cell death and, either directly or indirectly, the development of the marginal vascular sinus within the limb. These reciprocal interactions between ectoderm and mesoderm represent· the cornerstone of the Saunders-Zwilling hypothesis in which the

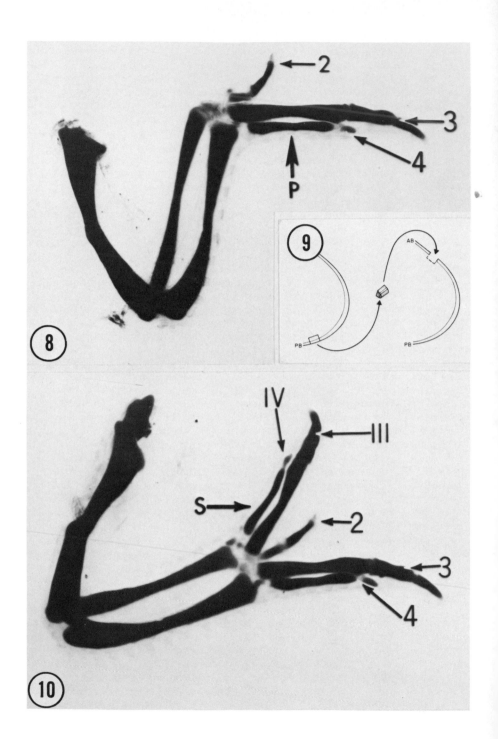

Figure 8. Normal 11 day chick wing skeleton. The (P) indicates the posterior limb border, and digits 2, 3 and 4 are labelled. Notice the feather germs (small bumps) along the posterior border. Figure 9. Drawing showing surgical procedure. A piece of posterior border (PB) is cut out of one limb bud and grafted to the anterior border (AB) of another. The presence or absence of ectoderm does not change the result, which is shown in Figure 10. Figure 10. Skeleton of a chick wing duplication 7 days after the procedure outlined in Figure 9 was carried out. S indicates the duplicated parts. From top to bottom in the micrograph there are supernumerary digits IV and III, a shared digit 2 and the host digits 3 and 4. Notice the feather germs along the "new" posterior border of the duplication.

****

apical ridge plays an indispensable outgrowth inductor activity on the underlying mesoderm.

It should be mentioned that Amprino and co-investigators (4) have pointed out that Saunders' experiments may be interpreted differently than originally suggested in that the postulate of an inductive substance may not be required to explain the effects of the ridge. However, the experiments of Cairns (8) provide compelling evidence that the apical ectodermal ridge is a source of morphogenetic substance required for normal limb development.

Cairns noted that following removal of the ridge, a wave of cell death passes through the distal mesoderm beginning at the anterior border about 3 hours following the operation. Necrotic mesodermal debris disappears and healing of the ectoderm commences about 14-16 hours after excision of the ridge. In marked contrast, limb mesoderm placed in culture without adjacent apical ectoderm begins to degenerate progressively in all regions of the explant after 10-12 hours. Mesoderm capped with an apical ridge exhibits little, if any, necrosis during a 24 hour culture period. However, in the absence of ectoderm (or any other non-ridge ectoderm), cell death develops within 10 hours of incubation. Clearly, the apical ectodermal ridge protects subridge mesodermal cells from necrosis during its active period in limb development, and only the apical ectoderm appears to exhibit this capability.

Furthermore, Cairns demonstrated that the protective ability of the ridge does not require close contact between interacting tissues. Ridges (with some mesoderm attached), suspended at a distance of more than 1 mm from a mesodermal explant, were effective in protecting the mesodermal cells from degeneration and necrosis for at least 2-3 hours after control explants lacking proximity to ridge tissue had died. Clearly, a diffusible factor is involved which mediates the ectodermal-mesodermal relationship.

However, to guard against concluding that the apical ectodermal ridge is programmed to provide specific, informative signals to subjacent mesoderm dictating the stepwise development of limb

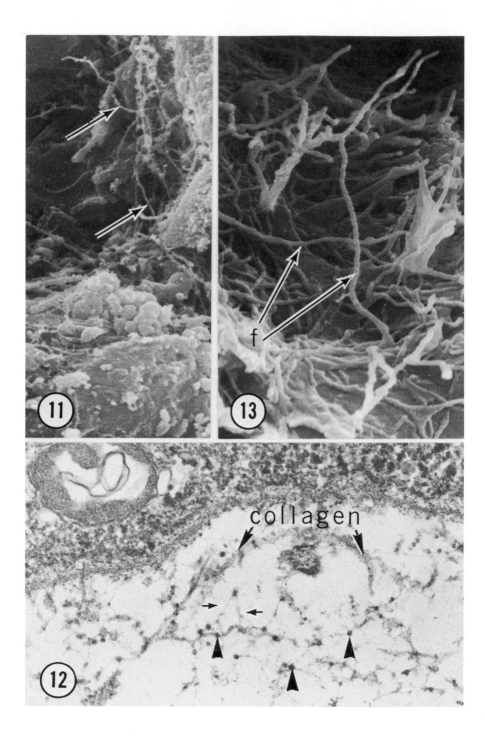

Figure 11. Scanning electron micrograph of the extracellular
matrix in the region immediately beneath the apical ridge of a
mammalian limb bud. Arrows indicate collagen fibrils which are
associated with a thin but continuous basal lamina (cf., Figure
12). X20,000.
Figure 12.   Thin section of limb bud specimen stained with
ruthenium red to reveal matrix components in addition to collagen
fibrils.   Electron   dense   particles   (larger   arrows)   are
approximately 10-15 nm in diameter, stain with ruthenium red and
are thought to be proteoglycan aggregates within the limb matrix.
Thin filaments (smaller arrows) are some 3.5-5.0 nm in diameter
and may be hyaluronic acid linking the proteoglycan aggregates.
In addition, other non-banded filaments are also present. It is
in such a structured milieu that limb mesenchymal cells exhibit
early morphogenetic properties and, ultimately, differentiation
into specific limb parts. X 70,000.
Figure 13.   Scanning electron micrograph of mesenchymal cell
surfaces immediately beneath the apical ridge. Cellular processes
(filopodia, _f_) extend both towards the epithelial surface and
towards adjacent cells within the limb mesoderm.   In addition,
processes are known to penetrate deep into the limb mesoderm,
forming contacts with other cells considerably removed from the
immediate subridge zone (cf., Figures 27 and 28). X 20,000.

                    ****

parts, it is appropriate to mention the experiments of Rubin and
Saunders (64). These investigators demonstrated that there is no
change in the influence of the apical ectodermal ridge on
underlying mesenchyme during limb development in   that   the
inductive effects of an early ridge are indistinguishable from
those generated by a later ridge grafted to the bud of a similar
stage host. Although the architecture of the ridge is affected by
the   subjacent,   stage-specific mesoderm, the possibility of the
specification of more distal parts by changing signals from the
apical ridge is precluded.   In addition, these investigations
demonstrated that the ultimate loss of the ability of the apical
ectoderm to respond to inductive mesodermal grafts and, in turn,
to influence subjacent mesoderm is the result of changes that
develop in the ectoderm with progressive developmental age
independent of the underlying mesoderm.

The Extracellular Matrix

    All of the aforementioned events in the development of normal
limbs, which require epithelial-mesenchymal and mesenchymal-
mesenchymal interactions, take place in and across a complex
molecular domain, loosely termed the extracellular "space" or,
more correctly, extracellular matrix. At least two components of
the extracellular matrix, collagen and proteoglycan, are known to
play important roles in the control and regulation of certain

developmental processes; viz. cell migration, polarity and chondrogenesis within the limb. Again, the reader is referred to more comprehensive reviews on the influences of the extracellular matrix on gene expression and cell and tissue interactions (e.g., 75).

The collagens to be considered at this time are the relatively well characterized Types I, II and III collagen and the more controversial Type IV (58). Type I collagen, characteristic of nearly all connective tissues, may be characterized as a hybrid molecule since its three polypeptide chains include two $\alpha 1(I)$ chains plus an $\alpha 2$ chain. Each of the constituent chains of all collagens exhibit a molecular weight of some 95,000 Daltons and contain slightly more than 1,000 amino acid residues. In contrast, Type II collagen is composed of three identical $\alpha 1(I)$ chains and is found principally in hyaline cartilages. The Type III collagen molecule is composed of three identical chains, termed $\alpha 1(III)$, and is usually found in concert with Type I fibers in the dermis, major blood vessels and the uterine wall. In addition, a Type IV molecule, less well characterized but distinct from the other three types, is found in several basement membranes.

During early development, mesenchymal cells in the central region (core, cf., Fig. 7) of a chick embryo limb undergo differentiation into cartilage, and from cartilage into bone. Linsenmayer et al. (48) have demonstrated that each transition is characterized by the deposition of a new, histologically distinct type of collagen within the extracellular matrix. The mesenchyme of the early limb bud produces a Type I collagen (two $\alpha 1$ chains plus 1 $\alpha 2$ chain), whereas slightly later in development, the prechondrogenic core of the bud begins to elaborate Type II collagen (three identical $\alpha 1(II)$ chains). As the bony components of the limb appear, collagen synthesis returns to a Type I molecule.

The other major matrix components, the proteoglycans, are large, highly hydrated compounds that are entrapped in the collagen network (59). They consist of a protein core to which chains of glycosaminoglycans are laterally attached. A unique feature of proteoglycans is their ability to form multimolecular aggregates with molecular weights on the order of 50-100 million Daltons. Such aggregates are common to the matrix of the earlier chick limb bud (25). In addition, Hardingham and Muir (29) discovered that proteoglycans interact with the glycosaminoglycan, hyaluronic acid, in such a way that many proteoglycan molecules may become bound to a single chain of hyaluronate which acts as a thread linking proteoglycan molecules together. In the early chick embryo, Solursh (78) has demonstrated that hyaluronic acid is the major glycosaminoglycan produced by mesenchymal cells with smaller amounts of chondroitin sulfate and heparan sulfate also produced. More recently, Vasan and Lash (93) have shown that during the differentiation of limb cartilage, the proportion of aggregated forms of proteoglycan increases, whereas the monomeric forms decrease. They suggest that the appearance of aggregate formation is due to the synthesis of a stable binding site on the core protein of the proteoglycan molecule which is specific for hyaluronic acid. Clearly, differential gene expression by mesenchymal cells for these proteins and glycosaminoglycans takes place as differentiation of the limb progresses.

From a structural standpoint, considerable differentiation of the extracellular matrix accompanies the development of amphibian (39, 90), avian (35, 69, 70, 76), mammalian (7, 34) and human (37, 38) limbs. In order to visualize components of the matrix with either light or electron microscopes, it is generally necessary to fix and stain the matrix with some polycationic element; e.g., ruthenium red (49), which together with glutaraldehyde and osmium tetroxide preserves and facilitates the imaging of the small glycosaminoglycan and proteinaceous structures of embryonic extracellular matrix.

To leave the chick embryo for the moment, the matrix of the early human limb bud exhibits collagen fibrils (Figs. 11 and 12) which exhibit a 63-64 nm banding pattern (Fig. 12); non-banded filaments some 10-15 nm in diameter (Fig. 12); ruthenium red positive particles, 12-15 nm in diameter (Fig. 12) and attenuated threads, 3.5-5 nm in diameter (Fig. 12) which appear to connect particles, fibrils, filaments and the subepithelial basal lamina. It is in such a structured milieu that mesenchymal cells reside; those cells immediately beneath the ridge extending filopodia (Fig. 13) towards the overlying, inductively active apical ectodermal ridge (dissected away in Fig. 13). Figure 14 illustrates the close association achieved by mesenchymal cell processes with the basal lamina of the apical ridge. However, it is important to note that at no point in development of the vertebrate limb are these processes known to penetrate the basal lamina and to contact directly the plasma membranes of overlying ridge cells.

Although it is difficult to make an accurate correlation of structure seen in electron micrographs with normal molecular composition in vivo (due to the dehydration of specimens during preparation for microscopy), it is probable that the ruthenium red positive particles present in the limb matrix illustrated in Fig. 12 represent proteoglycan aggregates. The thin filaments (3.5-5.0 nm threads) may be composed of the glycosaminoglycan, hyaluronate. Incubation in testicular hyaluronidase, an enzyme which digests hyaluronate, chondroitin and chondroitin sulfate, removes both of these structural components of the matrix (37), suggesting their proteoglycan/glycosaminoglycan nature.

The general structural organization of human limb matrix does not change significantly until formation of the hand plate occurs and the future interdigital zones are delineated. At that time, a striking reorganization of collagen fibrils develops beneath the thinning apical ridge which is directly over those zones which will form interdigital spaces (Fig. 15). Clusters of fibrils extend at right angles from the basal lamina deep into the extracellular matrix. These features appear to accompany those cellular events which lead to cell death and phagocytosis within

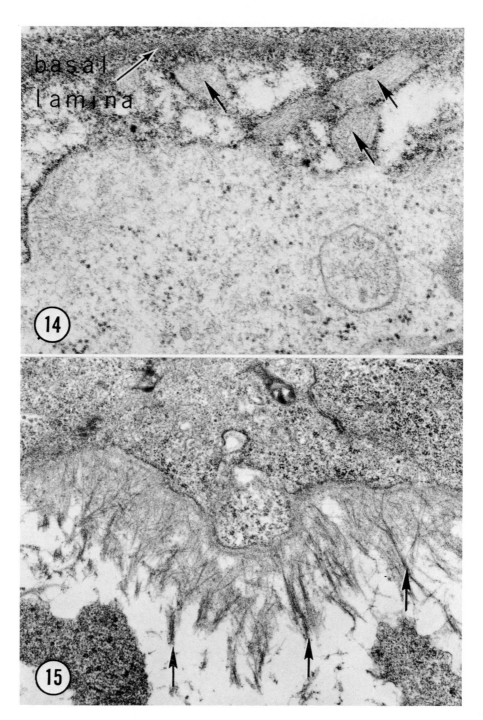

basal
lamina

14

15

Figure 14. Micrograph of the epithelial-mesenchymal interface following staining with ruthenium red. Processes (arrows) of mesenchymal cells (Figure 13) penetrate the sublaminar matrix to establish intimate association with the basal lamina. It is important to note that processes do not penetrate the basal lamina to contact the basal surfaces of ridge cells. X 75,000.
Figure 15. Considerable reorganization of collagen fibrils (arrows) accompanies the early development of the interdigital zones in primates, including man. Cell death in the mesoderm contributes to the formation of the interdigital space. X 35,000.

****

the developing interdigital space. These general features of matrix organization within the developing human limb in the early subridge and later interdigital zones are summarized in Figure 13.

Functionally, the role of the extracellular matrix in the morphogenesis of limbs is far from clear even though differentiative events are known to correlate with the stepwise progression of developmental events within limbs. By studying hyaluronate metabolism at discrete stages in development, Toole (87, 88, 89) has suggested correlations between hyaluronate synthesis and cell migration and between hyaluronidase activity and cell differentiation. He suggests that a hyaluronate-rich extracellular matrix provides a beneficial milieu for mesenchymal cell migration and proliferation, and also may prevent precocious differentiation. In addition, several investigators (for example, see 47) have proposed that the interactions of proteoglycan and collagen may be an important controlling event in deposition of cartilage matrix. Furthermore, taking clues from a number of morphogenetic systems, glycosaminoglycans are implicated in the regulation of proliferation (11, 42); migration (61, 94); maintenance of morphogenetic structures (6); and cellular differentiation (53, 54).

Of particular interest to this discussion are the observations of Holmes and Trelstad (31) and Trelstad (91) who noted that a shift in cell polarity (primarily the position of the Golgi apparatus) develops in the mesenchyme during mouse limb morphogenesis which occurs at a time when there is an apparent increase in the amount of extracellular matrix, especially in the region below the basal lamina subjacent to the apical ridge. It must be stressed that this is only a correlation. However, it is possible that this orientation represents an initial and essential positioning of cells in preparation for the secretion of an oriented matrix. This is in contrast to the theory that matrix secretion causes cell orientation (27). In addition, it is equally intriguing to speculate that the polar positioning of organelles in mesenchymal cells immediately beneath the apical ridge may be a structural reflection of secretory events required to maintain the epithelial-mesenchymal interactions which direct and regulate the morphogenesis of the vertebrate limb.

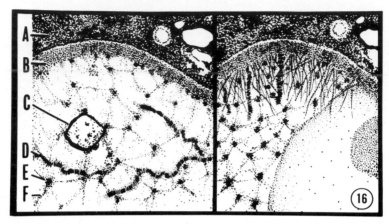

Figure 16. Schematic diagram illustrating differences in structural organization of matrix components during limb development in human embryos. The panel on the left shows features characteristic of subridge matrix during early stages of limb development, whereas the panel on the right summarizes the appearance of matrix during late stages of development when interdigital and digital individuation occurs. A. Epithelial cell; B. Basal lamina; C. Mesenchymal cell process; D. Collagen fibril; E. Proteoglycan aggregate; F. Hyaluronic acid.

****

Structural Specializations Which May Facilitate and Regulate Intercellular Communication

From the preceding discussion, it is clear that considerable experimental effort has been expended in attempting to define the nature of mesodermal induction and maintenance of ectodermal thickening and the reciprocal induction by the apical ridge of progressively defined limb parts. In addition, it has been unclear until recently whether structural features develop which could facilitate and regulate morphogenetic communication (i.e., signalling) between cells both in ectodermal and mesodermal tissues. To this end, we have examined the fine structure of limb mesoderm in developing chick limbs (41) in addition to the cytoarchitecture of the apical ridge and adjacent dorsal and ventral ectoderm in two orders of birds (20), five orders of phylogenetically divergent mammals (20) and man (40), using the techniques of transmission electron microscopy, freeze fracture and scanning electron microscopy. We have discovered the development of a subcellular structure, the gap ("communicating") junction (see 80 for review), which distinguishes the inductively active apical ectoderm from adjacent dorsal and ventral ectoderm. In addition, we have learned that mesodermal cells in the subridge, core, anterior and posterior borders of developing chick limbs have the structural capability for electrotonic and metabolic coupling (23) during a critical period of morphogenesis. We will consider first the structural and physiological features of gap junctions and their appearance in the development of the apical ridge. Second, we will inquire whether cells in the limb mesoderm exhibit differences in membrane structure which indicate the potential for communication only in specific morphogenetic zones or throughout the entire mesoderm.

In the human embryo, the apical ridge begins to form about 26 days post-fertilization (60). During this early period (cf. Figs. 3 and 4) a uniform, two layered epithelium (including the outer periderm) develops into a stratified epithelium consisting of some 4-5 layers and covered by an outer, attenuated layer of periderm. Figure 17 illustrates the external surface of the apical ridge from a human embryonic limb bud revealing a close cell-cell association with numerous small processes extending into the amniotic fluid. However, during this period, the peridermal cells develop extensive tight junctions (zonula occludens) which seal the apical surfaces of the periderm (22) and effectively separate the amniotic cavity from intercellular compartments within the apical ridge and dorsal and ventral ectoderm (Fig. 18 illustrates a tight junction between ridge cells in a comparably staged quail embryo). In addition, Staehelin (80) has suggested that tight junctions facilitate the maintenance of osmotic gradients between, and within, epithelial compartments. We believe that compartmental sealing in combination with the development of extensive gap junctions (Figs. 20, 22 and 23) within the ridge, create a unique opportunity for electrotonic and metabolic coupling within the ridge. No other region of limb ectoderm exhibits this extensive capability for coordination of intercellular signalling during a precise period of morphogenesis.

In addition, the position of gap junctions within the ridge is directly correlated to the manner in which thickening occurs. Specifically, avian embryos develop an apical ridge in the form of a pseudostratified columnar epithelium (Fig. 21), whereas mammals develop a true stratified epithelium (Fig. 19) at the distal tip of limb buds. In birds, gap junctions assemble primarily along the lateral, basal borders of cells (Fig. 22). All of these cells abut a continuous basal lamina. Few, if any, junctions are observed to form at other, more apical, cell surfaces. In contrast, mammals form gap junctions at all apposed cellular surfaces (Fig. 20) throughout the multilayered epithelium which forms ridge tissue. It is important to note that both forms of ridge tissue acquire junctions distributed in such a manner as to achieve the potential for coupling between all cells within the ridge.

It should be clear from examining Figures 20 and 23 that gap junctions are localized plaques or maculae where apposing membranes are separated by a 2-4 nm space (63) and which are composed of numerous small 8-9 nm particles within the plane of the lipid bilayer. During freeze-fracturing, most particles remain with the cytoplasmic half of the cell membrane (Fig. 20)

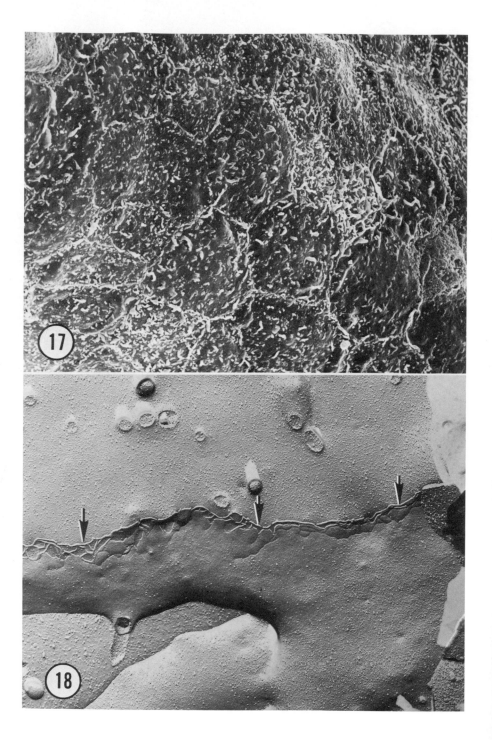

Figure 17. External surface of the apical ectodermal ridge. Cells are closely apposed to form a "cobblestone" appearance. Short projections (microvilli) are present at both regions of intercellular contact and on exposed surface abutting extraembryonal fluids. X 1,000.

Figure 18. Freeze-fracturing reveals extensive tight junctions (zonulae occludens) between cells which form the outer surface of the apical ridge in both avian and mammalian embryos. These junctions (arrows) effectively separate the interior of the ridge from the environment external to the limb and, in addition, may facilitate the inductive nature of the ridge by forming an enclosed, functional "compartment." X 40,000.

****

whereas the exoplasmic (outer) half of the fractured membrane reveals a characteristic hexagonal pattern of pits (e.g., see also Fig. 28).

The gap junction has been observed during embryogenesis (13, 26, 63, 92) but its functional significance is far from clear. In limbs, our observations indicate that these communicating junctions increase both in peripheral dimension and quantity in the apical ectodermal ridge during a period when epithelial-mesenchymal interactions essential to normal morphogenesis occur. Thus, compared to adjacent epithelia, the external surfaces and plasma membranes of cells in the apical ectodermal ridge are different in their response to environments created by the subjacent mesoderm. In addition, as cell degeneration and necrosis initiate the ultimate demise of the apical ridge in most vertebrate species (Figs. 24 and 25), gap junctions also exhibit reduction in size and component subunits, in addition to a reduced distribution within the thinning epithelium (see Fig. 26 for summary). Clearly, it is premature to speculate on the precise function of gap junctions within this inductively active epithelium. However, it seems reasonable to point out that the abundance of gap junctions in the apical ectodermal ridge makes it likely that apical ridge cells are extensively coupled, both metabolically and electrotonically. In addition, we would propose that the gap junctions are required for ridge cells to act in concert to perform their directive functions. To this end, recent unpublished results by Fallon and Sheridan (in progress) have shown that Lucifer Yellow dye can be transferred between cells of the apical ridge yet appears not be be transferred between the ridge and cells of the adjacent dorsal and ventral ectoderm, supporting the suggestion that the unique potential for metabolic and electrotonic coupling within the ridge is requisite for the normal inductive activities of that tissue.

In turning our attention to regions of mesoderm with known morphogenetic roles (cf. Fig. 7), it must be reemphasized that no direct intercellular contact has been observed between the

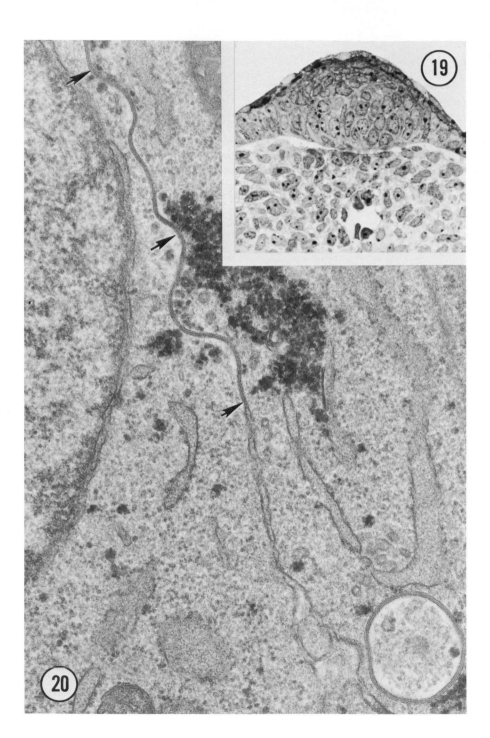

Figure 19. Light micrograph of the apical ridge typical of mammalian embryos. The epithelium thickens to form a stratified tissue capped by a layer of peridermal cells (cf., Figure 21) (reproduced from reference 40). X 500.

Figure 20. Gap junctions (arrows) develop between ectodermal cells as apical tissues thicken. The junctions reach maximum size and achieve greatest distribution during the period when the ridge is thickest and most active. Subsequently, in association with the decline of the ridge, junctions are reduced in size and number. It is important to note that in mammals all cells of the stratified epithelium are coupled with gap junctions, suggesting that electrotonic and metabolic communication is required during the period of inductive activity within the ridge (reproduced from reference 40). X 50,000.

****

interacting epithelium and mesenchyme of the limb. As exciting as this possibility is in attempting to explain the structural means by which information is transmitted between interacting tissues, signalling is apparently accomplished via the matrix which we have already discussed. However, it is fundamental to problems of spatial patterning within limb mesoderm during morphogenesis to elucidate structural mechanisms which mediate intercellular communication between mesenchymal cells of the limb bud.

For this investigation, we elected to return to the chick embryo since the regions of mesoderm with known morphogenetic roles are well characterized. Figure 27 reveals the interior of the plasma membrane of a typical mesenchymal cell. Three gap junctions are present, each characterized by aggregates of particles, approximately 8-9 nm in diameter, and portions of attached outer membrane segments from apposed cells. An hexagonal pattern of pits is apparent in this surface. Although precise configuration of cell-to-cell association is uncertain, it is probable that junctions illustrated in Fig. 27 are between apposed bodies of mesenchymal cells. We have observed, on occasion, gap junctions which are transected by narrow channels which form small, separate domains of particles within the larger periphery of the complete junction. It is noteworthy that gap junctions with this dispersed lattice arrangement appear to be most prevalent in the subridge mesoderm.

In addition, gap junctions are observed at all potential sites of cell-to-cell contact between mesenchymal cells in the limb mesoderm. Junctions form between both the apposed tips of cell processes (Fig. 28) and the sides of filopodia which are in contact. Junctions also form at the tips of processes which traverse the extracellular matrix and contact the bodies of neighboring mesenchymal cells. Upon examining the subridge region with scanning electron microscopy (e.g., see Fig. 13) we found that processes not only extend short distances between cells but may also extend several micrometers through the extracellular matrix. Thus, there is contact and potential coupling of cells

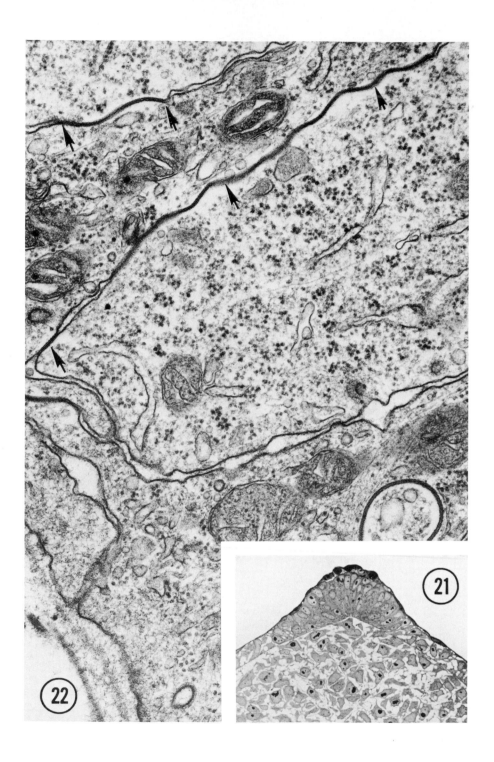

Figure 21. In contrast to mammals, avian embryos form a ridge which is a pseudostratified, columnar epithelium capped by a layer of periderm. All basal cell surfaces contact a continuous basal lamina (reproduced from reference 20). X 400.

Figure 22. Although, similar to the ultrastructure of the mammalian ridge, all cells within the avian apical thickening are coupled by gap junctions (arrows). It is important to note that most, if not all, gap junctions between avian ridge cells are located along the basal surfaces of cells within the pseudostratified tissue (reproduced from reference 20). X 35,000.

****

several cell diameters distant from one another in the subridge mesoderm (the "progress zone"). This is less common in other regions of the limb mesoblast where numerous, shorter cellular projections extend to neighboring, more densely packed cells. It should be emphasized that although processes are often observed in close association in all parts of the limb bud, gap junctions are not always observed at points of apparent contact.

In addition, Table I presents data generated from analyses of electron micrographs of a minimum of seven replicas from each region of limb mesoderm indicated in Fig. 7. By counting the number of gap junctions observed in the total number of cells examined in each area, it is clear that numbers of gap junctions between cells of the mesoderm do not vary widely. It should be noted that a slight decrease in the number of junctions was apparent in the posterior border of the limb (the zone of polarizing activity) which may reflect changes preceding death of cells in the posterior necrotic zone. In addition, the average number of particles in individual gap junctions varies little when comparisons are made among regions.

Although we do not observe major variance between distribution and size of junctions in the various morphogenetic regions of limb mesoderm, one must consider that the initiation of pattern and ultimately differentiation may be related to the assembly and maintenance of gap junctions which permit constant electrotonic or metabolic signalling between cells. Alternatively, interruption or reduction of signals either mediated or controlled by gap junctions may be a principal component in the mechanisms of differentiation. In this context it is reasonable to hypothesize that gap junctions are regulating as well as communicating structures for intercellular signals in the developing limb and that the apical ridge may ultimately condition the strength of the signal. Tight coupling may be the basis for maintaining the embryonic nature of the subridge whereas too rapid uncoupling, as a result of ridge removal, may bring about cell death in the subridge mesoderm. In addition, such changes in signals through gap junctions may be an underlying mechanism in establishing the cell behavior which leads to differentiation as proposed in the progress zone theory of development (84).

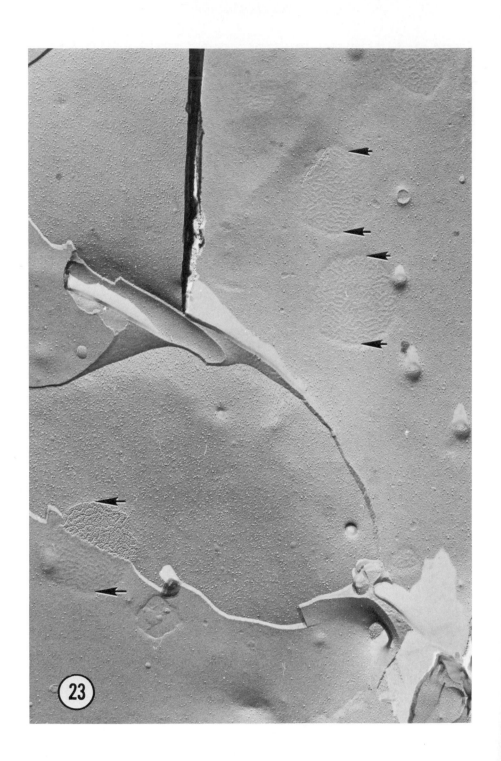

Figure   23.   Freeze-fracturing   reveals   the   intramembrane
organization of gap junctions (arrows) within the apical ridge of
a quail wing bud.   Particles which form each junction are
organized   into   smaller   aggregates   separated   by   narrow,
discontinuous channels. Note also that individual cells assemble
multiple junctions with adjacent cells within the ridge.   X
40,000.

****

Conclusions and Perspectives

Since the early discovery of primary induction by Spemann and
Mangold (79), investigators have been both intrigued and perplexed
in search of an understanding of the mechanisms by which inductive
interactions between developing tissues occur.   In the past twenty
years, the vertebrate limb has become a well-characterized,
developmental system which permits not only an experimental
approach to analyzing theoretical modeling, but a biological
system which permits the investigator to approach problems on the
molecular and cellular nature of tissue interactions. The apical
ectoderm should now prove to be a useful system for studying the
development, function and demise of cellular junctions potentially
active in intercellular communication. In addition, the various
morphogenetic regions of limb mesoderm and the associated matrix
provide the investigator with opportunities to provide questions
of continual or intermittent signalling between cellular regions
during pattern formation and signalling.   The limb system now
demands attention of investigators using techniques for cell
biology, immunology, electrophysiology and molecular biology to
focus on the underlying molecular and supramolecular events which
progressively effect the establishment of normal vertebrate limbs.

Figure 24. A mammalian ridge is shown which is nearing the end of
its inductive period. Arrows denote cell death which contributes
to thinning of the ridge and the final establishment of a
continuous fetal epidermis (reproduced from reference 40). X 500.
Figure 25. Thin section through a mammalian apical   ridge
revealing electron-dense, necrotic cells present in the ridge
during the early stages of its degeneration. Necrotic debris is
contained in phagocytic vesicles of nondengenerating epithelial
cells. A gap junction (arrows) is also present (reproduced from
reference 40). X 10,000.

****

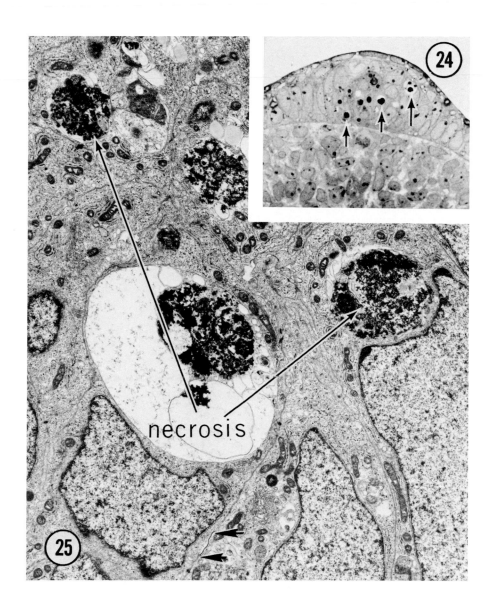

necrosis

Table 1.

Gap Junctions Between Limb Mesoderm Cells

	Tip	Core	Anterior Border	Posterior Border
Number of specimens examined	11	10	11	12
Number of replicas examined	8	9	7	8
Gap junctions observed/total number of cells examined	31/256	7/82	16/183	11/151
Number of junctions observed/ 100cells	12.1	8.5	8.7	7.3
Average number of particles/ gap junction	42.4+7.6	38.3+5.2	37.4+6.5	34.5+4.7

Data represent the total number of gap junctions observed/total number of cells examined in a
minimum of seven replicas of each region of limb mesoderm

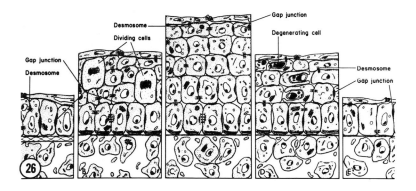

Figure 26. Schematic diagram illustrating progressive alterations
of structure during development and demise of the human apical
ectodermal ridge. In Panel A, epithelial (above) and mesenchymal
cells (below) are separated by a complex double-layered basal
lamina, the layers being cross-linked by additional components of
the lamina. Shortly, the lamina will develop a single-layered
morphology typical of most epithelial basal laminae. Panel B,
many dividing cells are seen and the ridge thickens. Gap
junctions become more prevalent and microfilaments traverse the
basal cytoplasm of cells at the base of the ridge in a plate
perpendicular to the long axis of the ridge. These microfilaments
persist until the ridge disappears. The ridge epithelium then
thickens to five to seven layers of cells (Panel C); gap junctions
are well-developed and distributed throughout the ridge (in marked
contrast to nonridge limb ectoderm); and desmosomes and tight
junctions are prevalent. In Panel D, degeneration of cells is
evident; necrotic cells are contained in phagocytic vacuoles
within neighboring cells; and the ridge begins to flatten. By
this stage, gap junctions in the apical epithelium are sparse and
are of lesser diameter than in the definitive ridge. Thus, a
morphologically distinct apical ectodermal ridge is no longer
present. The apex of the limb is covered by two cell layers
typical of human embryonic epidermis (Reproduced from reference
40).

****

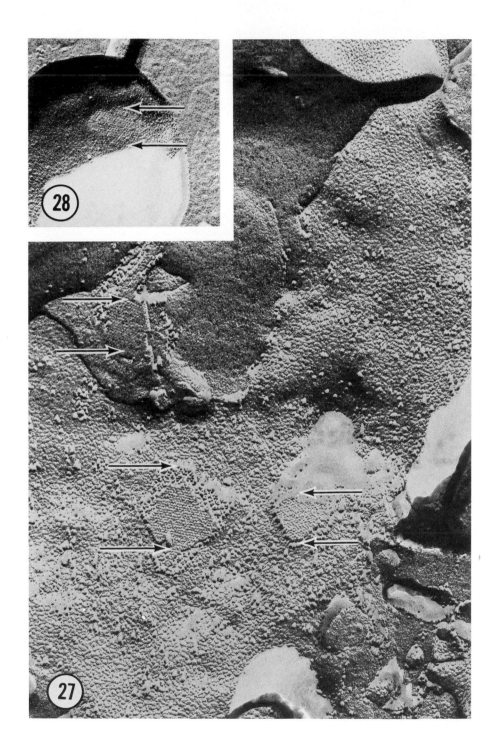

Figure 27. Replica of a freeze fractured cell in subridge mesoderm. Three gap junctions are characterized by aggregated particles and an hexagonal pattern of pits in the attached outer membrane fragment of the apposed cell (Reproduced from reference 41). X 90,000.

Figure 28. Freeze-fracturing reveals the intramembrane organization at the tip of a process extending from a cell within the limb mesoderm. The outer half of the cell membrane is exposed, revealing an hexagonal pattern of pits (arrows) characteristic of gap junctions. It is probable that all mesodermal cells in the limb bud are coupled via gap junctions (see Table I). However, it is not known whether all junctions are equally permeable to the transfer of ions and metabolites during the several morphogenetic events which form the limb (Reproduced from reference 41). X 85,000.

****

ACKNOWLEDGEMENTS

Grateful acknowledgement is made to Ms. B. Kay Simandl and Mr. Bradley D. Perdue for technical assistance; to Ms. Lucy Taylor and Mr. Michael Norviel for assistance with illustrations; to Ms. Suzanne Newell for preparation of the typescript; and to the National Institutes of Health and the National Science Foundation for grant support (AgOOl9l; HD70407; GB24704; and GB40506). In addition, we wish to thank Dr. John W. Saunders, Jr.,; the Wistar Press; Academic Press; and the Company of Biologists, Ltd.; for granting permission to reproduce previously published illustrations and micrographs.

REFERENCES

1. Agnish, N. D. and D. M. Kochhar (1977): Dev. Biol., 56:174-183.
2. Ahrens, P. B., M. Solursh, R. S. Reiter, and C. T. Singley (1979): Dev. Biol., 69:436-450.
3. Amprino, R. (1965): In: Organogenesis, edited by R. L. de Haan and H. Ursprung, pp. 255-281, Holt Rinehart and Winston, New York.
4. Amprino, R. and M. E. Camosso (1955): C. R. Ass. Anat., 42:197-203.
5. Balcuns, A., M. T. Gasseling, and J. W. Saunders, Jr. (1970): Amer. Zool., 10:323.
6. Banerjee, S. D., R. H. Cohn, and M. R. Bernfield (1977): J. Cell Biol., 73:445-463.
7. Berczy, J. (1966): Z. Anat. Entwicklungsgesch., 125:295-315.
8. Cairns, J. M. (1975): J. Embryol. Exp. Morph., 34:155-169.
9. Cameron, J. A. and J. F. Fallon (1977): Dev. Biol., 55:320-330.
10. Chevallier, A., M. Kieny, and A. Mauger (1977): J. Embryol. Exp. Morph., 41:245-258.
11. Cohn, R. H., J. J. Casseman, and M. R. Bernfield (1976): J. Cell Biol., 71:280-294.
12. Crosby, G. M. and J. F. Fallon (1975): Dev. Biol., 46:28-39.
13. Decker, R. S. and D. S. Friend (1974): J. Cell Biol., 62:32-47.
14. Dhouailly, D. and M. Kieny (1972): Dev. Biol., 28:162-175.
15. Ede, D. A., J. R. Hinchliffe, and M. Balls (1977): Vertebrate Limb and Somite Morphogenesis. The Third Symposium of the British Society for Developmental Biology, Cambridge University Press, Cambridge.
16. Faber, J. (1971): Adv. Morph., 9:127-147.
17. Fallon, J. F. and G. M. Crosby (1975a): J. Exp. Zool., 193:449-455.
18. Fallon, J. F. and G. M. Crosby (1975b): Dev. Biol., 43:24-34.
19. Fallon, J. F. and G. M. Crosby (1977): In: Vertebrate Limb and Somite Morphogenesis, edited by D. A. Ede, J. R. Hinchliffe, M. Balls, Cambridge University Press, pp. 55-69.

20. Fallon, J. F. and R. O. Kelley (1977): J. Embryol. Exp. Morph., 41:223-232.
21. Fallon, J. F. and S. D. Thoms (1979): Anat. Rec., 193:534.
22. Farquhar, M. J. and G. E. Palade (1963): J. Cell Biol., 17:375-412.
23. Gilula, N. B., O. R. Reeves, and A. Steinbach (1972): Nature (London), 235:262-265.
24. Goetinck, P. F. (1966): Current Topics in Developmental Biology, 1:253-283.
25. Goetinck, P. F. and J. P. Pennypacker (1977): In: Vertebrate Limb and Somite Morphogenesis, edited by P. A. Ede, J. R. Hinchliffe, and M. Balls, pp. 139-159, Cambridge University Press, Cambridge.
26. Gould, R. P., A. Day, and L. Wolpert (1972): Exp. Cell Res., 72:325-336.
27. Gould, R. P., L. Selwood, A. Day, and L. Wolpert (1974): Exp. Cell Res., 83:287-296.
28. Gruneberg, H. (1963): The Pathology of Development, John Wiley and Sons, New York.
29. Hardingham, T. E. and H. Muir (1972): Biochem. Biophys. Acta, 279:401-405.
30. Hascall, V. C., T. R. Oegema, and M. Brown (1976): J. Biol. Chem., 251:3511-3519.
31. Holmes, L. B. and R. L. Trelstad (1977): Dev. Biol., 59:164-173.
32. Jacob, M., B. Christ, and H. J. Jacob (1979): Anat. Embryol., 157:291-309.
33. Janners, M. Y. and R. L. Searles (1971): Dev. Biol., 24:465-476.
34. Jurand, A. (1965): Proc. Roy. Soc. London Ser. B., 162:387-405.
35. Kaprio, E. A. (1977): Wilhelm Roux Archives, 182:213-225.
36. Kelley, R. O. (1973): J. Embryol. Exp. Morph., 29:117-131.
37. Kelley, R. O. (1975): J. Embryol. Exp. Morph., 34:1-18.
38. Kelley, R. O. (1977): In: Vertebrate Limb and Somite Morphogenesis, edited by D. A. Ede, J. R. Hinchliffe, and M. Balls, Cambridge University Press, Cambridge, pp. 267-280.
39. Kelley, R. O. and J. G. Bluemink (1974): Dev. Biol., 37:1-17.
40. Kelley, R. O. and J. F. Fallon (1976): Dev. Biol., 51:241-256.
41. Kelley, R. O. and J. F. Fallon (1978): J. Embryol. Exp. Morph., 46:99-110.
42. Kelley, R. O., G. C. Palmer, H. A. Crissman, and J. H. Nilson (1977): J. Cell Sci., 28:237-250.
43. Kieny, M. (1960): J. Embryol. Exp. Morph., 8:457-467.
44. Kieny, M. (1971): Annales d'Embryologie et de Morphogenèse, 4:281-298.
45. Kieny, M. (1972): Colloque International sur le Dévelopment du Membre, Grenoble.
46. Kosher, R. A., M. P. Savage, and S. -C. Chan (1979): J. Embryol. Exp. Morph., 50:75-97.

47. Lee-Owen, V. and J. C. Anderson (1976): Biochem. J., 153:259-264.
48. Linsenmayer, T. F., B. P. Toole, and R. L. Trelstad (1973): Dev. Biol., 35:232-239.
49. Luft, J. H. (1971): Anat. Rec., 171:369-415.
50. MacCabe, A. B., M. T. Gasseling, and J. W. Saunders, Jr. (1973): Mech. Aging Devel., 2:1-2.
51. MacCabe, J. A. and B. W. Parker (1976): Dev. Biol., 54:297-303.
52. MacCabe, J. A., J. W. Saunders, Jr., and M. Pickett (1973): Dev. Biol., 31:323-335.
53. Markwald, R. R., T. P. Fitzharris, and W. M. Adams Smith (1975): Dev. Biol., 42:160-180.
54. Markwald, R. R., T. P. Fitzharris, H. Bank, and D. H. Bernanke (1978): Dev. Biol., 62:292-316.
55. Milaire, J. (1962): In: Advances in Morphogenesis, edited by M. Abercrombie and J. Brachet, Vol. 2, pp. 180-209, Academic Press, New York.
56. Milaire, J. (1965) : In: Organogenesis, edited by R. L. de Haan and H. Ursprung, pp. 283-300, Holt Rinehart and Winston, New York.
57. Milaire, J. and J. Mulnard (1968): J. Embryol. Exp. Morph., 20:215-236.
58. Miller, E. J. (1976): Mol. Cell Biochem., 13:165-192.
59. Muir, H. and T. E. Hardingham (1975): In: Biochemistry of Carbohydrates. MTP International Review of Science, edited by W. J. Whelan, pp. 153-222, University Park Press, Baltimore.
60. O'Rahilly, R. and Gardner, E. (1975): Anat. Embryol., 148:1-23.
61. Pratt, R. M., M. Larsen, and M. C. Johnston (1975): Dev. Biol., 44:298-305.
62. Raynaud, A. (1972): Collogue International sur le Dévelopment du Membre, Grenoble.
63. Revel, J., P. Yip, and L. L. Chang (1973): Dev. Biol., 35:302-317.
64. Rubin, L. and J. W. Saunders, Jr. (1972): Dev. Biol., 28:94-112.
65. Saunders, J. W., Jr. (1948): J. Exp. Zool., 108:363-403.
66. Saunders, J. W., Jr. and M. T. Gasseling (1963): Dev. Biol., 7:64-78.
67. Saunders, J. W., Jr. and M. T. Gasseling (1968): In: Epithelial-Mesenchymal Interactions, edited by R. Fleischmajer and R. E. Billingham, pp. 78-97, Williams and Wilkins, Baltimore, MD.
68. Saunders, J. W., Jr. and C. Ruess (1974): Dev. Biol., 38:41-50.
69. Searls, R. L. (1965): Dev. Biol., 11:155-168.
70. Searls, R. L., S. R. Hilfer, and S. M. Mirow (1972): Dev. Biol., 28:123-137.
71. Searls, R. L. and M. Y. Janners (1971): Dev. Biol., 24:198-213.

72. Searls, R. L. and E. Zwilling (1964): Dev. Biol., 9:38-55.
73. Slack, J. M. W. (1977a): J. Embryol. Exp. Morph., 39:151-168.
74. Slack, J. M. W. (1977b): J. Embryol. Exp. Morph., 39:169-182.
75. Slavkin, H. C. and R. C. Greulich, editors, (1975): Extracellular Matrix Influences on Gene Expression, Academic Press, New York.
76. Smith, A. A., R. L. Searls, and S. R. Hilfer (1975): Dev. Biol., 46:222-226.
77. Smith, J. C. (1979): J. Embryol. Exp. Morph., 52:105-113.
78. Solursh, M. (1976): Dev. Biol., 50:525-530.
79. Spemann, H. and H. Mangold (1924): Arch. Entw. Mech. Org., 100:599-638.
80. Staehelin, L. A. (1974): Int. Rev. Cytol., 39:191-283.
81. Summerbell, D. (1974): J. Embryol. Exp. Morph., 32:651-660.
82. Summerbell, D. (1977): J. Embryol. Exp. Morph., 40:1-21.
83. Summerbell, D. (1979): J. Embryol. Exp. Morph., 50:217-233.
84. Summerbell, D., J. H. Lewis, and L. Wolpert (1973): Nature, 244:492-496.
85. Thornton, C. S. (1968): Advan. Morphog., 7:205-249.
86. Tickle, C., D. Summerbell and L. Wolpert (1975): Nature, 254:199-202.
87. Toole, B. P. (1972): Dev. Biol., 29:321-329.
88. Toole, B. P. (1973): Am. Zool., 13:1061-1065.
89. Toole, B. P. (1976): In: Neuronal Recognition, edited by S. H. Barondes, pp. 275-329, Plenum Press, New York.
90. Toole, B. P. and J. Gross (1971): Dev. Biol., 25:57-77.
91. Trelstad, R. L. (1977): Dev. Biol., 59:153-163.
92. Trelstad, R. L., E. D. Hay, and J. Revel (1967): Dev. Biol., 16:78-106.
93. Vasan, N. S. and J. W. Lash (1979): J. Embryol. Exp. Morph., 49:47-59.
94. Weston, J. A., M. A. Derby, and J. E. Pintar (1978): Zoon, 6:103-113.
95. Wolpert, L. (1969): J. Theor. Biol., 25:1-47.
96. Wolpert, L. (1971): Curr. Top. Devel. Biol., 6:183-224.
97. Wolpert, L. and J. H. Lewis (1975): Fed. Proc., 34:14-20.
98. Zwilling, E. (1949): J. Exp. Zool., 111:175-187.
99. Zwilling, E. (1961): In: Advances in Morphogenesis, edited by M. Abercrombie and J. Brachet, pp. 301-330, Academic Press, New York.
100. Zwilling, E. (1964): Dev. Biol., 9:20-37.
101. Zwilling, E. and L. Hansborough (1956): J. Exp. Zool., 132:219-239.

Morphogenesis and Pattern Formation,
edited by T. G. Connelly et al.,
Raven Press, New York © 1981.

Tooth Development and Dental Patterning

Edward J. Kollar

*Department of Dental Medicine, University of Connecticut Health Center, Farmington,
Connecticut 06032*

DEDICATION

Soon after this paper was delivered, our colleague and my dear friend Dr. Beatrice Garber of the University of Chicago died. Bea worked in the area of morphogenesis since her student days with professor Paul Weiss. She was well known to many developmental biologists here and abroad. Bea Garber was also the most magnanimous person any of us has known. I am indebted to her because when I was a young colleague in Professor Moscona's laboratory she gave me her friendship and guidance. It has been a great honor to have worked with Bea and it will always be a magnificent experience to have known her. I dedicate this paper to her memory.

The dentition shares with the limb, spinal column, and several other organ systems a structural dependence on complex spatial patterning of the subunits into functional organ systems. As in all of these examples, there are several levels of pattern maintenance in any dentition. For example, individual teeth must be initiated in specific functional patterns in the mandibular and maxillary arches. Teeth must display right- and left-handed symmetry as well as upper and lower counterparts that are structurally compatible. Within the dental row, a variety of individual tooth shapes (incisors, molars, etc.) have evolved for versatile masticatory function. In addition, the deposition of the hard tissues, enamel and dentin, must be precisely patterned in each tooth so that function is enhanced. Consider, for example, the precision of enamel deposition in the rodent incisor. The labial aspect of the incisor is heavily enameled while the lingual surface is not. This differential distribution of hard tissue permits the rodent to maintain chisel edges on the occluding upper and lower incisors. Molars, on the other hand, display completely enameled occlusal cusp patterns.

These complex patterns at the organ, tissue and cellular levels arise through a series of stages during embryogenesis and neonatal growth. The tooth begins as a downgrowth of epithelial cells from the basal layer of the oral epithelium associated with a condensation of mesenchymal cells, the dental papilla, which condenses adjacent to the epithelial bud. The epithelial bud lengthens and expands to form a bell-shaped enamel organ. The inner surface of this enamel organ will ultimately deposit enamel proteins that subsequently calcify to become mature enamel. However, enamel cannot be deposited until a layer of dentin has been laid down by the differentiating odontoblast found in the dental papilla adjacent to the epithelial cells on the inner surface of the enamel organ. While this sequence has been known since the early part of the last century, the causal relationship between the interacting tissues has been investigated intensively only in the last two decades.

Inductive Tissue Interactions

While considerable understanding of tooth morphogenesis has been achieved in the past, there is also some confusion that stems in part from a tendency to relate all other experimental models to each other (12, 30). At the outset, the distinction should be made that the ectoderm appears to have a more stringent requirement for tissue interactions with specific areas of the mesenchyme in order to express differentiated states. In contrast, the endodermal and mesodermal layers very early acquire a predetermination toward certain kinds of differentiation. The classic experiment of producing exogastrulae in amphibians clearly demonstrates the inability of the ectoderm to self differentiate in the absence of a mesenchymal component. Thus, attempting to apply data obtained from experiments with pancreas rudiments or developing somites may prove to be more confusing than illuminating.

In contrast, the ability of the mesodermally or ectomesenchymally (neural crest) derived stroma to elicit specific differentiated tissues and specific gene products from the ectoderm has been demonstrated repeatedly. This ability to evoke new genetic expression -- especially in the integument -- has been referred to as directive inductive influences (25 and Saxén, this volume). These tissue-specific responses are in contrast to other tissue interaction in which the differentiated product can be elicited by a variety of exogenous (even non-biological) stimuli. Such interactions have been termed permissive influences (25 and Saxen, this volume). Permissive interactions most often expedite the expression of a previously determined (protodifferentiated) tissue or exaggerate the synthesis of a product typical of the tissue. These models are often of a very low level of structural organization or may even be considered as single-cell models.

In contrast, in the skin and oral mucosa, there are several examples in which a labile epithelial tissue can be instructed or directed to pursue a new developmental course and to express a new gene product (18, 19, 21).

In all of these interactions there is an element of reciprocal interaction. That is, appropriate function in the mesodermal stroma may depend on an epithelial covering and, in turn, the specific activity of the epithelium can be related to the source of the underlying stroma. During tooth development, in addition to clear evidence that the mesenchymal papilla initiates tooth development, the presence of a specific epithelial component, the enamel organ, is necessary in order to permit dentin formation in the mesenchyme. In turn, the presence of a layer of dentin signals the start of enamel protein synthesis in the epithelium. Thus, during tooth development, there is an instructive influence from the mesenchymal component to form an enamel organ followed by a permissive influence from the epithelium to the mesenchymal component for continued expression which then signals epithelial cell function. A similar relationship exists in limb development (Kelley and Fallon, this volume).

Experimental evidence has unraveled some of these relationships. When epithelial enamel organs are enzymatically separated from mesenchymal dental papillae, tooth morphogenesis is halted. Neither of the components is able to differentiate normally; the isolated epithelium cornifies and dies and the denuded dental papilla, at best, may deposit random spicules of bone. On the other hand, if the two components are reassembled, tooth morphogenesis begins de novo and a recognizable tooth is formed (16). The ability of tooth buds to recover from experimental insult has permitted us to ask questions about the control of tooth development and the determinants of tooth shape.

The Role of the Dental Mesenchyme in Tooth Development: Control of Tooth Initiation and Tooth Shape

When isolated dental mesenchyme is recombined with non-dental epithelium, the dental mesenchyme can initiate enamel organ histogenesis and can evoke the expression of genetic information for enamel protein synthesis in these epithelia. Integumental epithelium from the developing foot (18), epithelium from the oral vestibule (17), gingival epithelium from the edentulous diastema of embryonic mice (19) and even oral epithelium from embryonic chicks (21) respond to the influence of the dental mesenchyme and participate in dental morphogenesis and secrete enamel matrix.

Figure 1 illustrates a fully formed crown with dentin and enamel matrices harmoniously displayed as a molar tooth. This tooth is the product of a combination of oral epithelium from the diastema recombined with a molar dental papilla (19). Note that the details of morphogenesis are complete; even enamel-free areas

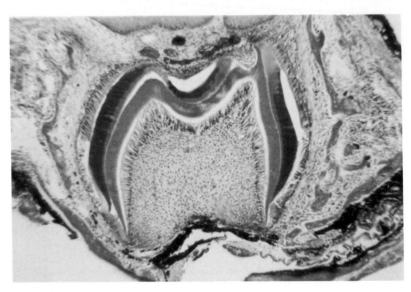

FIG 1. A well formed molar tooth has formed in a graft comprised
of embryonic mouse diastema epithelium reassociated with isolated
embryonic mouse molar papilla.

****

at the cusp tips have been specified by the dental papilla.   This
figure illustrates that the dental papilla can initiate tooth
development from an edentulous epithelium and that the shape of
the tooth is determined by the source of the dental mesenchyme.
Other experiments (16) in which the enamel organs and dental
papillae from incisors and molars were exchanged demonstrated
that, as a general principle, the dental papilla determines the
details of morphogenesis. The ability to elicit morphogenesis and
to determine histologic patterns is also manifest in other skin
derivatives such as hair, feathers, vibrissae, etc. (19).   Sengel
and his collaborators (5, 27) have suggested from their studies
that the signal is biphasic.   First there is an inductive
influence that does not depend on species or class origin of the
tissue involved. This signal, then, must be phylogenetically
ancient and recognized by a variety of vertebrate groups. This
first influence determined the size, shape and location of
epithelial derivatives, but the responding epithelium can produce
only those structures compatible with the genotype of that
epithelium.   Thus, hair-inducing dermis from embryonic mice can
induce feathers from chick corneal epithelium (3) because the

chick genotype responds to the signal by expressing chick characteristics despite the fact that the signal originated in the mouse. Once this first step in the inductive process has established the epithelial derivative, Sengel (27) suggests that a second more specific signal for the details of morphogenesis is involved. While the data support the first patterning influence, there is little evidence to support the second.

The Nature of the Mesenchymal Influences

The initiation of tooth morphogenesis as well as the final shape of the tooth depends on a downgrowth and modeling of the epithelium into a definitive enamel organ. These early influences determine epithelial patterns and influence the shape of the tooth even before hard tissues replace the basement membrane. Fortunately, this modeling function of the mesenchyme can be altered experimentally and the major components of the mesenchymal stroma: the mesenchymal or fibroblast cell population, the extracellular collagens, and the proteoglycans can be perturbed resulting in aberrant tissue patterns.

Historically, Grobstein and Cohen (11) demonstrated that disruption of collagen fibers in the extracellular matrix by collagenase could prevent salivary gland morphogenesis. This method of altering the matrix depends, of course, on digestion of extracellular fibers and does not interfere with cellular function or with continued synthesis of new collagen.

Alternatively, it is possible to inhibit collagen synthesis intracellularly at the level of the ribosomes. Several agents are available to do this, but I will describe our experience with the antibiotic drug, tetracycline (14). This drug is able to chelate free ions and one of these is ionic iron. Iron is necessary during collagen synthesis as a co-factor to the enzymatic hydroxylation of proline in the growing peptide chain of procollagen, the intracellular precursor of the mature extracellular collagen fiber. If iron is depleted, collagen synthesis stops. Figure 2 illustrates an incisor tooth bud grown for six days in vitro. The tooth bud was explanted at the bell stage of development and after six days in vitro it has continued to develop. Cytodifferentiation of the epithelium and the mesenchyme has taken place. Figure 3, on the other hand, illustrates the effect of tetracycline added to a similar tooth bud at the time of explantation. Note that the epithelium is still present, but that cytodifferentiation has been stopped; the stroma is virtually destroyed.

One of the remarkable advantages of tooth morphogenesis as an experimental model is the capacity for recovery even in the face of such devastating suppressions. If treated tooth germs are removed from the experimental medium containing tetracycline, and returned to control medium without the drug, the tooth buds recover and cytodifferentiation proceeds.

The involvement of iron in this sequence can be illustrated by adding an excess of ionic iron to the cultures in the continual

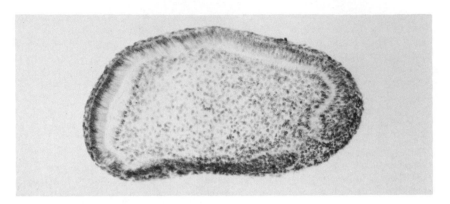

FIG.2   A 15-day old incisor tooth bud grown for six days _in vitro_.
Morphogenesis and cytodifferentiation are normal and advanced.

****

presence of tetracycline and noting that the effect of the drug is
circumvented. These cultures are indistingusihable from control
cultures (compare Figure 4 with Figure 2). Because tooth buds can
recover from severe inhibition an additional experiment was
attempted. In the presence of tetracycline at a dose sufficient
to severely inhibit morphogenesis, procollagen precursors of
fibrillar collagen were added exogenously to the cultures. Thus,
although the collagen secreting cells were no longer capable of
making indigenous collagen, the extracellular precursor product
was present. In the presence of exogenous collagen, these
inhibited tooth germs were identical to controls (Figure 5 and
compare with Figure 2 and 4). The data suggest that the
mesenchymal cells can process the procollagen and that the
epithelial cell can respond to the collagen in the stroma
irrespective of whether the collagen was deposited by dental
mesenchymal cells or not (14).

Local Stroma as the Inductive Substrate

For years the descriptions of the inductive stimulus as a
single, local, diffusible molecular signal has dominated our
thinking. But our data that the stroma models the epithelial
display and that the cells recognize exogenous sources of this
collagen suggest an alternative hypothesis.
The notion that epithelial cells respond to substrate molecules
and that the differentiation of epithelial cells can vary with the
nature of the substrate is well known. Recently, the limitation
of cell culture on fixed plastic or collagen substrates
has been emphasized (2, 6, 7, 22). The obvious interest in
analyzing cell cultures that are grown on collagen gels that have
been released from the culture dish has demonstrated that the

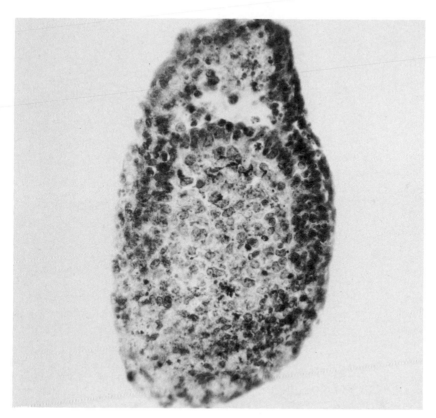

FIG. 3. A tooth bud similar to that illustrated in FIG. 2 at the time of extirpation has been grown for 6 days in the presence of 75 μg of tetracycline/ml of culture medium. Note the suppression of cytodifferentiation and the retarded and aberrant morphology.

****

degree of cellular attachment, the constraints of two-dimensional cultures, and the alteration of cell shape in cell cultures can dramatically bias cellular behavior and genetic expression. When cells grown on collagen gels are released from the plastic substrate a dramatic change in cell shape is noted in a very short time. Morphological changes in cell organelle organization follows and then synthesis of characteristic differentiated products are secreted or processed (28, 29). The transformation of the collagen from a restrictive platform to a substrate that acts as a stromal bed and permits diffusion at the cells' basal surface unleashes unsuspected cellular activity. The change in cell shape certainly preceeds biochemical expression of genetic information. The shape of the cell is certainly a prerequisite,

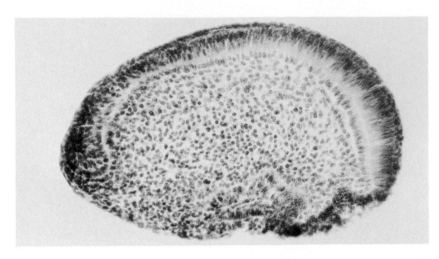

FIG. 4. This tooth has been grown in the presence of tetracycline and an excess of iron. The effect of the drug is circumvented and development is normal.

****

if not a causally linked determinant, of cell function and phenotype. The importance of devising and analyzing substrates that mimic normal stromal configurations is becoming increasingly obvious.

There are now five genetically distinct collagens found in varying proportions in various tissues which are associated with epithelial induction. In addition, the interaction of the glycosaminoglycans and fibronectin with the collagens is being described (15). Thus, the suggestion is made that the stroma and extracellular matrices underlying specific regions of the epithelia can be distinctly individual when the various molecular species are combined in a multiplicity of permutations and proportions. Thus, molecular patterning of the stroma locally may provide specifically different substrates for epithelial cells. The reaction of the epithelial cells to these distinct molecular patterns is then expressed as altered cellular behavior. Cell plasma membrane organization can be altered and intracellular cytoskeletal elements are modified by interactions with the substrate. These events ultimately result in selection of different modes of behavior at the biochemical and genetic levels.

Is there enough variation in the molecular patterning to account for the numerous stromal-specific activities seen during embryogenesis? The crude analogy might be made that four nucleotides can be combined in a sufficiently large number of variations to code for the entire genetic information contained in the organism. It is already known that cells do respond to

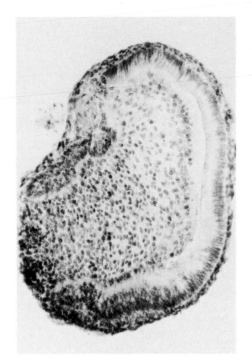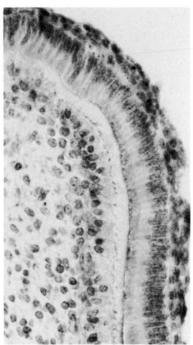

FIG. 5. If tetracycline is present but, in addition, exogenous procollagen is added, development is normal. Morphogenesis (A) is normal in all aspects and cytodifferentiation (B) has proceedednormally. Dentin is present and there are indications the enamel protein is being secreted.

****

foreign substrates. By changing cell shape such important functions as DNA synthesis and specific protein synthesis can be altered (9, 29). Thus, the availability of a reasonably small number of stromal components ubiquitous in all the animal kingdom, may account for the precise regional molecular patterning in the embryo.

While this hypothesis raises a number of unanswered ancillary questions, the basic premise is amenable to experimental verification. Experimental disruption of the stroma with specific inhibitors that alter the stroma should continue with the exogenous addition of matrix components. Indeed, the literature contains a number of studies examining the effects of diazo-oxo-norleucine (DON) an inhibitor which alters glycosaminoglycan synthesis (13). This agent alters tooth development presumably by affecting the mesenchymal synthesis of glycosaminoglycan molecules. But, the effects of adding exogenous glycosaminoglycans has not been reported.

In addition, however, artificial matrices should be constructed with a view toward experimentally mimicking the natural stroma (23). Past work suffered from using collagens of variable purity and fibrillar form. These data contribute little to unmasking the instructive nature of natural stromal substrates. Artificial matrices composed of components that mimic as closely as possible the components of the native stroma can be constructed. Such work is underway (23, MacCallum and Lillie, personal communication) and may prove to be a new model for epithelial-stromal interaction.

I have ignored thus far one important element in the communication between the epithelium and the mesenchymal stroma. That is the role of the basal lamina. Its structure, complexity, and functional role cannot be taken up here but are discussed by Bernfield (this volume and 10). The importance of this structure in maintaining epithelial patterns, of conferring stability to the basal cells, and as an interface in communication between epithelium and mesenchyme adds another element to the micropatterning seen locally in the embryo. Indeed, the experimental studies of tissue interactions focus on the light microscopic basement membrane which, of course, is an association of basal lamina and the immediately adjacent stromal elements.

The complexity of the basal lamina is gradually unfolding. There are two discrete species of collagens (IVa, IVb) in the lamina densa and a combination of proteins and glycoproteins (laminin, BM-1 glycoprotein) in the lamina lucida. Thus, a similar variety of components as seen in the stroma and that can be varied in proportion, composition and organization exist at this level of basement membrane organization. The highly organized nature of these components in mammary gland (10) and the alterations of the basal lamina during culture indicate an influence of the stroma on optimal basal lamina formation.

The interaction of the basal lamina and the immediately subjacent stromal elements further intensifies our suggestion that the limited elements in the basal lamina and the stroma may provide substrate information that obviates the need for specific inductive signals.

Needless to say, the cellular component of the stroma should not be overlooked. Because it is important that these cells provide the source of native collagen and proteoglycans, there is another function of the cells that needs to be considered in this view of the stroma as a determinant of epithelial shape. That is the role of extracellular proteases that expedite epithelial migration into the stromal bed. A recent study of Bode and Dziadek (1) demonstrated that the levels of extracellular proteases in the developing embryo are maximal in the mesoderm at the time of morphogenesis just when such activity would be expected to function in determining the shape of complex organ rudiments. Note also the identification of a neutral pH hyaluronidase and its role during gland morphogenesis as discussed by Bernfield (this volume). Physical pressure cannot be the driving force for epithelial invasion. There must be a cooperative sequence of stromal reorganization simultaneous with epithelial invasion. The result of course is an epithelial invasive display typical of complex rudiments such as tooth buds, hair follicles, or glandular acini.

Is the Inducer Diffusible?

Consider the very precise organization of epithelial differentiation. The surface integument and the oral mucosa provide ample evidence that the patterns of cellular stratification and keratinization can interface abruptly. Within a 1.6 mm border the epithelium can change to dramatically distinct cellular expressions (26). The vermillion border of the lip which abuts the facial skin and the border between the gingiva and the alveolar mucosa are two examples of the abruptness of epithelial specificity. The discrete localization of these epithelial micropatterns argues strongly against a diffusible or easily transmissable factor in the stroma as the inductive signal. Some recent evidence from Fisher and Solursh (8) and Noden (24) indicates that the local stromal environment is very stable, that stromal areas expand not by random cellular migration but by expansion of a local cellular and extracellular mass. Thus, extracellular matrix components modify the activities of ectopically transplanted mesenchyme cells. Once the local micropatterns are established in the developing embryo, the cellular and extracellular matrix micropatterns can maintain their identities as local tissue-specific inductive stromata. Local maintenance of epithelial structure in the adult organism is merely a historical expression of local patterns established in the underlying stroma during early embryogenesis.

It is essential to note that the inductive tissue interactions that we have described for the embryo continue to operate throughout the life of the organism. Maintenance of pattern and stability of structural form are in part due to stromal influences not unlike those described as operating in tooth morphogenesis. The importance of other directive influences in the genital tract and their influences on adult structure have been reviewed by Cunha et al. (4).

Establishment of Overall Patterns in the Dentition

Although the local stromal and basal lamina micropatterns may account for some of the discrete regional differences in epithelial differentiaton there is still another level of pattern that exists in the organism. In some cases, the entire organ system must be organized into overall functional groupings of similar segmented but separate subunits. How does the embryo organize the segmented series of tooth buds into the appropriate occlusal masticatory pattern?

Earlier, as an example of the directive role of the embryonic dental mesenchyme, I selected an experimental combination of edentulous epithelium from the diastema (that separates the incisor from the first molar of the mouse dentition) and a molar dental papilla (see Fig. 1). That predictably toothless space is a functional requirement in rodents but it can produce a tooth bud from the overlying epithelium if it is influenced experimentally by tooth mesenchyme. Thus, the normal and expected absence of teeth suggests that during development an active dental mesenchyme is never established in this region. Why? What determines the appearance of an incisor region mesially, and then, following a toothless region, the appearance of a molar region?

We have preliminary evidence that in the craniofacial region the sensory innervation may play a decisive role in organizing the dentition as well as other epithelial derivatives. I do not attempt to apply this idea to other spatially segmented and patterned organ systems in the body. But, in the head, the nervous system plays a very strong role in organizing bilateral sense organs.

Note, for example, that both the teeth and the sensory vibrissae follicles are innervated by the sensory components of the trigeminal ganglion and in both cases about one-half day before the tooth buds or the vibrissae epithelial buds become visible the innervation approaches the site of the future structure. Our experimental evidence so far is preliminary (20) but the relationship between the presence of the innervation and the ability to develop teeth is enticing.

The details of the relationship of the innervation to the development of a competent embryonic rudiment are not known. Once the rudiment is established the innervation is not necessary since older tooth buds and vibrissae follicles can be explanted to organ culture in the absence of innervation without impairment of the development. Nonetheless, the importance of the innervation may be related to the initiation of the embryonic rudiment.

How the innervation functions is not known. Whether the innervation is merely trophic in the sense that it enhances the interactions operating during the very early stages of initiation, or whether there is a directive role of the nerve fibers initiating the epithelial and mesenchymal cell population that permanently retains the information to produce a tooth or vibrissae follicle is not known. Clearly, since both vibrissae and teeth demonstrate this relationship with the trigeminal innervation, specificity of the interaction cannot be claimed; it must be a more generalized interaction. Nonetheless spatial specificity so common in the nervous system may be reflected in the initiating events of the embryonic end organs.

This specificity is dramatically demonstrated by the vibrissae. The vibrissae are tactile sensory organs distributed in precise spatial patterns on the snout which are projected to barrels of nerve cells in the sensory cortex (33, 34). The spatial distribution of the two components is very tightly correlated in this system in particular and is genetically controlled.

SUMMARY

Induction: Initiation, Histogenesis, Cytodifferentiation

These observations when considered as a whole suggest that the entire concept of tissue differentiation, pattern formation and induction should be redefined. I repeat my earlier qualification; the developing ectoderm and its array of specialized structures and regional specificities (19) requires a stringent set of conditions for differentiated function at all levels of organization. It is in the ectoderm and its derivatives that the evidence for directive tissue interactions finds its strongest and most unequivocal demonstrations. The evocation of enamel synthesis from non-dental epithelia and across Class lines in the oral epithelium of the chick embryo cannot be considered a potentiation of a protodifferentiated cell population. Nor, as is often the case in other systems, can it be treated as an exaggerated synthesis of products already being secreted by the cells involved in the interaction. New genetic information is expressed in response to an appropriate tissue interaction.

Induction as it is traditionally described usually implies transmission of some specific instructions. Often these have been described as a specific molecule that transmits information to a responding tissue whose entire genome is an open switchboard waiting for the appropriate combination to be tapped. Yet, inductive influences (from the mesenchyme) in fact, seem to be general in nature and very ancient since the information can be interpreted across wide phylogenetic lines (21). The response is specific only in so far as the genetic information in the responding genome (in the epithelium) permits compatible structural and enzymatic proteins to be produced.

In the context of this discussion, I will define embryonic induction as that process which evokes stable, persistent morphological structures that in turn expedite the utilization of gene products in predictable sequences. The nature of the inductive signal is not known and has been the central issue of developmental biology since the Mangold-Spemann experiments first exposed the phenomenon. But, it is the device for organizing and synchronizing the appearance of vertebrate form. The signal is not specific in that there is a distinct molar inducer or a unique salivary gland inducer, etc. In fact the inducing tissue for hair is recognized by chick epithelium and the response is the development of chick-specific structures (3, 21). Rather, the inductive signal is more general in nature; it is the response that is specific and it is determined by the specific genetic information that is deployed in the responding cell.

In part the difficulty in arriving at a workable hypothesis for the mechanism of induction stems from a tendency to oversimplify the process. Clearly, induction is not a single event that concerns itself only with gene expression for unique specialized products when cytodifferentiation takes place. Gene expression for a characteristic enzymatic or structural protein is the final event in a sequence of interactions.

During tooth development it is obvious that initiating events occur very early in embryogenesis to establish epithelial and mesenchymal sites of toothness or other organ rudiments and these are established in organized spatial patterns. The initial inductive events somehow establish stable cell populations that retain the information necessary for tooth development for long periods in pre- and post-natal life. Cells can recover from inhibition because they remember their morphogenetic histories. Part of that information enables the mesenchyme to direct specifically the histogenesis of the individual teeth. Specific information that supports incisor or molar tissue organization is expressed long after the initiating events have occurred. The first stages of the inductive process is, indeed, a stable restriction of the cells' developmental capabilities. The bias toward a more limited set of responses occurs at this point.

Finally, after considerable interaction and histodifferentiation has occurred, the cells of the inner dental epithelium and the odontoblast layer of the mesenchyme differentiate and secrete characteristic proteins. This final stage of developmental expression is very tightly linked to the previous histodifferentiative events since experimental uncoupling of the interacting tissues stops development. Certainly, there is evidence for communication between the epithelial and mesenchymal cells during this phase (31). But, the inductive event as thought of in the traditional sense probably occurred during the initiating phase when stable changes in the cells take place that permit the subsequent series of interactions resulting in odontogenesis.

The complexity of this final stage should be emphasized. Thesleff (32) points out the anti-fibronectin fluorescent staining disappears in areas of odontoblast differentiation but persists in more immature areas of the tooth bud. Thus, the gradient of cellular differentiation in the tooth bud is reflected in a change in the fibronectin of the basement membrane.

In addition, a complex reorganization of the pre-ameloblasts occurs in the epithelium in response to this cue from the odontoblast layer. The basal lamina breaks down, the Golgi apparatus and the nucleus reverse their polarity, and then enamel matrix proteins are secreted. Note that a "lumen" is created by this maneuver so that a former epithelial basal cell is transformed into a glandular cell. Enamel protein is secreted into a space once occupied by the basal lamina. This cellular transformation may be unique in epithelial differentiation.

The sequence of differentiation that began earlier with events that established stable dental patterns now ends with a complex and unique epithelial specialization. The intervening substrate, tissue and cellular interactions result in tooth morphogenesis.

ACKNOWLEDGEMENTS

The author acknowledges the support of the National Science Foundation (PCM76-19975) and the University of Connecticut Research Foundation. Special thanks to Ms. S. Pearson who contributed enormously to the typing and editing of this manuscript.

REFERENCES

1. Bode, V. C. and M. A. Dziadek (1979): Dev. Biol., 73:272-289.
2. Chlapowski, F. J. and L. Haynes (1979): J. Cell Biol., 83:605-614.
3. Coulombre, J. L. and A. J. Coulombre (1971): Dev. Biol., 25:464-478.
4. Cunha, G., L. W. K. Chung, J. M. Shannon and B. A. Reese (1980): Biology of Reproduction, 22:19-42.
5. Dhouailly, D. (1975): Wilhelm Roux's Arch., 177:323-340.
6. Emerman, J. T., S. J. Burwen and D. R. Pitelka (1979): Tissue and Cell, 11:109-119.
7. Fisher, M. and M. Solursh (1979a): Exp. Cell Res., 123:1-14.
8. Fisher, M. and M. Solursh (1979b): J. Embryol. Exp. Morph., 49:295-305.
9. Folkman, J. and A. Moscona (1978): Nature, 273:345-349.
10. Gordon, J. R. and M. R. Bernfield (1980): Dev. Biol., 74:118-135.
11. Grobstein, C. and J. F. Cohen (1965): Science, 150:626-628.
12. Hay, E. D. and S. Meier (1978): In: Textbook of Oral Biology, edited by J. H. Shaw, E. A. Sweeney, C. C. Cappuccino and S. M. Miller, pp. 3-23, Saunders, Philadelphia.
13. Hurmerinta, K., I. Thesleff and L. Saxen (1979): J. Embryol. Exp. Morph., 50:99-109.
14. Kerley, M. A. and E. J. Kollar (1980): Amer. J. Anat., in press.
15. Kleinman, H. (1980): In: Current Research Trends in Prenatal Craniofacial Development, edited by R. Pratt and R. L. Christiansen, Elsevier - North Holland, in press.
16. Kollar, E. J. and G. Baird (1969): J. Embryol. Exp. Morph., 21:131-148.
17. Kollar, E. J. and G. Baird (1970a): J. Embryol. Exp. Morph., 24:159-171.
18. Kollar, E. J. and G. Baird (1970b): J. Embryol. Exp. Morph., 24:173-186.
19. Kollar, E. J. (1972): Am. Zool., 12:125-135.
20. Kollar, E. J. and A. G. S. Lumsden (1979): J. Biol. Buccale, 7:49-60.
21. Kollar, E. J. and C. Fisher (1980): Science, 207:993-995.
22. Lillie, J. H., D. K. MacCallum and A. Jepsen (1980a): Exp. Cell Res., 125:153-165.

23. Lillie, J. H., D. K. MacCallum and A. Jepsen (1980b): Abstr., Second Internat. Congress Cell Biology, in press.
24. Noden, D. (1980): In: Current Research Trends in Prenatal Craniofacial Development, edited by R. Pratt and R. L. Christiansen, Elsevier-North Holland, in press.
25. Saxén, L. (1977): In: Cell and Tissue Interactions, edited by J. W. Lash and M. M. Burger, pp. 1-9, Raven Press, New York.
26. Schroeder, H. E. and M. Amstad-Jossi (1979): Cell Tissue Res., 202:75-97.
27. Sengel, P. (1976): Morphogenesis of Skin, Cambridge University Press, London.
28. Shannon, J. M. and D. R. Pitelka (1977): J. Cell Biol., 77:32a.
29. Shannon, J. M. and D. R. Pitelka (1980): In Vitro., in press.
30. Slavkin, H. C. (1979): J. Biol Buccale, 6:189-203.
31. Thesleff, I. (1977): In: Cell Interactions in Differentiation, edited by M. Karkinen-Jasskelainen, L. Saxen, L. Weiss, pp. 191-208, Academic Press, London.
32. Thesleff, I. (1980): In: Current Research Trends in Prenatal Craniofacial Development, edited by R. Pratt and R. L. Christiansen, Elsevier-North Holland, New York, in press.
33. Welker, C. (1971): Brain Res., 26:259-275.
34. Woolsey, T. A. and H. van der Loos (1970): Brain Res.,

Morphogenesis and Pattern Formation,
edited by T. G. Connelly et al.,
Raven Press, New York © 1981.

The Development of Laminated Pattern in the Mammalian Neocortex

Verne S. Caviness, Jr., M. Cecilia Pinto-Lord, and Philippe Evrard

*Department of Neurology, Eunice Kennedy Shriver Center,
Waltham, Massachusetts 02154*

The neocortex is an extensive sheet of neurons which lies at the surface of the mammalian cerebral hemispheres (32). This structure plays a central role in the most complex functions of the human nervous system: language, cognition and memory (21, 22). It has a regular, laminate architecture which evolves through an elaborate sequence of developmental events. The present review is concerned with the developmental history of this remarkable architectural pattern. The discussion draws heavily upon comparative studies of the neocortex in normal and <u>reeler</u> (<u>rl</u>) mutant mice. This mutation, associated with a systematic anomaly in the laminar architecture of the neocortex (6), highlights cellular interrelationships upon which normal neocortical development is critically dependent (7, 11). Observations and principles based upon studies in mice are complemented by work on the developing neocortex in other species, particularly in primates (36, 37).

STRUCTURE OF THE NEOCORTEX

The Normal Neocortex

The normal neocortex is constructed of six parallel planes, or laminae, which vary in only relatively minor ways from region to region (4, 5). A narrow molecular layer (layer I) formed principally of neuronal dendrites and axons but also containing scattered neuronal somata, lies at the surface (Fig. 1A). The five subjacent laminae, by contrast to layer I, are each richly populated by neuronal somata. Each of these is dominated by neurons of a specific class. By neurons of a class we mean neurons having a similar morphologic configuration as well as having similar patterns of afferent and efferent connections.

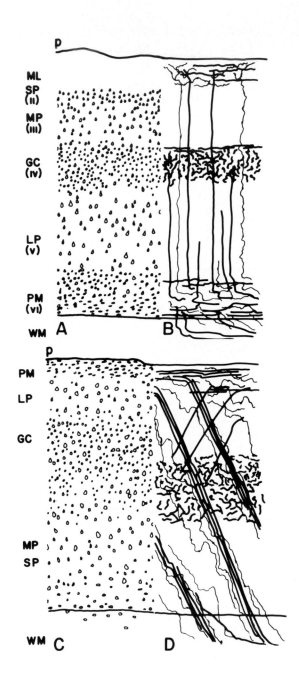

ML
SP
(II)
MP
(III)
GC
(IV)
LP
(V)
PM
(VI)
WM

A   B

p
PM
LP
GC
MP
SP
WM

C   D

FIG. 1. Cell and fiber patterns of normal (A, B) and <u>reeler</u> (C, D) neocortex. Polymorphic (PM), large pyramidal (LP), granule (GC), medium pyramidal (MP) and small pyramidal (SP) cells are ordered from deep to superficial in the normal (A) but superficial to deep in the mutant (C) cortex. Normal neocortical layers are designated by Roman numerals in A. Large fiber fascicles enter the zone of PM cells in the depths of the normal (B) but ascend to the superficial plane of the mutant (D) cortex. see text for further details.

****

From superficial to deep in the cortex, these neuronal classes and their respective laminae are: small pyramidal neurons (layer II), the medium-sized pyramidal neurons (layer II), the granular or stellate neurons (layer IV), the large pyramidal neurons (layer V), and the polymorphic neurons (layer VI). The small and medium-sized pyramidal cells of layers II and III make the major contribution to connections between neocortical regions within the same and between the two cerebral hemispheres (23, 49, 50, 53). The large pyramidal neurons of layer V give rise to descending, subdiencephalic projections while the polymorphic neurons of layer VI project upon the thalamus (7, 51). The stellate neurons of layer IV are local circuit neurons (29): their axons are distributed in a restricted fashion within the cortical sector in which the neuron soma resides.

Large fiber fascicles pass between the neocortex and subcortical structures (Fig. 1B). Within the cortex, they enter a tangentially coursing fiber stratum in the depths of layer VI. Additional fiber strata are encountered at higher cortical levels particularly in layer I and overlapping layers III and IV. In addition, fibers pass singly or in small fascicles, in radial fashion throughout all levels of the neocortex.

The Reeler Neocortex

The neocortex of the mutant contains cellular populations and fiber systems which are homologous with those of the normal neocortex (6, 7). Remarkably, however, there is a systematic inversion in the relative positions in the radial dimension of the cortex that are occupied by the various neuronal classes and fiber strata (6, 12). Thus, polymorphic neurons occupy the superficial plane of the cortex in the mutant, that is, the level normally given to the molecular layer (Fig. 1C). Large pyramidal cells lie immediately subjacent while small and medium-sized pyramidal cells predominate in the depths of the cortex. Granular interneurons predominate at an intermediate neocortical level. Although neurons are laminated by class in <u>reeler</u> in this way, it should be emphasized that laminar segregation is less rigorous with more overlap of adjacent neuronal classes in reeler than in the normal cortex. Further, a number of neurons of a class may be dramatically out of register with other neurons of the same class (7).

Large fiber fascicles also pass between subcortical structures and the neocortex in the mutant (Fig. 1D). The trajectory of these fascicles in reeler, unlike those in the normal animal, traverses the full width of the cortex (6). At the superficial plane of the cortex, the axons enter a tangential fiber stratum, which like its counterpart in the normal animal, courses through the zone occupied by polymorphic neurons. As in the normal animal, a cortical stratum of ramifying fibers lies at the cortical level occupied by granular interneurons (10). A tangential fiber stratum, homologous with that passing through layer I of the normal neocortex, has not yet been identified in the mutant neocortex. As in the normal animal, radially directed fibers pass through all levels of the mutant neocortex.

Despite the fact that axons follow aberrant trajectories in the neocortex of reeler, the major afferent systems appear to be topologically equivalent to their normal counterpart (11). Further, the axons of these systems terminate among the same neuronal classes in reeler as they do in the normal cortex (6, 10, 11, 15).

NEOCORTICAL DEVELOPMENT

Overview

Development of the cerebral neocortex proceeds through two broad epochs, each served by a different sequence of cellular events (19, 36, 37). The first of these is the epoch of cytogenesis -- or cell generation, and histogenesis -- or the assembly of cells and fiber systems into laminar order within the cortex. The events occurring during this first epoch are the principal focus of the present discussion. They proceed in a relatively compressed time frame. In the rodent, they are largely accomplished during the third or final week of gestation and continue for only a few days into the first postnatal week (2).

Cytogenesis and histogenesis are succeeded by a more extended, second epoch of neuronal differentiation and growth. Once in position at the end of their migrations, neurons elaborate their schematic and dendritic surfaces (28, 39) and make synaptic contact with terminals of converging axons (1). The second epoch continues through the first postnatal month in rodents. As cortical neurons achieve their full size and the surrounding neuropil becomes fully constituted during this period of time, the five cellular layers of the neocortex, established during the first epoch, acquire their definitive character (40).

Cytogenesis and Neuronal Migration

Contrary to expectation, perhaps, neurons are not formed in the relative positions which they will occupy in the adult neocortex. Remarkably, the neurons of the neocortex are generated instead in a pseudostratified epithelium (41, 42) which lines the ventricular cavity at the inner surface of the developing cerebrum (47). In terms of size of the young neuron at the end of its last mitotic division, this generative epithelium lies a great distance from the developing cortex. In order to find its correct position, the young postmitotic neuron must migrate as a freely motile element across an extraordinarily complex, extended terrain known as the intermediate zone (IZ). The young neuron appears to be critically dependent for guidance in this journey upon the assistance of a non-neuronal cell class, the "radial glial cell" (34, 35). The somata of radial glia cells are located near the ventricular lining of the developing cerebrum. From the soma, an elongated process extends radially to the outer surface of the cerebrum where a distal expansion contributes to the investing, limiting glial membrane.

The young, postmitotic neuron migrates along the radially extended fiber to its cortical destination. In the course of its ascent, it has a fusiform configuration with radially extended leading and trailing processes. Prior to its entry into the cortex, the cell enlarges slightly (38) and the axonal process emerges from the inferior pole of the cell (44). Otherwise, the cell undergoes no visible differentiation prior to the completion of its migration.

This mechanism of transfer of the young neuron assures an orderly topologic transformation of the two tangential dimensions of the generative epithelium upon the two tangential, or surface dimensions of the cortex (36, 37). That is, cells formed at "adjacent points" in the generative epithelium will be brought to lie at "adjacent points" in the tangential dimensions of the neocortex (Fig. 2).

This topologic transformation is achieved normally in reeler. Thus, it appears, neurons are generated at the normal time and at the normal rate; they migrate across the IZ in the sequence in which they are generated and they are guided in their migrations by radial glial fibers (6, 13, 45) (Pinto-Lord, Evrard and Caviness, unpublished observations). It is only after the young neuron enters the plane of the developing cortex that the developmental anomaly, associated with the mutation at the reeler locus, becomes apparent. That is, the systematic inversion in the radial order of neurons with respect to the temporal sequence in which they are generated (6, 13) appears to come about as a consequence of events occurring after the cell enters the cortex.

Laminar Order of Successive Neuronal Cohorts:
The Initial Lamination Patterns

The majority of neurons of the cerebral cortex of the mouse are generated between embryonic day 11 (E11) and embryonic day 17 (E13) (2, 6, 13). The maximum rate of generation continues from E12-14. The earliest formed cells complete their migrations by

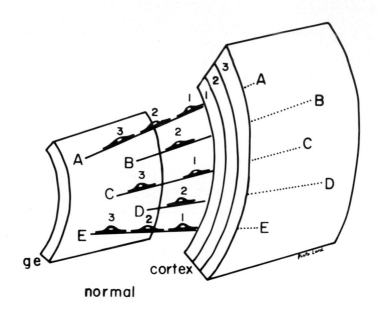

normal

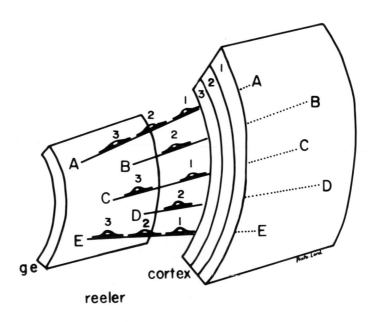

reeler

FIG. 2. Schematic representation of the transformation of generative epithelium (ge) upon the neocortex in normal and reeler embryos. In both genotypes there is an orderly "point-to-point" (A-E), or topologic, transformation of the tangential dimensions of the epithelium upon the tangential, or surface, dimensions of the cortex. Successive generations of cells (1-3) are ordered in an inside-out sequence in the radial dimension of the normal but in outside-in sequence in that of the mutant cortex.

****

E13 and the last shortly after the time of birth.

The earliest arrivals (E13) are distributed diffusely in the superficial plane of the cerebral wall in a fashion that is indistinguishable in normal and reeler embryos (6). Within 24 hours, between E13-14, with the arrival of increasing numbers of additional cells, this "primordial" cortex becomes laminated (Fig. 3). From the outset, the pattern of lamination is abnormal in reeler (6, 33). Thus, in the normal animal (Fig. 3A), two laminae housing relatively few neuronal somata -- an outer molecular layer and a deep stratum referred to as the subplate (SB) (25) -- bracket a lamina which is densely packed with neuronal somata --the cortical plate (CP). In reeler (Fig. 3B), by contrast, the CP forms subjacent to a zone which contains a low density of neuronal somata -- the superplate (SP). For reasons to be considered later, the SP bears close structural homology with the SB of the normal neocortex. The CP of the mutant, in turn, is partitioned into inner and outer tiers by a plexiform zone which emerges at an intermediate level of the cortex by E14. This plexiform stratum -- the intermediate plexiform zone (IPZ) -- is. crossed by additional plexiform planes which span the SP and the IZ.

Intracortical Movement of Successive Neuronal Cohorts

The primary neuronal cohort, that generated on E11, is distributed at the end of its migration in diffuse fashion at the superficial level of the cerebral wall (Fig. 4A). Dramatic differences characterize the pattern of redistribution of these neurons in the two genotypes over the next 24 hours as the CP emerges (6, 44; Caviness, unpublished observations). In the normal animal, this primary cohort is partitioned into two subpopulations: a small contingent which remains in the molecular layer superficial to the CP and a larger contingent which comes to occupy the SB below the CP (Fig. 4B). In reeler, by contrast, the neurons of the E11 cohort remain together in the SP above the CP. Only exceptional cells of this cohort come to be in subjacent positons, below or within the CP.

Cohorts of neurons generated subsequently, on E12 or later, are

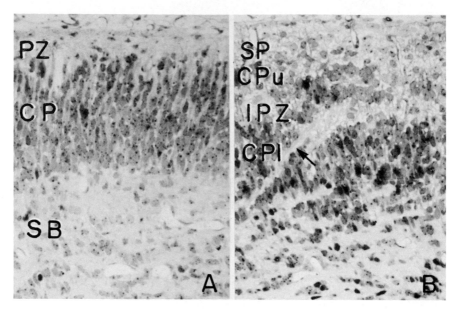

FIG. 3. Micrographs of the normal (A) and <u>reeler</u> (B) developing neocortex of E16 embryos. Lamination scheme in the normal is molecular layer, or plexiform zone, (PZ); cortical plate, (CP) and subplate, (SB). In the <u>reeler</u>, the lamination scheme is superplate, (SP); upper and lower tiers of the cortical plate, (CPu) and (CPl), respectively; and intermediate plexiform zone, (IPZ). 1 μm sections, toluidine blue, X 247.

****

directed to the CP in both the normal and <u>reeler</u> (Caviness, unpublished observations). In the normal animal, the neurons of successive cohorts bypass positions occupied by neurons of earlier formed cohorts in their ascent through the cortex (Fig. 4C). Eventually, they arrive at the interface of the CP and the molecular layer where their migrations are arrested. At this cortical level, the cell appears to encounter an impediment to further outward movement.

Throughout its ascent, the migrating cell appears to remain applied to, and to some extent coiled around, the intracortical segment of the radial glial fiber (Pinto-Lord, Evrard and Caviness, unpublished observations). It is evidently able to interpose itself between the radial glial fiber and the somata or dendrites of postmigratory cells which lie along its migratory path (Fig. 5, 6). In fact, the surface of the radial glial fiber appears to be the only corridor of ascent through the developing

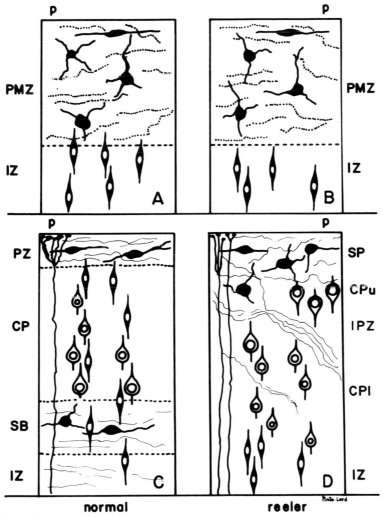

FIG. 4. Schematic representations of the developing neocortex prior to (A, B) and after (C, D) the emergence of the cortical plate in normal and reeler neocortex. Prior to the appearance of the cortical plate, postmigratory cells in the postmigratory zone (PMZ) are distributed diffusely in a manner indistinguishable in the two genotypes. Successive cohorts of neurons crossing the intermediate zone (IZ) are able to penetrate the PMZ and establish a cortical plate subjacent to the external plexiform zone (PZ) in the normal but not in the mutant cortex. Successive cohorts of cells transmigrate positions occupied by predecessors and ascend fully to the PZ in the normal cortex. They terminate their ascent as they approach the positions occupied by preceding cohorts in the mutant cortex. Radial glial fibers (at the left in C and D) span the IZ and cortex of both genotypes.

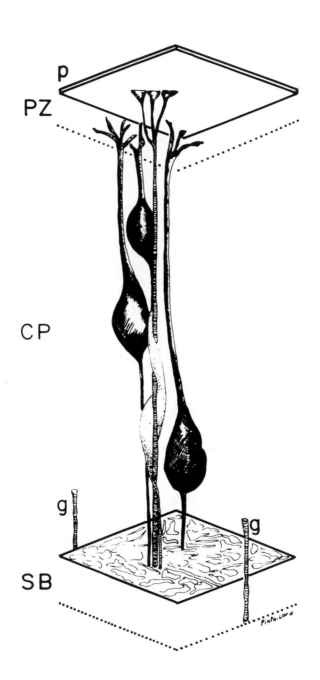

p

PZ

CP

SB

g

g

Pinto-Lord

FIG. 5. Normal neocortex. A migrating cell (stippled) ascends the intracortical segment of a radial glial fiber (g). It interposes itself between the fiber and postmigratory cells (shaded in black) which it encounters in its ascent.

****

cortex (Pinto-Lord, Evrard and Caviness, unpublished observations).

Once the cell completes its migration, it appears to become fixed in position with respect to tangentially adjacent members of the same cohort and also with respect to radially adjacent members of preceding cohorts (Caviness, unpublished observations). The somata of neurons which migrate along the same, or along a cluster of closely adjacent, radial glial fibers become grouped into compact columnar aggregates, aligned in the radial dimension of the cortex (Fig. 7; Pinto-Lord, Evrard and Caviness, unpublished observations). Large numbers of apical dendrites, developing at the termination of migration from the leading migratory process are brought into apposition with each other, external to the columnar array of neuronal somata (Figs. 7, 8). Because the dendritic fascicles lie external to the columnar aggregates of somata, those arising from the somata of adjacent columns abut upon each other giving rise to a dendritic "compartment" which is continuous throughout the cortex. The columnar aggregates of neuronal somata are isolated from each other within the continuous dendritic volume.

The intracortical movements of successive cohorts of migratory cells are radically abnormal in <u>reeler</u> (Fig. 4D). In particular, it appears that neurons of a cohort are unable to ascend beyond the positions occupied by neurons of the preceding cohort (Caviness, unpublished observations). This pattern is evident as early as the arrival of the first cohort of neurons which come to constitute the CP in the mutant. Unlike their normal counterparts, these first neurons of the CP are unable to penetrate the primordial zone of postmigratory cells. Thus, this latter population of cells does not come to be partitioned into deep and superficially lying subpopulations as occurs in the normal animal. Similarly each successive cohort of cells ascends to the position occupied by the prior cohort where its migration is arrested. Particularly at later stages of cortical histogenesis in <u>reeler</u>, there is an increasing degree of overlap between adjacent cohorts, however.

The nature of the impediment to migration which the young neuron encounters in the zone occupied by the prior cell cohort has not been identified. It is not yet known for example, if the impediment may be visualized in electron micrographs. Whatever the specific nature of the impediment, its consequence is clear: a systematic inversion in the radial order within the cortex of successively generated cohorts of neurons.

Once migrations are completed, neurons in <u>reeler</u>, like their counterparts in the normal animal, become fixed to tangentially and radially adjacent elements (Caviness, unpublished

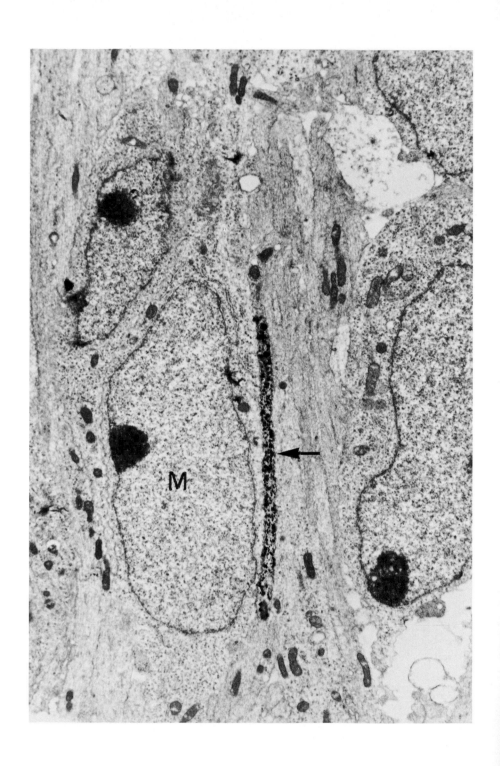

FIG. 6. Electron micrograph of a migrating cell (M) ascending in apposition to the intracortical segment of a radial glial fiber, impregnated by the rapid Golgi method (arrow), X 9020

****

observations). The extent to which the somata of neurons migrating along closely adjacent radial glial fibers come to be aggregated into radially aligned columns in the mutant is not yet known. Nor is it clear as yet to what extent in reeler the apical dendrites arising from cells affiliated with adjacent radial glial fibers merge to form a dendritic volume continuous throughout the cortex.

Commitment to Neuronal Class

The foregoing observations illustrate the sequence of events through which neurons of the same cohort become aligned in the cortex at the end of their migrations. It is a corollary of these observations that cells which are members of the same cohort are also members of the same neuronal class. Although one might postulate that class is "induced" or "imposed" secondarily upon the post-migratory cell by factors which impinge upon it from its milieu, this appears not be be the case. An additional set of observations from studies in reeler is pertinent to this point. Thus, the majority of large pyramidal cells, cells formed at a maximum rate on E13, lie superficially in the outer part of the reeler cortex. A few cells typical of this class are, however, "misplaced" at deeper cortical levels (Mangini, Lemmon and Pearlman, and Caviness and Frost, unpublished observations). Despite being out of register with respect to other members of their cohort, these large pyramidal cells resemble the registered cells with respect to the general character and size of their somata and dendritic arbors and spines. Further, they, like other members of their cohort, give rise to subdiencephalic projections. The neighbors of the large pyramidal cells which lie "out of place" in the depths of the mutant cortex are typical medium-sized pyramidal cells (6). These give rise to a different set of connections -- the callosal and other corticocortical projections (15).

Evidently, these cells retain the principal attributes of their class despite isolation from other members of their cohort. Presumably, therefore, commitment to class antedates, and does not depend upon, entry of the cell into the cortex. Commitment might be determined as early as the time that the neuron undergoes its final mitotic division. The various cell classes are formed in sequence at each "point" in the generative epithelium. The class of a given cell might be an inevitable consequence --inevitable in terms of the activity of its genome -- of when in this sequence it is generated (3).

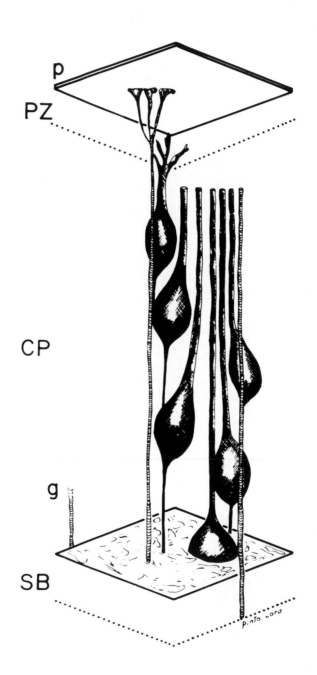

p

PZ

CP

g

SB

FIG. 7. Normal neocortex. The somata of postmigratory cells remain closely apposed to radial glial fibers. Their apical dendrites, directed away from the radial glial fiber, become fasciculated with others arising from neurons affiliated with an adjacent radial glial fiber.

****

Laminar Order of Neocortical Afferents
Early Arriving Afferents : The MA System

Monoaminergic (MA) axons are the earliest afferents of extrinsic origin, yet identified, to arrive within the rodent neocortex (26, 43) (Caviness and Korde, unpublished observations). They enter the cortex of both normal and reeler mice as early as El4 but do so only after the cortical plate has emerged (Caviness and Korde, unpublished observations). That is, they enter the cortex only after the differential laminar structure and migration patterns characteristic of each genotype have become established.

The pattern of deployment of this early afferent system within the cortex appears to be dependent upon intracortical cues. Though structurally homologous, these cues lie at quite different depths of the neocortex in reeler and normal embryos (Fig. 9). Thus, these fibers ascend as large fascicles which pass directly to the zone occupied by the earliest formed, the polymorphic, cells (Caviness and Korde, unpublished observations). Only after they achieve the level of the cortex occupied by these cells do the fascicles break up into single fibers and become part of a tangential fiber system. In the normal animal the encounter between axon fascicles and polymorphic cells occurs in the SB, that is, in the depths of the cortex. In reeler, by contrast, the fascicles follow an obliquely ascending trajectory across the full width of the cortex and encounter the zone occupied by polymorphic cells at the most superficial level of the cerebral wall.

In both genotypes, single axons derived from the larger fiber fascicles are also directed into the plexiform strata. At this early stage of development, these strata are formed principally by apical dendrites of pyramidal cells (33). In neither genotype is there a propensity of the MA axons to branch among the densely packed somata of pyramidal cells in the CP. Thus, in the normal animal, MA fibers ascend radially from the SB to the molecular layer. There is little evidence of arborization as it crosses the CP. In reeler, the ascending fiber fascicles give off collaterals as they ascend through the plexiform strata. These collaterals do not penetrate beyond the plexiform strata among the neuronal somata of the cortical plate, however.

Late Arriving Afferents : The Class I
Thalamocortical and Callosal Systems

Two major afferent systems are known to penetrate the neocortex somewhat later in development than the MA systems. These are the

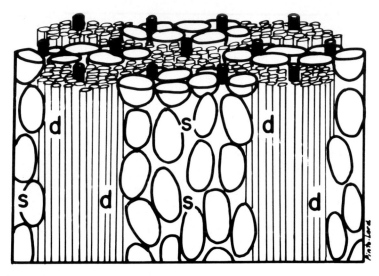

FIG. 8. Schematic representation of normal neocortical dendritic (d) and somatic (s) compartments. Neuronal somata are aggregated into micro-columns, isolated from each other by a consolidated volume of apical dendrites which is continuous throughout the neocortex. Radial glial fibers (shaded in black), isolated from each other, ascend axially through both the somatic micro-columns and dendritic fascicles.

****

Class I thalamocortical axons (axons which terminate principally in layers III/IV and to some extent in layer VI) and the callosal afferent system. The former system reaches the cortex late in gestation in both normal and reeler mice (Lund and Caviness, unpublished observations) as in other rodents (30, 52). The latter systems arrives early in the postnatal period of development in the normal animal (22, 50) and, though not verified experimentally as yet, presumably also in reeler.

Class I thalamocortical axons have as their targets the polymorphic cells in the depths of the cortex as well as the granule cells and medium-sized pyramidal neurons at mid-cortical levels (17). Like MA afferents, the class I thalamocortical afferents ascend to the cortex in large fascicles which continue to the cortical level occupied by polymorphic cells -- in the depths of the normal animal but superficially in the cortex of reeler (10, 11). The fascicles become diffused as single fibers in the tangential plane occupied by these cells and remain at this level for approximately one week before penetrating to midcortical levels to achieve their secondary cellular targets in layers III and IV. The direction of penetration is from below in the normal animal but from above in the reeler.

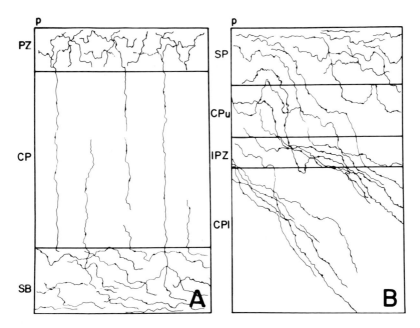

FIG. 9. Pattern of intracortical deployment of monoaminergic axons in the developing normal (A) and reeler (B) neocortex. Fascicles of fibers ascending from the subcortical level are directed initially to the zone occupied by polymorphic cells in the subplate (SB) deep in the normal but to the superplate (SP) at the superficial plane of the reeler neocortex. There is rich arborization among the consolidated apical dendrites of pyramidal cells in the external plexiform zone (PZ) of the normal as well as in the intermediate plexiform zone (IPZ) of the mutant cortex. No arborization occurs among the densely consolidated neuronal somata of the cortical plate (CP) of either genotype.

****

Callosal afferents become deployed in a fiber plane under target sectors of cortex early in the postnatal period (22, 50). They penetrate the cortex only after a delay of several days. These targets are the small and medium-sized pyramidal cells which lie superfically in layers II and III of the normal animal but in the depths of the reeler cortex.

THE CLASS II THALAMOCORTICAL AFFERENTS - A QUESTION

The time of entry of the final, presently recognized, class of afferent axons of extrinsic origin to the neocortex, the class II thalamocortical afferents (axons diffusely distributed to all cortical layers (17), is unknown. These afferents arise principally from the intralaminar and ventromedial nuclei but

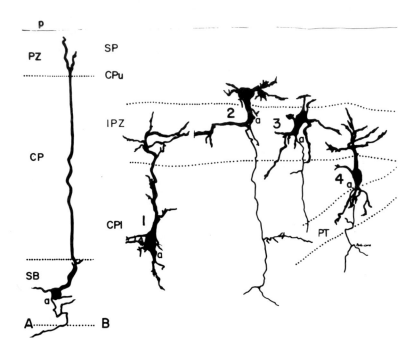

FIG. 10. Dendritic arborization with respect to axonal strata in the developing normal (A) and reeler (B) developing neocortex. In the normal, the relationship of postmigratory cell to axonal strata is uniform. The apical dendrite ascends to branch within the PZ; somatic dendrites sprout into the SB. The relationship of postmigratory cell to axonal strata is varied in the mutant. Polar dendritic systems may ascend (1) or descend (2) to the IPZ. Where the cell is bracketed between two plexiform planes (4) it may direct a polar dendritic system to each. Where the cell lies within a plexiform zone (3), dendrites issue radially from the cell soma. In both genotypes, axons (a) descend.

****

also, to some extent it appears, from virtually all nuclei of the thalamus (9, 17, 19). The pattern of intracortical deployment of this system is virtually the same as that of the MA axons, and there are arresting parallels in the regional patterns of distribution of subsets of thalamic and MA systems (16, 18, 27). For example, the dopaminergic system has a regional distribution identical to that of class II axons arising from the medial dorsal nucleus of the thalamus; the serotonergic and noradrenergic systems are approximately congruent in their regional distributions with the class II axons arising in the intralaminar and ventromedial nuclei of the thalamus.

Axon Targeting Mechanisms

Axon systems, afferent to normal and reeler neocortex, appear to have specific cell classes as their targets. Comparative studies reviewed above indicate that afferent axons readily penetrate the cortical levels occupied by their respective target cells whether these cells are in normal position or in abnormal position in reeler. The phenomenon is consistent with a mechanism of axon guidance implemented by diffusible substances which originate from target cells and which are perceived as a gradient by growing axons. It is not consistent with a mechanism dependent upon fixed positional cues along the axon trajectory itself such as "molecular instructions" in the surfaces of cells or "preformed channels" between cells (48). Admittedly late arriving axons which share primary cellular targets with early arriving afferents might be directed to these primary targets by fasciculation along earlier axon trajectories. However, these late entering axon systems eventually penetrate more deeply into the cortex to reach cellular targets which they do not share with the early arriving neocortical afferents. Again, attraction along a gradient of diffusable substances would appear the most plausible mechanism to implement such a phenomenon.

Pyramidal Cell Configuration

During the early phases of cortical development, dendrites appear to grow only towards and within axon strata in both normal and reeler neocortex (33). The different positional interrelationships of postmigratory neurons and axon strata in the normal and reeler neocortex are associated with dramatic differences in the configuration and the alignment of neurons within the neocortex (Fig. 10). In the normal animal, for example, there is uniformity in the positional relationships of the postmigratory pyramidal cell and the principal early axonal strata of the molecular layer and the SB. Thus, the pyramidal cell completes its migration with its leading migratory process directed into the molecular layer. Its soma eventually abuts upon and lies within the SB. The apical dendrite, realized by transformation of the leading migratory process, ascends and develops within the molecular layer while the basal dendrites, emerging from the cell soma, expand within the SB.

In reeler, by contrast, the apical dendrite may ascend or descend to the IPZ, depending upon the position of the cell soma with respect to this fiber stratum. On the other hand, if the cell soma is bracketed by the IPZ and an ascending plexiform plane, the neuron may have two major polar dendritic systems ascending and descending to these respective axonal strata. Finally, a cell fully submerged within the IPZ appears to achieve a stellate configuration with multiple dendrites radiating in a spherically symmetric fashion from the soma into the surrounding axonal bed.

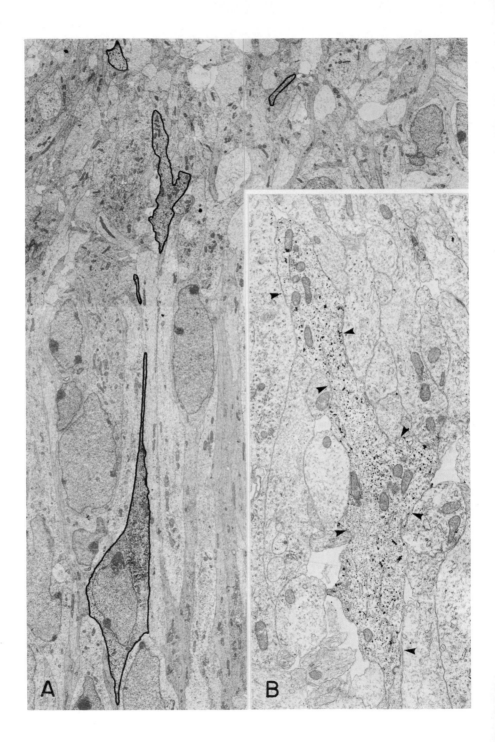

FIG. 11. Electronmicrograph of a postmigratory pyramidal cell (A) impregnated by the rapid Golgi method (outlined in India ink). The apical dendrite arborizes in the depths of the external plexiform layer. X 3,100. In B the arborization (outlined by arrow heads), is seen at higher magnification. There are no recognizable synaptic junctions along the plasma membrane. X 10,300.

****

The close correlation between the direction of dendritic growth and the positional relationship of the cell soma to surrounding axonal strata underscores the importance of a trophic influence of axons upon dendritic growth and differentiation (33). Dendritic growth and differentiation proceeds in the neocortex of both genotypes well before synaptogenesis occurs to any significant extent (Pinto-Lord, Evrard and Caviness, unpublished observations). Synaptic junctions are not observed upon growing terminal segments of dendrites (Fig. 11). Presumably, therefore, the trophic action of axons upon dendrites is mediated by diffusible substances. It is thus probable that axons and dendrites exert potent trophic actions upon each other.

CONCLUDING COMMENTS

The foregoing sections have reviewed the steps through which a pseudostratified epithelium, comprised of undifferentiated dividing cells and lining the developing cerebral wall, is transformed into the cerebral cortex. The final structure is composed of multiple neuronal classes, ordered by class into laminae. The construction of the cerebral cortex involves in the first instance an orderly "point-to-point", or topologic, transformation of the two tangential dimensions of the epithelium upon the two tangential dimensions of the cerebral cortex. In the second instance, it involves an orderly transformation of the temporal sequence in which neurons are generated within the epithelium into the positional order of neuronal classes in the radial dimension of the cortex. Axons entering the cortex are deployed with respect to the laminar positions of their specific cell targets. The dendrites of target cells, in reciprocal fashion, are elaborated in such a way as to conform to the position of their specific afferent systems.

In the course of this developmental sequence, each young neuron undergoes a series of dramatic changes in its state and behavior. The undifferentiated dividing cell is transformed into a postmitotic, migrating cell which is committed to differentiate later into a cell of a specific class. It terminates its migration and becomes fixed in a position to which it appears to attract afferent axons. It responds to the presence of these axons by elaborating its receptor surfaces.

As the cell proceeds through this sequence, it enters into close relationship with a succession of similar as well as unlike neighboring cells. Its relationship with other dividing cells and with the radial glial cell are transient. The relationship eventually achieved with postmigratory neuronal somata and dendrites and with afferent axons arising from more distally located cell somata will be enduring ones.

It is a central tenet of developmental neurobiology that the sequential transformations in the state and activity of the cell are responses to signals emanating from, or properties of, other cells. For example, the dramatic changes in state or in direction of movement of growth might be triggered by diffusible substances emanating from one cell population and influencing another. Peptides (8) or non-peptide transmitters (24) are plausible agents of this type of interaction. The sustained contacts between adjacent cell populations, on the other hand, such as the temporary contact between radial glial fiber and migrating cell or the permanent relationship between postmigratory cells might be mediated by high affinity binding between the surfaces of the adjacent cells (46). Glycoproteins and glycolipids, integral to the plasma membranes of cells, have been plausibly suggested as agents of this type of interaction (31).

The capacity of cells to interact with each other via such mechanisms does not in itself assure the formation of the cerebral cortex from a population of undifferentiated, dividing cells, however. From the outset and throughout the entire history of cortical histogenesis, the opportunity for favorable cellular interactions to occur derives from the spatial patterns of deployment and the temporal succession of encounters between cellular elements responsive to each other. Further, structural constraints may act as impediments to unfavorable variations in cell position and possibly also, to unfavorable directions of dendritic and axonal growth. Predictably, these factors no less than the molecular agents of cellular interactions, are indispensable to the realization of the laminate pattern of the mammalian cerebral cortex.

REFERENCES

1. Aghajanian, G. K. and F. E. Bloom (1967): Brain Res., 6:716-727.
2. Angevine, J. B., Jr. and R. L. Sidman (1961): Nature (Lond.), 192:766-768.
3. Bisconte, J. C. and R. Marty (1975): J. Hirnforsch., 16:55-74.
4. Brodmann, K. (1909): Vergleichende Lokalisationslehre der Grosshirnrinde in Ihren Prinzipien Dargestellt auf Grund des Zellenbaues. J. A. Barth, Leipzig.
5. Caviness, V. S., Jr. (1975): J. Comp. Neurol., 164:247-264.
6. Caviness, V. S., Jr. (1976): J. Comp. Neurol., 170:435-448.

7. Caviness, V. S., Jr. (1977): In: Society for Neuroscience Symposia, Vol. 2, edited by W. M. Cowan and J. A. Ferrendelli, pp. 27-46, Society for Neuroscience, Bethesda.
8. Caviness, V. S., Jr. (1980): In: Neurosecretion and Brain Peptides: Implications for Brain Function and Neurological Disease, edited by J. B. Martin and K. Bick (in press). Raven, New York.
9. Caviness, V. S., Jr. and D. O. Frost (1980): J. Comp. Neurol., (in press).
10. Caviness, V. S., Jr., D. O. Frost, and N. L. Hayes (1976): Neurosci. Lett., 3:7-14.
11. Caviness, V. S., Jr. and P. Rakic (1978): Ann. Rev. Neurosci., 1:297-326.
12. Caviness, V. S., Jr. and R. L. Sidman (1973): J. Comp. Neurol., 147:235-254.
13. Caviness, V. S., Jr. and R. L. Sidman (1973): J. Comp. Neurol., 148:141-152.
14. Caviness, V. S., Jr. and R. S. Williams (1980): In: Mental Retardation: The Search for Cures, National Association for Retarded Citizens (in press).
15. Caviness, V. S., Jr. and C. H. Yorke, Jr. (1976): J. Comp. Neurol., 170:449-460.
16. Fallon, J. H. and R. Y. Moore (1978): J. Comp. Neurol., 180:545-580.
17. Frost, D. O. and V. S. Caviness, Jr. (1980): J. Comp. Neurol., (in press).
18. Fuxe, K., B. Hamberger, and T. Hokfelt (1968): Brain Res., 8:125-131.
19. Herkenham, M. (1980): Science, 207:532-535.
20. Geschwind, N. (1965a): Brain, 88:237-294.
21. Geschwind, N. (1965b): Brain, 88:585-644.
22. Ivy, G. O. and H. P. Killackey (1979): Neurosci. Abs., 5:164.
23. Jacobson, S. and J. Q. Trojanowski (1974): Brain Res., 74:149-155.
24. Kasamatsu, T., J. D. Pettigrew, and M. Ary (1979): J. Comp. Neurol., 185:163-182.
25. Kostovic, I. and M. E. Molliver (1974): Anat. Rec., 178:395.
26. Levitt, P. and R. Y. Moore (1978): Brain Res., 139:219-231.
27. Lewis, M. S., M. K. Molliver, J. H. Morrison, and H. G. W. Lidov (1979): Brain Res., 164:328-333.
28. Lorente de Nó, R. (1933): J. Psychol. Neurol. (Leipzig), 45:381-438.
29. Lorente de Nó, R. (1938): In: Physiology of the Nervous System, edited by J. F. Fulton, pp. 291-340. Oxford University Press, New York.
30. Lund, R. D. and M. J. Mustari (1977): J. Comp. Neurol., 173:289-306.
31. Moscona, A. A. (1974): In: The Cell Surface in Development, edited by A. A. Moscona, pp. 67-99. Wiley, New York.
32. Nauta, W. J. H. and H. J. Karten (1970): In: The Neurosciences Second Study Program, edited by F. O. Schmitt,

pp. 7-26.

33. Pinto Lord, M. C. and V. S. Caviness, Jr. (1979): <u>J.</u> <u>Comp.</u> <u>Neurol.</u>, 187:49-70.
34. Rakic, P. (1971): <u>Brain</u> <u>Res.</u>, 33:471-476.
35. Rakic, P. (1972): <u>J.</u> <u>Comp.</u> <u>Neurol.</u>, 145:61-84.
36. Rakic, P. (1978): <u>Postgrad.</u> <u>Med.</u> <u>J.</u>, 54:25-40.
37. Rakic, P. (1980): In: <u>The</u> <u>Cerebral</u> <u>Cortex</u>, edited by F. O. Schmitt and F. G. Worden (in press), MIT Press, Cambridge.
38. Rakic, P., L. J. Stensaas, E. P. Sayre and R. L. Sidman (1974): <u>Nature</u> <u>(Lond.)</u>, 250:31-34.
39. Ramon y Cajal, S. (1960): <u>Studies</u> <u>on</u> <u>Vertebrate</u> <u>Neurogenesis</u>, translated by L. Guth, Charles C. Thomas, Springfield.
40. Rice, F. L. and H. van der Loos (1977): <u>J.</u> <u>Comp.</u> <u>Neurol.</u>, 171:545-560.
41. Sauer, F. C. (1935): <u>J.</u> <u>Comp.</u> <u>Neurol.</u>, 63:13-23.
42. Sauer, M. E. and B. E. Walker (1959): <u>Proc.</u> <u>Soc.</u> <u>Exp.</u> <u>Biol.</u> <u>(N.Y.)</u>, 101:557-560.
43. Schlumpf, M., W. J. Shoemaker and F. E. Bloom (1977): <u>Neurosci.</u> <u>Abs.</u>, 3:118.
44. Shoukimas, G. M. and J. W. Hinds (1978): <u>J.</u> <u>Comp.</u> <u>Neurol.</u>, 179:795-830.
45. Sidman, R. L. (1968): In: <u>Physiological</u> <u>and</u> <u>Biochemical</u> <u>Aspects</u> <u>of</u> <u>Nervous</u> <u>Integration</u>, edited by F. D. Carlson, pp. 163-193. Prentice-Hall, Englewood Cliffs.
46. Sidman, R. L. (1974): In: <u>The</u> <u>Cell</u> <u>Surface</u> <u>in</u> <u>Development</u>, edited by A. A. Moscona, pp. 221-253. Wiley, New York.
47. Sidman, R. L. and P. Rakic (1973): <u>Brain</u> <u>Res.</u>, 62:1-35.
48. Singer, M., R. H. Nordlander and M. Egar (1979): <u>J.</u> <u>Comp</u> <u>Neurol.</u>, 185:1-22.
49. Wise, S. P. (1975): <u>Brain</u> <u>Res.</u>, 90:139-142.
50. Wise, S. P. and E. G. Jones (1976): <u>J.</u> <u>Comp.</u> <u>Neurol.</u>, 168:313-344.
51. Wise, S. P. and E. G. Jones (1977): <u>J.</u> <u>Comp.</u> <u>Neurol.</u>, 175:129-158.
52. Wise, S. P. and E. G. Jones (1978): <u>J.</u> <u>Comp.</u> <u>Neurol.</u>, 178:187-208.
53. Yorke, C. H., Jr. and V. S. Caviness, Jr. (1975): <u>J.</u> <u>Comp.</u> <u>Neurol.</u>, 164:233-246.

Morphogenesis and Pattern Formation,
edited by T. G. Connelly et al.,
Raven Press, New York © 1981.

Discussion of Sections I and II

SMITH: I find this just fascinating; I heard you once in London and have been thinking about it ever since. One of the questions that has come up concerns what you think is primarily involved in governing the growth of the muscle and the tendons. Do you feel that in some way cartilage is the primary thing here?

WOLPERT: Not absolutely. There are few interactions after cells leave the progress zone. I should have emphasized that there is a phase of coordinated growth so that the growth of the muscles and the tendons, we would argue, is determined by the cartilage, and we have quite good evidence for that. If ever you shorten the cartilaginous elements, for example, if you put on a teratogen so that the cartilage is short, you'll find the muscles and the tendons just beautifully coordinately shortened in the same way. In other words, one would say that the muscle was simply dragged out by the cartilage, and it simply follows along with the cartilage, and that's how you get the coordination.

SMITH: I have a second question along the same vein. How does muscle come to be where it is from the standpoint of origin and insertion? I've been impressed in some cases of abnormal morphogenesis, where there are missing parts in a limb, that the muscles and tendons seem to be hooked up about as well as one could imagine they might be. Would you comment on that in more depth?

WOLPERT: Well, we don't have a great deal more evidence from experiments with chicks that would absolutely conform with what you are saying. First of all, if you look at mirror image duplications for example, sometimes you lose a cartilaginous element but you don't lose the muscles, and they will simply hook up to what's available. You can see this best if you do the following experiment. You do a dorso-ventral inversion of the hand of the distal part of the limb so that you now have ventral tendons coming along to meet dorsal tendons. They simply join up with whatever is closest. That would be the answer to your question and that will be true of muscles too. That is why I say that there is little local interaction. They don't like to end in dead air: they will join up with whatever is closest to them.

SMITH: The other one that has been intriguing, which you haven't yet commented on, was in regeneration, the impact of the nerve roots and all. I appreciate that you didn't bring that up, and I'd like to hear your thoughts on it.

WOLPERT: That is really dangerous territory. Dr. Carlson is the authority here. First of all, it is important to realize, and I don't think that anyone here would argue, that the pattern is not dependent on the nerves. Marcus Singer has shown that any old nerves will do. My own personal feelings, and we have one tiny paper on this, are that the role of the nerves is in relation to the vascular system. I think it is as lousy an hypothesis as anybody else's, but I personally believe it to be true. That is, that the blastema remains avascular in a denervated limb, and no blood, no growth.

JACOBSON: I'm Row 11-Seat 5 in positional value. It seems to me that a theory that says that a cell may do anything or nothing in response to its positional value is basically untestable and it has an epicyclic effect.

WOLPERT: I'm sorry, that is not what I said. I don't think that that's the sort of model that one's actually proposing, because first of all, its developmental history makes a great deal of importance for the cell. In general, in certain pattern forming systems, the cells' behavior will depend upon position, and in fact this position will actually be graded, and if you think that all I said is epicyclic, I can say absolutely nothing.

BOOKSTEIN: I'm very intrigued by some of Arthur Winfrey's recent work that shows that there is a lot of information in the singularity of the coordinate system. I was wondering what you might think the role of singularities would be in these coordinate systems, because the Cartesian case is very highly specialized both in the mathematics and in the real world.

WOLPERT: I honestly don't know Art Winfrey's recent stuff. If you believe in coordinate systems, then you regard boundary regions as singularities. That's absolutely critical. In other words, a great deal of thinking about positional information actually requires you to consider what your boundary regions are, and how these are set up. It turns out, for example, that if we look at compartments in insects, one of their functions may be that a boundary region can only be established where two compartments meet: that you have a cooperative process. I don't know if that will relate to what Art Winfrey means or not. Also, I think that Winfrey and others have shown that the differences between a Cartesian and a polar coordinate system are not as severe as perhaps those of us who are less sophisticated think.

CARLSON: Excuse me, could you do one thing of the benefit for the non-mathematicians in the audience, and define what you mean by the term singularity?

WOLPERT: Not me, not me.

BOOKSTEIN: A singularity is a place like the center of the polar coordinate system where two positional values you think you've been carrying around with you as a cell, one of them doesn't have a value anymore and you really have a different kind of information there than you have in Row 11-Seat 5 for instance. You don't know your row anymore.

WAELSCH: In the last model you showed, which was that of Meinhardt, is there any correlation between the genes? You said one batch of certain genes. Are they related in any way to each other?

WOLPERT: It's too early to say. I cannot speak for Hans Meinhardt, but perhaps what he would say is that he could make use of the system to make quite a lot of sense, he would argue, of the bithorax system of E. B. Lewis in Drosophila. I think it's just too early to tell. I think we are just too ignorant once you get inside the cell. I think it's just a beginning. I cannot answer that question, I'm sorry.

RIZKI: The last model you presented is actually Curt Stern's on the double extra sex comb (esc) in Drosophila. In this case you get an extra sex comb on the second and third pairs of legs. He interprets this on the basis of a threshold response of the mutant gene.

WOLPERT: If I had been allowed to use insect material I would have referred to Curt Stern's work. My normal talk, in fact does exactly that, because his idea of prepatterns is very similar, but not identical to what I've been talking about.

SMITH: Prof. Wolpert indicated that cell numbers seem to be critical I'd like to ask Dr. Saxen if it is critical in the processes of induction that one have a proper number of cells in order to have it take place?

SAXÉN: The cell number seems not to be critical during induction. You can get the induction with very few cells. But it is critical for differentiation. It has been known for quite a while that there is what is known as a "critical mass" below which the cells will not form any organ. But, for the induction itself a critical mass is not necessary.

WOLPERT: Did the diffusion — mediated induction (directed induction) of the CNS really give you more that just neural structures, or can you get regional neural structures by diffusion? My prediction would have to be that you don't. Partly because I know the answer.

SAXÉN: That was not a fair trick because you know the answer. No, the answer really is that we get only forebrain derivatives, not regionalization. There is a trick by which you can get it, but you really need contacts. Are you pleased for some reason?

WOLPERT: Since I want to argue that directive induction is a similar process, then it would fit with any other directive one that you have, where you actually have to have contact probably via the matrix.

PIESCO: How do you reconcile the fact that Thesleff has been unable to get odontoblast differentiation with matrix basement membrane? Would you consider that it could still be a diffusion phenomenon?

SAXÉN: With regard to the second part of your question, I think that it can hardly be a diffusion, because then filters would not prevent it as they do in the kidney system. I don't think it's a diffusion. You're absolutely right even if the results are, to my knowledge unpublished, that Thesleff has tested various matrices without any success, so obviously it requires a living inductor cell as well. Maybe there has to be a constant turnover of the matrix or the surface molecules. There is one report in the literature that those matrices may induce ameloblast differentiation, but we haven't been able to reproduce it.

PIESCO: I also wanted to ask what role you think heterotypic contacts play in the tooth situation? After the odontoblasts differentiate, the ameloblasts eliminate the basal lamina entirely and there are heterotypic contacts, but it seems that the ameloblasts are differentiated before these contacts are formed.

SAXÉN: The truth really is that we are not quite sure when the ameloblasts differentiate. Maybe I should explain what the question was about, because I showed a continuous basal membrane between the interacting tissues. At a later stage, after the odontoblasts have differentiated, there are discontinuities in the basement membrane and direct cell contact between the two interactants. It has been suggested that this second step could be contact-mediated. There is no conclusive evidence for this. The only thing I can say is that Thesleff's studies are mostly on odontoblast differentiation. But you are right, there are contacts. We have seen the contacts later on, but whether they mediate the second step or not, that I don't know.

POOLE: I wanted to ask about the primary induction and how sure you can be that it is not really an induction of some matrix material, such as hyaluronic acid, which isn't well preserved in preparations for scanning or transmission electron microscopy.

There could be matrix filling the pores but you just can't detect it in the EM preparation.

SAXÉN: I agree that this is a possiblity. At least I think that actual cell processes are excluded. But then it is a matter of definition of how the material travels through the pores that are 12 microns long. Your material would perhaps crawl through them, whereas I'm speaking about diffusion, so while it's not excluded that there is some large molecular material, we haven't seen it.

MADERSON: Lauri, in reference to Lewis' question, hasn't a report come from your lab that if you study the ultrastructure of primary induction in vivo, in fact during what you would call spino-caudal induction, if you were doing experimental work, you do actually get direct cell contact between the chordamesoderm and the overlying neural plate?

SAXÉN: I think you are summarizing two papers, only one of which comes from our laboratory. I didn't want to go into the details because I know what Lewis wanted me to reply. But the fact is that if you do some tricks, if you precultivate the tissues, then keep them in contact for longer periods, occasionally you get processes through big holes. In those cases you also get caudal structures. So I left it out because I'm not convinced yet that this suggests that you need contact for the regional or secondary step of the primary induction.

MADERSON: I inferred that's what Lewis wanted it to be.

SAXÉN: Right, that's true.

MADERSON: You didn't give him what he wanted, but in fact, you could have.

SAXÉN: I gave him half of what he wanted. Now, the second paper is from the Berlin group, where they see processes at the late stages of invagination. So these two fit together, you are right.

STEINBERG: Lauri, you showed a slide of the famous Spemann experiment in which the dorsal lip of the blastopore of either an early or late gastrula was implanted into the blastocoele. The resulting induction was specific for the region. What would have been the anterior archenteric roof induces a head structure, and what would have been the posterior archenteric roof induces a trunk structure. I noticed in the slide that the head that results, the secondary head, lay in the head region and the secondary trunk lay in the trunk region, so that there was a matching up of the antero-posteriority of the induced structure with that of the head. Is that a general property of these systems or just of that particular case?

SAXÉN: Well, it's hard to say. I'm going to disappoint you again. (LAUGHTER). You are absolutely right, and there is in this kind of experiment the difficulty that the host fields may have an influence. I may say you get the very same results if you use what we call the sandwich technique where you take only the ectoderm from two graft gastrulae and put the inductor between those. In this case you exclude the host effect totally. You still get the very same result. At least the result is not due to the site of the implant.

STEINBERG: That settles that question, but when the experiment is done the way Spemann did it, is that generally the observation? I have some recollection that there was some comment in the old papers that this was so. I'm asking another question then: given that a secondary structure is differentiating now, does it seek its appropriate level within the host?

SAXÉN: I don't think this has been systematically studied, but together with my former teacher Toivonen, we have performed a few thousand of these experiments and at least it's not a striking phenomenon. However, no statistics have ever been made on the level of the differentiation. For instance, if you use a caudal type inductor it's almost a random distribution where the secondary structure develops. Does this answer your question?

CARLSON: Just one comment on this point. In some regenerating systems there does seem to be a rather interesting tendency towards level-seeking.

CUNHA: Just a comment to put these inductions, both permissive and directive, in a broader context. There is evidence today that these inductions are not just embryonic inductions. They are events that begin during embryonic life and continue into adult life. It has been known for quite some time that in order for an adult epithelium to function normally, mesenchyme or stroma may act as a permissive inductor allowing that epithelium to do its thing. Perhaps with a fully differentiated epithelium, something as simple as a collagen matrix may substitute for the living stroma. We have recently demonstrated, which I think is now the first one of its type, a directive induction involving adult epithelium. One can take an epithelium from the urinary bladder of an adult mouse or rat, and this can be reprogrammed to form something that looks like, and indeed biochemically is, prostate. These inductions are not restricted to this period and I think that one of the implications of this is that alterations or abnormalities of epithelial function or morphology in adulthood, the so-called preneoplastic or neoplastic states, expressed within the epithelium, may have an etiology based on an alteration in the underlying stroma. Would you like to comment on that as well?

SAXÉN: Not really, but I would like to say one thing since

Dr. Cunha is in the audience. Our chairman promised that I would deal with pathological implications of inductive processes. I had to omit this because of the shortness of time, but references to Dr. Cunha's excellent work are included in my manuscript.

PAULSEN: In the models where it appears that contact is necessary, is there any indication that a minimum area of surface contact between the cells is necessary?

SAXÉN: If there is a minimum contact area, we haven't yet reached it. But the time required for the completion of the induction is a function of the contact area. The larger the contact area is, the shorter the time until the induction is complete. This was published in 1979.

PAULSEN: Is there any indication that there is some sort of rearrangement of the components of the membrane that takes place in this contact, or do you expect it to be simply a transfer of molecules through the contact?

SAXÉN: The present hypothesis is that it is an interaction of surface-associated molecules, but the evidence is inconclusive. We are working on that at present.

BERNFIELD: I just want to point out that the elegant studies using filter imposition between tissues can demonstrate that contact is not required, but I don't think they can allow us to say that contact is required or necessary. You mentioned, Lauri, some studies which you've done using inhibitors and other conformitors of interposition, and I'm wondering whether you have any evidence which would help us in deciding whether or not contact is necessary?

SAXÉN: No, I can't think of any absolutely final proof except what I showed earlier. There is extremely good correlation between contact formation and induction. I couldn't, of course, bring all the results here, but you can also correlate the ingrowth of various inductor tissues and the completion of induction. Those which grow only through larger holes don't induce with the smaller holes. There is plenty of circumstantial evidence, but you are right. Unfortunately I can't really see how you can get the final anser to that. Perhaps what I should say is that we have now demonstrated with many techniques that there is a discontinuity of the basal membrane at the inductive tip.

WOLPERT: I'd like to make some comments on the points raised by Drs. Saunders, Stocum and Iten. John, the point that different tissues can act as a polarizing region is just what one would expect. There is nothing that is special about the polarizing region. The whole philosophy of signals, and Ed Kollar's work supports this, is that these are common things. The things that are interacting are widespread and common, and they have no bearing on whether it's a polar coordinate system or not. Also, I don't think it is quite fair to say that any tissue will act as a polarizing region. We've tried lots of tissues that don't, and I think it may turn out that those tissues that do, have something in common. For example, Hensen's node, another signalling region, also does it. Just want to make that point clear.

I simply don't understand David Stocum when you say that the progress zone isn't a model with very specific predictions. It may be wrong, and I'm prepared to think that, but it makes absolutely specific predictions. They're not easy to guess test. I could tell you tests that we could do which, if they come out in a specific way, would show the model to be totally wrong. So I must take strong exception to that. Do you want me to tell you what the experiment is? Indeed, very simple 'tis. Where's the chalk? You are hiding the chalk. The experiment that would show that the model is absolutely wrong would be to lift the apical ectodermal ridge and put in a thin sliver of proximal mesenchyme here, just beneath the ridge with some sort of backing. If you take that bit of sliver and put it in here, and if that gave you a normal limb, then the progress zone model would have to be all wrong. It's a difficult experiment to do because in order to get a normal limb this would have to expand to make the progress zone. One would, therefore, predict that proximal structures would have to be missing.

STOCUM: What I'm saying is that the results of that kind of experiment would provide us with no more than what we already know must be going on there. It would simply demonstrate that.

WOLPERT: I find that extraordinary. What do you think the answer to that experiment is? You mean whichever way it turns out it fits your model? (LAUGHTER). Well, I can tell you it disproves mine, therefore, I claim I have a model.

I'm going to comment on the results of Dr. Iten. First, with regard to the polarizing region and the question of the ulna, the following points are important. Both Iten and I have shown that you can get an extra ulna in a situation in which the polarizing region cells play no role whatsoever. For example, you can irradiate the polarizing region with 10,000 rads, as Jim Smith has done, and you still get this extra ulna. Now the question of whether you get ulna-radius-ulna is simply a matter of the time when you put in the polarizing region. If you put it in early, you'll get ulna-radius-ulna. If you do it at a slightly later stage, because the limb hasn't got time to widen, you'll get ulna-ulna. Now, I don't believe that your results are really in any way contradictory with changing positional value.

I now want to give some further evidence that the signal from the polarizing region may be a diffusible morphogen. Firstly, we have carried out experiments grafting two polarizing regions. Grafting a polarizing region opposite somite 16 gives the standard duplication of digits 4 3 2 2 3 4. We have then grafted in a second polarizing region at various positions along the antero-posterior axis in order to see how close they can be placed such that digit 2 still forms. On an intercalation model two digit 2's should always form if there is host tissue between the polarizing regions. Amata Hornbruch found that when the second polarizing region was opposite somite 18 no digit 2 formed in 50% of the cases. We interpret this as being due to the concentration of the morphogen being above the threshold for digit 2. Secondly, Jim Smith has found that if the widening that occurs following the graft of a polarizing region is prevented with x-irradiation, digit 2 is again lost. The reason is similar: the host and grafted polarizing regions are too close together. Thirdly, Larry Honig has provided direct evidence for long range interaction. He grafted a polarizing region to the anterior margin and also replaced the wing bud tissue adjacent and posterior to the graft, with leg bud tissue. The leg bud tissue responds by forming toes. The question was whether the signal from the polarizing region could propagate across the leg tissue and still signal the more posterior wing tissue to form an additional digit 2. The answer is yes.

ITEN: The experiments that Prof. Wolpert alluded to were x-ray studies in which the donor limb bud is x-rayed with higher and higher doses of irradiation. The question I have for him about those experiments is: were the controls done in which quail wing buds that have received graded doses of x-rays up to 10,000 rads of gamma irradiation, grafted to the flank to see if they make any structures at all? We have done the same experiments, and we do not get attenuation; we get a variety of structures implying that cell survival for a certain period of time is variable. So as for losing a digit 4 and then losing a digit 3 as the extra digit next to the graft, we can't, in our hands do that.

WOLPERT: I'm just astonished, because in our hands we have hundreds of experiments with that because you can get that attenuation, for example, with Cheryl Tickle's reduction in the number of polarizing zones. So, we would interpret attenuation following x-irradiation as simply being due to the killing off of the number of polarizing regions.

BRINKLEY: Dr. Kollar, it appears that you are arguing causality of patterning by virtue of innervation. What directs the nerve to the specific vibrissae-forming area in the first place? Why not postulate that something inherent in the epithelial/mesenchymal previbrissae area attracts the nerve?

KOLLAR: The reason for not proposing that is cowardice. (LAUGHTER). I can test the hypothesis that it's going there and interacting and if it comes out negative then I must go back almost to the early stages where the ectoderm is just an ectoderm, and that's very difficult. It's possible, but I'd like to do the easy ones first.

ASHER: Is the abnormal stratification observed in the <u>reeler</u> neocortex also observed in the <u>reeler</u> retina?

CAVINESS: The retina is phenotypically normal.

DINSMORE: Dr. Kollar, you indicated that dentin-free collagen supported differentiation in your tetracycline-inhibited system. Do you have data on other types of precollagen that would substantiate the implied type-specific morphogenetic induction by matrix? Also, do teeth develop in denervated jaws?

KOLLAR: That's a broad range of questions. We specifically tried the dentin-free type collagen because it was available, and we did not try other types. The controls for that were albumin, serum, and high molecular weight proteins. They were negative. I can't tell you what kind of collagen specificity there is. I really don't think that is the crux of the issue when it's a combination and a proportion of a number of them. If one collagen did or didn't to a greater extent wouldn't bother me too much at this point. It's the combination of the souffle that were interested in.
       What was the other question? Denervation, yes. Well, that was one of the early experiments to find out whether there was indeed some sort of effect there. It's very difficult to denervate the embryo and have the embryo survive. Now with <u>in vivo</u> embryo culture techniques that may be possible, and that's coming, probably this summer. The alternative is to go back earlier and earlier in time, and cut off the mandibular segment before the nerve is down there, of course. If you do that, you don't get teeth. If you take a larger segment that includes the trigeminal region, then you get teeth in an increased number of cases. Also, the number of teeth you get when you take these segments varies chronologically. But, earlier and earlier in time you don't get them. So I think that was one of the reasons that sent us along that direction besides the biology of it. You shouldn't have to have sensory innervation.

WAELSCH: I have two questions for Dr. Caviness. 1). Are heterozygous reelers (+/re) perfectly normal in respect to the cellular organization of the neocortex? 2). What are the possible connections between the cellular abnormalities and the <u>reeler</u> symptoms?

CAVINESS: The heterozygote is indistinguishable from its genetically normal littermates by morphologic criteria. These are the only ones we've exercised. The recognizable phenotype is primarily a motor abnormality. There is a dystonic posturing, high amplitude action tremor, a reeling ataxia of gait. This is indistinguishable from the behavioral phenotype of a number of other mutants in which the cerebellum is devastated and they derive from problems of the cerebellum.

We don't know much about the forebrain function, but I should say that single cell receptive properties have been looked at in the visual cortex by both Ristrodrega and Perlman . Receptive field properties of a number of cells are normal with respect to size, molecularity and stimulus alignment requirement.

Morphogenesis and Pattern Formation,
edited by T. G. Connelly et al.,
Raven Press, New York © 1981.

Organization and Remodeling of the Extracellular Matrix in Morphogenesis

Merton R. Bernfield

*Department of Pediatrics, Stanford University School of Medicine,
Stanford, California 94305*

The extracellular matrix is the "stuffing" between cells of multicellular organisms. The matrix consists of fibrous proteins (principally the collagens) embedded in a gel containing polysaccharides (the glycosaminoglycans or proteoglycans), glycoproteins and interstitial fluid. The matrix between cells has evolved to enable individual cells to behave as integrated cell groups. Indeed, nearly every cell type is capable of producing these matrix molecules which they deposit into the extracellular space.

The extracellular matrix (ECM) is thought to play an important role in the formation of organisms and structures during development. There is a great number of studies of the matrix during morphogenesis and a vast literature has developed (52, 53, 63). Most of these studies are correlations between morphogenetic changes and alterations in the composition and organization of the extracellular materials, but some direct experimental evidence on how the matrix influences cellular behavior is now being obtained.

It has become increasingly evident that normal cellular behavior is dependent on the close association of cells with a supporting surface or substratum (39). Morphogenesis involves groups of cells and their coordinated changes in behavior lead to changes in tissue form. The in situ substratum for these cells is the ECM, including its specialization, the cell surface matrix. In this paper I will examine the hypothesis that cellular behavior during morphogenesis is regulated by the organization of the ECM and that this organization is modified by localized synthesis and deposition of materials, their assembly and orientation, and their removal. These processes, which result in reconstruction or remodeling of the in situ cellular substratum, are exquisitely controlled both temporally and spatially, and thus permit the specific changes in tissue form which occur during development.

In each organ there are both parenchymal and stromal elements contributing to its ultimate morphology. The stroma is composed

139

of loose connective tissue derived from embryonic mesenchyme and contains substantial ECM surrounding connective tissue cells. The parenchyma may be any of the major tissue types, for example epithelia, endothelia, muscle or nerve and is separated from the surrounding stroma by a specialization of ECM, the basal lamina. Nearly all organs develop due to interactions between their stromal and parenchymal elements. Our contention is that the interaction is reciprocal. A theme of this paper is that parenchymal and stromal tissues influence their own and the other's behavior during morphogenesis by modifying their and the other's ECM.

The ECM will be briefly defined but the focus in this paper will be on the basal lamina, a matrix closely associated with the surface of parenchymal cells. I shall review the data indicating that the basal lamina functions to maintain the morphology of epithelial organs, describe the evidence that the lamina undergoes remodeling at specific sites and times, suggest that this remodeling leads to changes in epithelial morphology and conclude with a general model for morphogenetic tissue interactions which involves the remodeling of the matrix by the interacting tissues.

The Extracellular Matrix

There are many recent reviews on ECM components, detailing the molecular characteristics and interactions of the collagens, proteoglycans and matrix glycoproteins and therefore only a very brief overview will be attempted here. While the importance of the collagens in the structural organization of the ECM has been known for years, analogous interest in the glycosaminoglycans and proteoglycans is more recent and the significance and abundance of the matrix glycoproteins has only very recently become evident.

Collagens (25, 26, 44, 45). The collagens are a group of proteins found in metazoan organisms which share the features of a triple helix, a coiled coil of three polypeptides, which imparts structural rigidity to the molecule. The collagens differ in the sequence of their polypeptide chains, and in their ability to form the fibrils and long fibers which are characteristic of the interstitial collagens. Other, non-fibrillar collagens are found closely associated with cell surfaces (Table 1).

The various collagens have similar mechanisms of synthesis, processing and secretion. Biosynthesis involves several post-translational modifications, including hydroxylations, oxidative deaminations and glycosylations of a precursor polypeptide, procollagen. Secretion of procollagen is accompanied by a processing in which peptides at both the amino- and carboxy-terminal ends of the molecule are removed by highly specific extracellular enzymes, the procollagen peptidases. This extracellular processing is required for fibrillogenesis and for the formation of stable intramolecular crosslinks in the mature fibril.

The intrinsic properties of the different collagens determine to a large extent the properties of the matrices of which they are

Table 1.

Types of Collagen

	Type	Subunits	Form	Location
Interstitial	I	$[\alpha 1 (I)]_2 \alpha 2$	Fibrils	Skin, bone, tendon, ligaments, (collagen vulgaris)
	II	$[\alpha 1 (II)]_3$	Fibrils	Cartilage, vitreous, notochord
	III	$[\alpha 1 (III)]_3$	Reticulin fibers	Fetal skin, blood vessels
Cell Surface	IV	$[\alpha 1 (IV)]_2 \alpha 2 (IV)$ (?)	Amorphous	Epithelial, endothelial basal lamina,
	V (A-B)	Disputed	Amorphous	muscle basal lamina, minor pericellular component

components. For example, type I forms the large coarse and strong fibers characteristic of tendons, while type III forms the fine reticulin fibers present in loose meshworks. The physical properties of the cell surface collagens are not known, but because of their secondary structure, they are likely to add a firm framework to the cell periphery.

The Polysaccharides (35, 40, 48). The polysaccharides of the ECM have evolved with the acquisition of multicellularity. Indeed, the simplest multicellular social organisms, the prokaryotic myxobacteria, secrete polysaccharides which cement the individual cells together into functional aggregates. The polysaccharides in vertebrate cells are the glycosaminoglycans in proteoglycans (Table 2). The glycosaminoglycans (GAG) are linear, well-hydrated polyanions which, except for keratan sulfate, contain a repeating disaccharide of an N-acetyl hexosamine and a uronic acid. There are several types of GAG, differing in the substituents on the disaccharide and the type of glycosidic linkage. They are able to bind many proteins and ions both specifically and non-specifically.

The nature and concentration of the GAG determine whether a matrix is loose (e.g., fluid in joint spaces), soft (semi-fluid "ground substance"), firm (cartilage) or rigid (tendons). Hyaluronic acid, the major GAG in the interstitial space, can be a

Table 2.

Matrix Polysaccharides: Glycosaminoglycans in proteoglycans
General formula: [N-Ac-hexosamine-uronic acid] -protein
(SO_4)

Type	Major Features	Location
Hyaluronic acid	Forms gels no protein no sulfate MW to 10^7	Ubiquitous in extracellular spaces cell surfaces
Chondroitin sulfate proteoglycan	Aggregates with hyaluronate MW to 4 X 10^4	Cartilage , bone, cornea
Heparan sulfate proteoglycan	Sequence complexity MW ca. 10^4 and 5 X10^4	Cell surfaces, basal lamina
Dermatan sulfate proteoglycans	Binds to collagen MW to 4X 10^4	Skin, heart valves
Keratan sulfate proteoglycan	Glycoprotein-like N-Ac-neuraminate	Cornea, cartilage, intervertebral disk

very long single chain which, because of its hydration and random coil conformation, occupies extraordinarily large molecular domains and readily forms gels that enclose substantial amounts of interstitial fluid. Multiples of the smaller polysaccharide chains, chondroitin sulfate and heparan sulfate, are covalently linked to proteins in proteoglycans. These proteoglycans tend to aggregate, forming highly hydrated globules which may interact with other matrix components. Cartilage proteoglycans, for example, form supermolecular aggregates with hyaluronic acid and certain cartilage-specific glycoproteins, as well as with type II collagen.

Matrix Glycoproteins (16, 37, 62). While a great variety of glycoproteins are found in the extracellular matrix, they have only recently been well-characterized. The major matrix glycoprotein is fibronectin (previously also known as Large External Transformation Sensitive protein [LETS] and Cell Surface Protein [CSP]). This molecule, found both on cell surfaces and in the ECM, functions as an adhesive protein, participating in the formation of cell surface adhesive plaques and possibly in the transmembrane organization of intracellular actin filament bundles. Fibronectin is a long, ellipsoidal disulfide bonded dimer which is insoluble at physiological pH. It has binding domains for collagen, hyaluronic acid and heparan sulfate proteoglycan, and thus may be involved in organizing the matrix into various ordered forms. Recently, laminin, a matrix glycoprotein found exclusively in the basal lamina of a number of parenchymal cells has been characterized (57). Although it is similar to fibronectin in size and disulfide arrangement and apparently interacts with other extracellular matrix constituents, it is located exclusively in the basal lamina.

The Cell Surface Matrix

With the exception of those cells circulating in the blood, all cells have molecules at their outer boundary which extend for various distances beyond the plasma membrane lipid bilayer. Indeed, by morphological criteria it is often difficult to define the boundary between the cell's plasma membrane and the ECM. Some of these molecules at the cell periphery are those generally ascribed to the ECM such as proteoglycans, hyaluronic acid and procollagen, while others are commonly thought to be cell surface components, such as fibronectin and other glycoproteins. The ECM might be considered to be a greatly extended part of the surfaces of the nearby cells, but the matrix constituents at cell surfaces are not always identical to those in the ECM. The cell surface matrix (CSM) is a distinct part of the ECM, operationally defined as that part of the ECM which is produced by the cell but cannot be removed from the cell by mechanical means (Table 3).

The surface matrix of stromal cells remains with the cells as a pericellular collection of materials when these cells are physically isolated, but remains in association with the in vitro substratum when such cells are removed from the substratum by detergent treatment. This cell surface matrix from fibroblasts in culture has been extensively studied by Culp (49), by Chen (11) and by Veheri (36) and their colleagues. These workers have shown that the CSM is rich in procollagen, fibronectin, hyaluronic acid and proteoglycans, all of which are found in abundance in the extracellular matrix. On these connective tissue cells, the CSM does not appear to be structurally arranged and can be removed from the cell periphery by treatment with proteolytic enzymes.

The CSM of parenchymal cells is different, especially in its organization, from the CSM of stromal cells. Wherever epithelial, endothelial, or muscle cells are adjacent to the connective tissue, their CSM is organized into a basal lamina. By electron microscopy, the basal lamina is seen to consist of two relatively uniform layers which conform closely to the contours of the basal cell surface (7). Contiguous with the superficial aspect of these layers is an ECM of varying thickness and density which, together with the basal lamina, constitutes the basement membrane. In

Table 3.

Cell surface Matrix

	Stromal Cells	Parenchymal Cells
Structure	Pericellular net of fibrils and filaments	Basal lamina of ordered globules and fibrils
Major Collagens	Types I and II procollagen	Type IV and V (A-B) Collagen
Major Polysaccharides	Hyaluronic acid Chondroitin sulfate (Heparan sulfate)	Heparan sulfate Hyaluronic acid (Chondroitin sulfate)
Major Glycoproteins	Fibronectin	Fibronectin Laminin

contrast to the basal lamina, the basement membrane is readily visualized by light microscopy.

With special staining procedures, the basal lamina of certain tissues shows a precise and highly regular ultrastructural organization (13, 29). This organization is seen as a two-dimensional tetragonal array of nearly uniform sized globules of GAG. This highly ordered pattern is an unusual arrangement, suggesting that one of the components of the lamina is asymmetric. The components of the basal lamina are similar to those in the extracellular matrix, containing specialized types of collagen, a variety of polysaccharides, as well as laminin and possibly, fibronectin. The type of GAG in the basal lamina apparently varies with the type of tissue and possibly with the developmental stage of that tissue (29).

The CSM has been suggested to serve as an exoskeleton for the cells, interacting with the plasma membrane and with the cytoskeleton (8). As Revel (47) and others (30) have found, when trypsin-treated stromal cells are plated on plastic or glass dishes, the cells do not associate directly with the surface of the artificial substratum. Rather, they deposit an amorphous matrix on the glass or plastic and adhere directly to these materials. Thus, cells carry this CSM, the substratum to which they are anchored, on their own plasma membranes. The production of a CSM substratum is more evident for parenchymal cells. When cultured on a gel of native type I collagen, mammary epithelial cells become polarized, deposit a basal lamina at their surfaces adjacent to the gel (23), and in the presence of the proper hormonal milieu, synthesize casein and lactose (22). When the epithelial cells are cultured on plastic, no lamina accumulates and the cells do not express these differentiated properties. Thus, there is evidence that the CSM, the basal lamina in this case, allows the cells to function physiologically.

Morphogenetic Cell Behavior

Morphogenesis involves the precise and organized arrangement of groups of cells into distinctive structures, the organs. Although the ultimate shape of each organ is unique, the types of cellular behavior involved in the formation of these structures is not. All morphogenesis can be viewed as resulting from the coordination in time and space of a limited repertoire of cellular behaviors: cell adhesion, cell proliferation, cell death and the changes in cell shape which lead to the locomotion of single cells and the movement of cell groups. Every cell, regardless of type, can express these behavioral properties. The unique structure of each organ, however, results from the expression of these behaviors in different groups of cells at different times, to different extents and at different sites. This view of morphogenesis contends that all cells perform similar morphogenetic functions and that structural differences between organs result from the regulation of these behaviors.

While each of these types of cellular behavior involves distinct organelles and cellular structures, with the exception of cell death, they each require the anchorage or at least the close association of the cell to a supporting surface or substratum. A major means of regulation of cellular behavior, therefore, would involve changes in the association of cells with their substrata, the cell surface and extracellular matrices. a great number of in vitro studies illustrates the relationship between morphogenetic cell behavior and cell association with a substratum. I shall mention only a few of these.

Change in Cell Shape. Anchorage of cells to a substratum determines their shape and their mobility. all cells in suspension, whether fibroblast, epithelial or neural, are rounded, although microvilli may project from the cell periphery (24). The rounded cells show a disorganized cytoskeleton and lack the bundles of actin microfilaments that are characteristic of these cells when on a substratum. When a suspended fibroblast is plated onto a substratum, the initial contacts are made via the microvillar extensions. Upon settling the cell spreads over the surface forming adhesive contacts to the substratum near its margin. As it spreads bundles of microfilaments begin to organize and these bundles terminate or insert into the cell membrane at the points of adhesive contact with the substratum. Indeed, as the cell spreads, cellular actin and cell surface fibronectin rearrange to become coincidentally distributed (38). With attachment, actin and tubulin synthesis are markedly stimulated. These changes are rapidly and completely reversible upon removal of the cells from the substratum (28).

The effect of the substratum on cell shape is also seen with epithelial cells. A number of epithelial cell types are flat when grown on the usual glass or plastic substrata. However, when cultured on fibrillar collagen gels, where they produce a basal lamina, they retain both their polarity and their normal columnar or cuboidal configuration (23). When epithelial cells are stripped of their basal lamina, the actin microfilament bundles which normally are subjacent to the basal plasma membrane become disorganized and lose their integrity (3). At the same time these cells round up. This change in epithelial cell shape occurring with a change in actin microfilament organization is formally identical to the changes in cell shape and filament organization observed with fibroblastic cells when losing and regaining their cell-substratum adhesions.

In vitro studies have shown that anchorage to a substratum also regulates cell movements (see 59 for review). The initial events in fibroblast locomotion are extension and subsequent adhesion of the long, thin filopodia or knee-like lamellipodia which form at the margin of spreading cells. This protrusion of the cell margin advances the leading edge of the cell and the cell actually translocates forward by an abrupt shortening and release of adhesions at the posterior end of the cell. Indeed, the rapid release of the posterior adhesions is thought to allow the formation of the forward protrusions (12). Thus, anchorage to the substratum mediates both changes in cell shape and in locomotion.

Cell Proliferation. When normal cells are plated onto a substratum to which they do not adhere, such as agar, they fail to proliferate (42). If they adhere poorly to a surface, such as bacteriological plastic, proliferation rates are markedly reduced. However, if cultured on the usual tissue culture substrata, they proliferate until no further free substratum is available, resulting in a confluent monolayer of non-dividing cells arrested in the G phase of the cell cycle. With adequate nutrition, these non-dividing cells will remain viable for weeks. If these cells are removed from the substratum and replated at low density, proliferation resumes. However, if they are removed and cultured in suspension where they do not contact the surface, or on agar, they do not proliferate. These cells may even die, despite apparently adequate nutrition (43). Thus, cells must be bound to a surface in order to divide, a phenomenon termed anchorage-dependence by Stoker et al. (56), and must have sufficient available surface in order to multiply; the concept of density-dependent regulation of growth (1).

Both anchorage to and the availability of a substratum regulate growth. This relationship between the substratum and growth has in vivo correlates. For example, in the epidermis, the capacity to synthesize DNA and to divide is restricted to the basal cells, those in contact with the natural substratum, the basal lamina. Following wounding of an epidermis, the basal cells adjacent to the wound migrate over the exposed connective tissue as a single sheet of contiguous cells. These cells either do not divide or divide at a very low rate, but a high proliferation rate occurs in those cells remaining adherent to the basal lamina at the wound margin (51).

The crucial effect of substratum anchorage and availability on cell proliferation may be brought about by their influence on cell shape (27). When cells which normally have a highly spread and flattened in vivo configuration are cultured at low density on a substratum of continually graded adhesiveness, those cells on the less adhesive surface are more spherical and fewer cells are in S phase. When the various adhesivities are compared, there is a good correlation between the degree of cell flattening, measured by average cell height, and the proportion of cells undergoing DNA synthesis.

Epithelial Morphogenesis

These examples provide evidence that the substratum may regulate morphogenetic cellular behavior. The in vivo substratum is the CSM which may itself be anchored to the extracellular matrix. Cell sheets constitute the bulk of embryonic tissues and incipient organs. A cell sheet is a layer of cells displaying integrated behavior which exists as a cohesive unit because of both firm intercellular adhesions (intermediate junctions and desmosomes) at their lateral surfaces and anchorage to a basal lamina. Most of those sheets are cell monolayers and they are epithelial sheets if they have one surface which borders a real or potential cell-free space. Expansion and folding of such sheets represent the sum of the changes in the individual cells in the sheet. The generation of structural forms by cell sheets includes gastrulation, neurulation and development of the brain, as well as formation of the gut and integument and their accessory epithelial organs. The formation of these latter epithelial organs has been used as an experimental paradigm for understanding the mechanisms involved in the morphogenesis of cell sheets.

Embryonic epithelial organs initially arise as a round budding of the cell sheet. The bud subsequently undergoes a distinctive pattern of folding and branching, which together with cell proliferation ultimately results in a morphology that is characteristic of the organ. This epithelial morphogenesis is completely dependent upon the close association of the epithelium with loose stromal tissue or mesenchyme (32). In the absence of the mesenchyme, growth and branching cease, the epithelium fails to develop, loses its shape and finally, its epithelial characteristics.

The development of the mouse embryo submandibular salivary gland, absolutely dependent on the epithelial-mesenchymal interaction, has provided evidence that the organization and remodeling of extracellular and cell surface matrix materials influence morphogenesis. The 12-day gland has a single epithelial bud surrounded by mesenchyme which by 13 days has formed a few lobules. These lobules grow and repetitively branch by formation of clefts, resulting within a few days in a highly branched tree-like structure (Fig. 1). The mesenchyme, which grows to a much

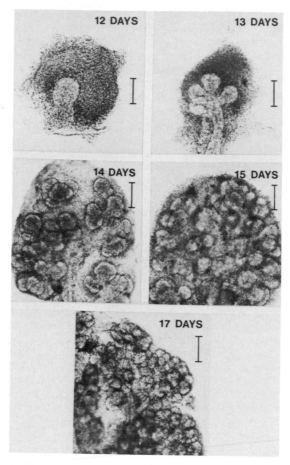

FIG. 1: Morphogenesis of the mouse embryo submandibular salivary gland. Photomicrographs of living whole glands at the ages indicated. Bar is 0.2 mm.

****

lesser extent, is distributed between and around the branched epithelial lobules and newly forming ducts. At the interface between epithelium and mesenchyme in the 13-day gland lies some amorphous extracellular materials, a well-defined basal lamina, and deposits of fibrillar collagen. These materials are not distributed uniformly over the epithelial surface (Fig. 2). The fibrillar collagen is in greater amounts in the clefts between lobules and on the stalk than at the distal aspects of lobules (33). The basal lamina encompasses the epithelium but is thinner and interrupted at the distal aspects of the lobules where contacts between epithelial and mesenchymal cells may be seen by electron microscopy (15).

The Basal Lamina Maintains Epithelial Morphology. The involvement of these matrix materials in morphogenesis has been examined by sequentially removing them with enzymes and replacing the epithelium in culture combined with fresh mesenchyme (3, 6, 7). Treatment of glands with highly purified collagenase and microdissection removes the mesenchyme, the amorphous materials and fibrillar collagen yielding an isolated epithelium retaining its basal lamina. Such epithelia maintain a normal ultrastructural appearance. When cultured with mesenchyme, the normal lobular morphology is maintained and with continued incubation, the epithelia will undergo branching morphogenesis. However, if the isolated epithelia are briefly treated with nannogram amounts of testicular hyaluronidase, which degrades the GAG in the lamina, the basal lamina is completely removed. These epithelia show a highly folded plasma membrane, disrupted cell junctions and disorganized actin filament bundles. When placed in culture with mesenchyme, they lose their lobular shape over 4-6 hours and form a spherical mass. They ultimately recover, however, and within 24 hours, an outgrowth buds from the mass from which branching morphogenesis will subsequently resume.

The cytological changes resulting from hyaluronidase treatment are completely reversed by culturing the epithelium in the absence of mesenchyme for as little as two hours. During this period, the epithelium covers nearly 70% of its surface with a newly deposited basal lamina. When these epithelia are cultured combined with mesenchyme, lobular morphology is maintained. Thus, the fibrillar collagen and amorphous materials are not responsible for maintianing the lobular morphology. Maintenance of normal cytoarchitecture and normal lobular morphology are dependent on the basal lamina, the cell surface matrix substratum for the epithelium.

Two other major conclusions are evident from these experiments. The basal lamina was completely removed by hyaluronidase treatment, indicating that the integrity of the lamina is dependent on its GAG. Secondly, although the mesenchyme is required for morphogenesis, it appears to be deleterious to epithelial recovery from loss of the lamina. If the mesenchyme reduces or slows the redeposition of the lamina, replacement of the lamina in the presence of mesenchyme would be insufficiently rapid to prevent the loss of morphology which occurs upon removal of the lamina.

Basal Lamina GAG Turnover Correlates with Morphology. This effect of mesenchyme on epithelial recovery could be related to normal morphogenesis. The mesenchyme may degrade laminar GAG, resulting in the thinning and interruptions of the lamina seen at the distal ends of the lobules. These disruptions in the epithelial cell substratum would produce modifications of cell shapes and possibly rates of cell proliferation, ultimately resulting in clefts or foldings of the epithelial sheet. This

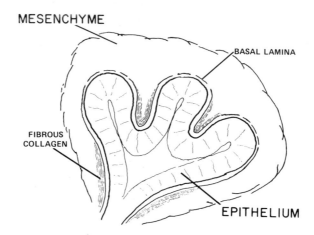

FIG. 2:   Distribution of extracellular materials on a 13 day mouse
embryo submandibular epithelium.   In this idealized   drawing,   the
epithelium   is   depicted   as   a   folded   sheet   of   cells   and the
interruptions in the lamina are exaggerated.   Reproduced from   (5)
with permission.

****

idea   suggests   that   laminar GAG is degraded at a greater rate at
the distal aspects of the lobules, the sites of new branching and
greatest rates of cell proliferation.

There   is   evidence   that   basal   laminar   GAG   turns   over   at
different   rates   depending   on   the   site   on   the   epithelium.
Histochemical   and   autoradiographic studies of the basal surfaces
of embryonic submandibular, sublingual, lung, mammary and ureteric
bud epithelia at various developmental stages show that the   total
amount   of GAG and the rate of labeled GAG accumulation differs at
different   sites,   consistently   reflecting the morphology   of   these
organs (Fig. 3).   At the stage of unbranched buds, total and newly
synthesized   GAG   are uniformly distributed.   However, with tissue
specific changes in morphology, more total GAG is at the   surfaces
of   the   clefts   and   lateral aspects of lobules and branches, the
morphogenetically quiescent sites, than at the distal   aspects   of
lobules   and branches, the sites where interruptions in the lamina
are seen ultrastructurally and where further branching will   take
place.   Substantially   greater   amounts of GAG in clefts have also
been observed by Cunha   and   Lung   (17)   in   embryonic   urogenital
epithelium   and   by   Solursh and Morriss (55) in embryonic neural
epithelium.   In   contrast,   after   brief   labeling,   labeled   GAG
accumulates   most   rapidly   at   the   distal   ends   of   lobules and
branches and least rapidly at the clefts.

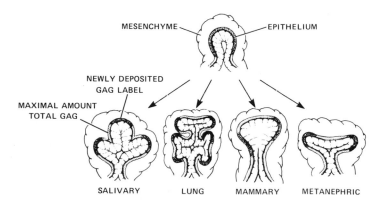

FIG. 3: Patterns of glycosaminoglycan distribution in several mouse embryo epithelial organs. Total GAG was assessed by Alcian Blue staining. Newly deposited GAG label was observed autoradiographically following two hours labeling with H-glucosamine into hyaluronidase-susceptible materials. Salivary represents the sublingual and submandibular epithelia, as they had identical distributions. See text for description. Modified from (5) and reproduced with permission.

****

Metabolic studies of submandibular epithelia reveal that these differences between sites are due to regional differences in GAG turnover (5). The regions were studied by labeling whole glands with glucosamine for various times, removing the mesenchyme with collagenase, and dividing the isolated epithelium into the stalk, lobules and the base which contains the clefts. Incorportion of label showed that the stalk is in the steady state with regard to GAG metabolism, whereas the lobules and base are not. The net amount of GAG accumulating in the lobules and base, a measure of the combined effects of GAG synthesis and loss, was determined from the incorportion of label into GAG and the specific activity of the glucosamine-containing precursor pools (Fig. 4). On a per epithelium basis, the lobules accumulate GAG at a greater initial rate than the base. However, with continued culture, GAG is lost from the lobules while it continues to accumulate in the base. This loss occurs despite no change in the incorporation rate or in the precursor specific activity, indicating that during culture the rate of GAG loss from the lobules must become greater than its rate of replacement. On the other hand, GAG continues to accumulate in the base, indicating that GAG synthesis exceeds loss at all times during the culture period. Regardless of any differences in the rate of GAG synthesis between base and lobules, because the base continues to accumulate GAG while the lobules do not, the rate of GAG degradation in the lobules must be greater

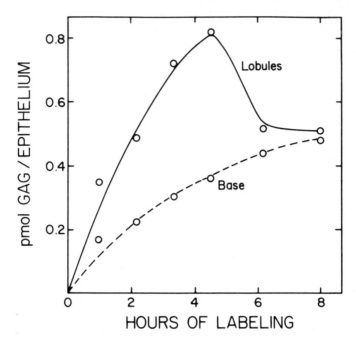

FIG. 4: Accumulation of glycosaminoglycan associated with the lobules and with the base. Whole glands were labeled for the indicated times and the mesenchyme was removed from the epithelia which retained its basal lamina. The base, which contained the clefts was then separated from the distal lobules and from the stalk. The pmol GAG (as disaccharide) were calculated from the ^{3}H-glucosamine incorporation levels and precursor pool specific activities in each set of fragments. See text for description.

****

than in the base.

The Mesenchyme Degrades Basal Laminar GAG. The reduction in the amount of GAG in the lobules is due to mesenchyme-mediated loss of laminar GAG. As previously noted, brief labeling of whole glands results in laminar GAG label primarily at the distal aspects of lobules. Removing the label and chasing shows that the GAG label is rapidly lost from these sites. However, if the epithelium is chased in the absence of mesenchyme, the rapid loss of laminar GAG label from the distal aspects of lobules is prevented. Incubation of mesenchyme with isolated epithelia containing labeled laminar GAG shows that this GAG loss is due to GAG degradation (54). In the presence but not the absence of mesenchyme, the media from these incubations accumulate a mixture of GAG fragments, including some of large molecular weight, as well as oligosaccharides and a small amount of N-acetyl-glucosamine. The release of large fragments suggests that the GAG on the epithelial surface may be cleaved extracellularly, prior to mesenchymal uptake and intracellular degradation of the GAG by lysosomal exoglycosidases.

An activity potentially capable of cleaving basal laminar GAG extracellularly is present in these glands and is developmentally regulated (2). This is a hyaluronic acid-degrading activity which is maximally active near neutral pH (pH optimum 6.5), is not sedimentable under conditions that pellet lysosomes, is found primarily in the mesenchyme and to a much lesser extent in the epithelium, and yields degradation products that are larger than the usual lysosomal hyaluronidase products. Interestingly, this neutral hyaluronidase activity increases during salivary morphogenesis from low levels at day 12, when the epithelium is a single round bud, to maximal levels at day 15, the period of most rapid branching, to low levels again at day 17 when branching morphogenesis has markedly slowed.

Thus, the basal lamina, which maintains epithelial morphology, is disrupted by mesenchymal degradation of its GAG. The disruptions in this epithelial substratum occur exclusively at the distal ends of lobules, where new clefts and branches form. The reason why the distal lobules show the greater rate of laminar GAG degradation is unclear. However, cell proliferation is rapid in the distal lobules; much faster than in the cells of the clefts. This difference in growth rate would cause the surface of the lobules to expand at a substantially greater rate than that of the clefts. This expansion enlarges the surface area to be covered by the pre-existing lamina, places the lobular surface in closer proximity to the mesenchyme and reduces the access of the mesenchyme to the surface of the clefts. This combination of factors might be sufficient to cause disruption of the lamina only on the lobules.

Collagen Stabilizes the Basal Lamina. In addition to differences in basal lamina integrity, the surfaces of the clefts and of the distal lobules differ in the amount of fibrillar collagen. A network of collagen fibers, presumably type I, covers much of the lamina on the clefts, but this collagen is nearly absent from the lamina on the distal aspects of lobules. The basis for this difference in collagen distribution is unclear. However, this distribution may play a significant role in morphogenesis because, as shown with mouse mammary epithelial cells, collagen reduces laminar GAG degradation and promotes the accumulation of a basal lamina (20).

Low passage cultures of the NAMRU mouse mammary epithelial cell line accumulate a basal lamina when cultured on a gel of type I collagen, but not on a plastic substratum. This basal lamina is ultrastructurally and, at least regarding its GAG, chemically analogous to the lamina found in mammary glands. Although the rate of GAG synthesis by these cells on collagen is identical to that on plastic, there is a substantial difference in the rate of

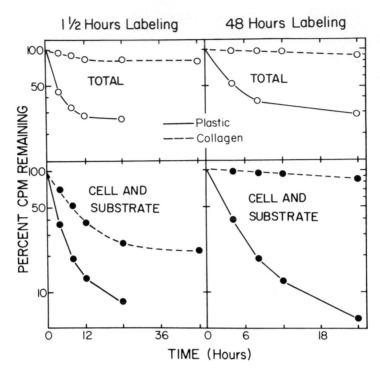

FIG. 5: Loss of S-GAG during a chase of mammary epithelial cells cultured on plastic (———) and collagen gels (– – –). Semilogarithmic plots of the percent ^{35}S-GAG remaining after 1.5 hours and 48 hours of labeling in the total culture (top) and in the cells plus their substratum (bottom). The collagen gel reduces the rate of total GAG degradation. Lengthening the labeling period has little effect on cell and substratum loss of GAG on plastic, but markedly reduces this loss in cultures on collagen. The slowly degrading cell and substratum ^{35}S-GAG pool is in the basal lamina (20). Modified from (20) and reproduced with permission.

****

GAG degradation. Compared to plastic, the GAG degradation rate in cultures on collagen is reduced more than 6-fold, suggesting that formation of a basal lamina in these cultures results from the collagen mediated reduction in laminar GAG degradation (Fig. 5).

Some of the GAG in the lamina is in a heparan sulfate-rich proteoglycan (18). This basal laminar proteoglycan is derived by an as yet unclear processing mechanism from a larger, less dense proteoglycan fraction found only with the cells. The basal laminar proteoglycan is not found within the cells and may be formed extracellularly, where it accumulates at the collagen-cell interface. In the absence of the collagen, the precursor is synthesized at a normal rate, but the processing is markedly diminished, the laminar proteoglycan does not accumulate and the precursor is degraded. Collagen apparently facilitates the conversion by the cells of a rapidly turning over cellular proteoglycan to a slowly degrading laminar proteoglycan. The mechanism by which collagen acts is unknown, but several matrix components bind to collagen, suggesting that it acts by organizing the laminar proteoglycan into a form more resistant to or less available for degradation.

Fibrillar collagen may be a physiological control of basal lamina assembly (19). In the submandibular gland, the fibrillar collagen near the epithelial surface is produced by the mesenchyme (4). Although not required for lamina formation, this collagen may stabilize basal lamina proteoglycans to degradation. Thus, because of the collagen distribution, the lamina on the clefts would be more stable than that on the distal lobules. Another influence of the mesenchyme on epithelial morphogenesis, therefore, may be its deposition of type I collagen which in turn stabilizes the basal lamina.

The Basal Lamina in Branching Epithelial Morphogenesis. These findings suggest a sequence for branching epithelial morphogenesis in which the critical element is the developmentally regulated changes in the assembly and remodeling of the basal lamina. The epithelium is responsible for the synthesis, deposition and organization of the lamina, whereas the role of the mesenchyme is to promote epithelial growth, degrade laminar GAG and deposit collagen on the epithelial surface. Epithelial growth in this sequence is the prime initiator of branching with differences in growth rate between regions determining the branching patterns. Changes in cell shape are mediated by actin microfilament contractility occurring initially at sites where the lamina is disrupted, due to loss of the substratum and possibly also to an influx of calcium ion resulting from the loss of GAG. In this scheme, direct contacts between epithelium and mesenchyme are a consequence rather than a cause of the morphogenetic events (50).

Where there is meager or symmetrical epithelial growth, as on the stalk or when the epithelium is a rounded bud, there is steady state production and degradation of laminar GAG, resulting in maintenance of an intact lamina and no changes in cell shape (Fig. 6). As the bud grows, however, it expands most rapidly at its distal aspects, causing GAG degradation at these sites to exceed GAG deposition, producing thinning and discontinuities in the lamina. The lamina interruptions cause the cells to change shape and these initial deformations induce contractions in adjacent cells, ultimately resulting in an invagination of the epithelial sheet. This early cleft would deepen because the cells adjacent to it continue to maintain their shape and to proliferate. Because of its reduced proximity to the mesenchyme and/or because of the deposition of fibrillar collagen, a complete basal lamina assembles on the cleft, providing a substratum for the cells

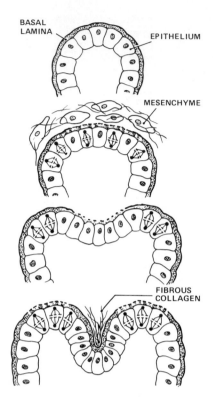

FIG. 6: Schematic model depicting a possible sequence of events
in branching morphogenesis. See text for description. Modified
from (7) and reproduced with permission.

****

within the newly formed cleft. Branching morphogenesis proceeds
as   each   newly   formed   lobule   grows and expands, initiating the
sequence of accelerated laminar GAG degradation, disruption of the
lamina and subsequent cleft formation.

MECHANISM OF MORPHOGENETIC TISSUE INTERACTIONS

The essential aspects of Grobstein's original proposal (31)
that the extracellular matrix mediates tissue interactions are
still valid. The additional aspects proposed here are that the
interacting   cells   reciprocally   influence   the   production,
organization and degradation of the other's extracellular and cell
surface matrix and that these alterations occur extracellularly by
mechanisms common to morphogenesis, reparative processes, and
possibly neoplasia.

In addition to tissue interactions, matrix remodeling also occurs in other morphogenetic events. For example, a major morphogenetic event is the shrinkage of cell-poor extracellular spaces as in the cornea and the paraxial space. Extensive work by Toole and his co-workers in several systems have shown that this change is associated with a precisely timed reduction in hyaluronic acid accumulation and the accretion of a lysosomal hyaluronidase, followed by the accumulation of chondroitin sulfate and, in the cornea and limb, of collagen (58). Similarly, selective disruption of the basal lamina allows migration of cells from a sheet as in the dispersal of mesenchymal cells from somites or neural crest cells from the neural fold (41). However, I will limit this discussion to the matrix remodeling involved in epithelial-mesenchymal interactions.

In epithelial-mesenchymal interactions, the epithelium apparently initiates the interaction by triggering the mesenchyme, following which there are multiple and reciprocal influences. For example, during the early development of several glandular epithelial organs, the initial budding of the epithelium is associated with condensation of the mesenchymal cells around the epithelial bud. Another example is the increase in collagen synthesis exhibited by mesenchyme when grown transfilter from developing epithelia (4). The requirement that mammary mesenchyme be adjacent to mammary epithelium before it will condense in response to testosterone (21) is another such phenomenon.

In each of these instances, the mesenchymal response subsequently affects the epithelium, completing the reciprocal interaction. The condensed salivary mesenchyme is able to degrade basal laminar GAG. Mesenchymal deposition of collagen on the epithelium, as previously noted, may stabilize the basal lamina. The mammary mesenchymal condensation is associated with the disruption of the mammary epithelial basal lamina which eventually leads to destruction of the epithelium. In each example, the mesenchymal response involves remodeling of an extracellular element.

Extracellular remodeling requires extracellular enzymes to perform the degradation. The best known of these are the collagenases, a group of zymogen enzymes which, when activated, are highly specific for the collagens (34). However, plasminogen activator, a less specific protease, and possibly elastase, an even more general protease, may also be involved (46). These enzymes are widely distributed neutral proteases acting extracellularly to cleave their substrates at a single or, at most, a few sites. Analogous enzymes which cleave glycosaminoglycans or proteoglycans have not been described although the hyaluronidase activity found in the submandibular mesenchyme may be a prototype for this class of enzyme (2).

These extracellular degradative enzymes may have a distinct role during morphogenesis. The extracellular and cell surface matrices of mature tissues are very stable and turn over quite slowly, often with a half-life of months. Indeed, basal laminae in adult organs are stable even in the presence of extensive

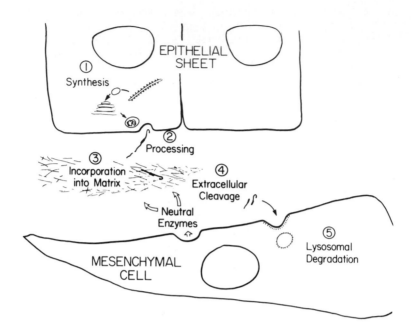

FIG. 7: The matrix remodeling model of epithelial-mesenchymal interactions. Although the events are numbered sequentially, the interaction is thought to be continuously reciprocal. See text for description.

****

cellular necrosis; they remain as extracellular scaffolds upon which new tissue boundaries will be established (60). This stability is inconsistent with the rapid changes in both tissue form and basal laminar integrity that occur during morphogenesis. In this situation, high local concentrations of highly viscous or insoluble matrix materials must be depleted. These molecules cannot be degraded by lysosomal hydrolases without their prior endocytosis, but because of these physical properties, endocytosis of the intact molecules is unlikely. Therefore, initial cleavage must be in the extracellular space. Although intracellular lysosomal degradation is subsequently involved, this reasoning indicates that the eseential modification of matrix molecules during morphogenesis occurs extracellularly.

The matrix remodeling model also requires extracellular regulation of matrix deposition. Processing of procollagen into collagen occurs by the action of extracellular procollagen peptidases (26). Indeed, this processing yields peptides which in turn may regulate procollagen production (61). The processing of basal laminar proteoglycan seems to be regulated by collagen (18).

Assembly of the molecules into an organized matrix, where they would be expected to be less susceptible to degradation, may be the function of the matrix glycoproteins.

A scheme summarizing the matrix remodeling hypothesis in epithelial-mesenchymal interactions is presented in Fig. 7. The synthesis and secretion of matrix molecules by the epithelium is followed by their processing which could occur extracellularly or at the cell surface. The predominant products of this processing are incorporated into the matrix while low molecular weight products could serve as a signal to the mesenchyme that the epithelium was proximate to it and/or was at a specific developmental stage. In response to this signal or to the presence of the epithelial matrix, the mesenchyme produces and secretes neutral enzymes which act on the matrix to form large, but soluble cleavage products. These are then taken up by the mesenchymal cell, possibly by receptor-mediated endocytosis, prior to degradation in the lysosomes (10). If receptors exist, these cleavage products might also signal the mesenchyme or epithelium in a fashion analogous to various polypeptide growth factors. The ultimate results of the interaction are a change in the matrix and an alteration in the morphogenetic behavior of the cells. This model, while speculative, makes several testable predictions.

CONCLUSIONS

I have tried in this brief review to indicate that cellular behavior during morphogenesis is linked to the dynamic changes occurring in the extracellular and cell surface matrix during morphogenesis. The matrix organization and remodeling discussed here are not unique to morphogenesis, but undoubtedly are general physiological processes. However, because the rapidity and precision of morphogenetic events are never again duplicated in an organism's life, the extent of these processes and therefore, their influence on cellular behavior may be evident in mature organisms only during the repair of injuries and the growth, invasion and metastasis of neoplasms.

ACKNOWLEDGEMENTS

The original research reported in this review was supported by grant HD06763 from the National Institutes of Health. I thank Shib Banerjee, Guido David, Joseph R. Gordon and R. Lane Smith for their expert collaboration, and M. Swenson-Rosenberg and J. Loew for assistance.

REFERENCES

1. Abercrombie, M. (1979): *Nature*, 281:259-262.
2. Banerjee, S. D. and M. R. Bernfield (1979): *J. Cell Biol.*, 83:469a.
3. Banerjee, S. D., R. H. Cohn, and M. R. Bernfield (1977): *J. Cell Biol.*, 73:445-464.

4. Bernfield, M. R. (1970): Develop. Biol., 22:213-231.
5. Bernfield, M. R. and S. D. Banerjee (1978): In: Biology and Chemistry of Basement Membranes, edited by N. A. Kefalides, pp. 137-148. Academic Press, New York.
6. Bernfield, M. R., S. D. Banerjee, and R. H. Cohn (1972): J. Cell Biol., 52:674-689.
7. Bernfield, M. R., R. H. Cohn, and S. D. Banerjee (1973): Amer. Zool., 13:1067-1083.
8. Bornstein, P. and J. F. Ash (1977): Proc. Natl. Acad. Sci. USA, 74:2480-2484.
9. Bragina, E. E., J. M. Vasiliev, and I. M. Gelfand (1976): Exp. Cell Res., 97:241-254.
10. Brown, M. S. and J. L. Goldstein (1979): Proc. Natl. Acad. Sci. USA, 76:3330-3337.
11. Chen, L. B., A. Murray, R. A. Segal, A. Bushnell, and M. L. Walsh (1978); Cell, 14:377-391.
12. Chen, W-T (1979): J. Cell Biol., 81:684-691.
13. Cohn, R. H., S. D. Banerjee, and M. R. Bernfield (1977): J. Cell biol., 73:464-478.
14. Comper, W. D. and T. C. Laurent (1978): Physiol. Rev., 58:255-315.
15. Coughlin, M. D. (1975): Develop. Biol., 43:123-139.
16. Culp, L. A., B. A. Murray and B. J. Rollins (1979): J. Supramolec. Struct., 11:401-427.
17. Cunha, G. R. and B. Lung (1979): In Vitro, 15:50-71.
18. David, G. and M. R. Bernfield (1979): J. Cell Biol., 83:469a.
19. David, G. and M. R. Bernfield (1979): J. Supramolec. Struct. Suppl., 3:199a.
20. David, G. and M. R. Bernfield (1979): Proc. Natl. Acad. Sci. USA, 76:786-790.
21. Durnberger, H. and K. Kratochwil (1980): Cell, 19:465-471.
22. Emerman, J. T., J. Enami, D. R. Pitelka, and S. Nandi (1977): Proc. Natl. Acad. Sci. USA, 74:4466-4470.
23. Emerman, J. T. and D. R. Pitelka (1977): In Vitro, 13:316-328.
24. Erickson, C. A. and J. P. Trinkaus (1976): Exp. Cell Res., 99:375-390.
25. Eyre, D. R. (1980): Science, 207:1315-1322.
26. Fessler, J. H. and L. I. Fessler (1978): Ann. Rev. Biochem., 47:129-162.
27. Folkman, J. and A. Moscona (1978): Nature, 273:345-349.
28. Goldman, R. D., M. J. Yerna, and J. A. Schloss (1976): J. Supramolec. Struct., 5:155-170.
29. Gordon, J. and M. R. Bernfield (1980): Develop. Biol., 74:118-135.
30. Grinnell, F. (1978): Int. Rev. Cytol., 29:65-102.
31. Grobstein, C. (1954): In: Aspects of Synthesis and Order in Growth, edited by D. Rudnick, pp. 233-256. Princeton Univ. Press, Princeton, New Jersey.
32. Grobstein, C. (1967): Natl. Cancer Inst. Monogr., 26:279-299.

33. Grobstein, C. and J. H. Cohen (1965): Science, 150:626-627.
34. Harris, E. D. and E. C. Cartwright (1977): In: Proteinases in Mammalian Cells and Tissues, edited by Barrett, pp. 249-283. Elsevier North-Holland Biomedical Press, Amsterdam.
35. Hascall, V. C. (1977): J. Supramolec. Struct., 7:101-120.
36. Hedman, K., M. Kurkinen, K. Alitalo, A. Vaheri, S. Johansson, and M. Hook (1979): J. Cell Biol., 81:83-91.
37. Hynes, R. O. (1976): Biochim. Biophys. Acta, 458:73-107.
38. Hynes, R. O. and A. T. Destree (1978): Cell, 15:875-881.
39. Letourneau, P. C., P. N. Ray, and M. R. Bernfield (1980): In: Biological Regulation and Control, edited by R. Goldberger, in press. Plenum Press, New York.
40. Lindahl, U. and M. Hook (1978): Ann. Rev. Biochem., 47:385-417.
41. Lofberg, J., K. Ahlfors and C. Fallstrom (1980): Develop. Biol., 75:148-167.
42. Martin, G. R. and H. Rubin (1974): Exp. Cell Res., 85:319-333.
43. Otsuka, H. and M. Moskowitz (1976): J. Cell Physiol., 87:213-220.
44. Prockop, D. J., K. I. Kivirikko, L. Tuderman, and N. A. Guzman (1979): New Engl. J. Med., 301:13-23.
45. Prockop, D. J., K. I. Kivirikko, L. Tuderman, and N. A. Guzman (1979): New Engl. J. Med., 301:77-85.
46. Reich, E. (1978). In: Biological Markers of Neoplasia: Basic and Applied Aspects, edited by L. Ruddon, pp. 491-498. Elsevier North-Holland, Inc., Amsterdam.
47. Revel, J. P., P. Hock, and D. Ho (1974): Exp. Cell Res., 84:207-214.
48. Roden, L. (1980): In: The Biochemistry of Glycoproteins and Proteoglycans, edited by W. J. Lennarz, pp. 267-371. Plenum Press, New York.
49. Rosen, J. J. and L. A. Culp (1977): Exp. Cell Res., 107:139-149.
50. Saxén, L. and E. Lehtonen (1978): J. Embryol. Exp. Morph., 47:97-109.
51. Sengel, P. (1976): Morphogenesis of Skin. Cambridge University Press, Cambridge.
52. Slavkin, H., editor (1972): The Comparative Molecular Biology of Extracellular Matrices. Academic Press, New York.
53. Slavkin, H. D. and R. C. Greulich, editors (1975): Extracellular Matrix Influence on Gene Expression. Academic Press, New York.
54. Smith, R. L. and M. R. Bernfield (1977): J. Cell Biol., 75:160a.
55. Solursh, M. and G. M. Morriss (1977): Develop. Biol., 57:75-86.
56. Stoker, M., C. O'Neill, S. Berryman, and V. Waxman (1968): Int. J. Cancer, 3:683-696.
57. Timpl, R., H. Rohde, P. G. Robey, S. I. Rennard, J-M Foidart, and G. R. Martin (1979): J. Biol. Chem., 254:9933-9937.

58. Toole, B. P., M. Okayama, R. W. Orkin, M. Yoshimura, M. Muto, and A. Kaji (1977): Soc. Gen. Physiol., 32:139-154.

59. Trinkaus, J. P. (1976): In: The Cell Surface in Animal Embryogenesis and Development, edited by G. Poste and G. L. Nicolson, pp. 225-329. North-Holland Publishing Co., Amsterdam.

60. Vracko, R. (1978): In: Biology and Chemistry of Basement Membranes, edited by Nicholas A. Kefalides, pp. 165-176. Academic Press, New York.

61. Wiestner, M., T. Krieg, D. Horlein, R. W. Glanville, P. Fietzek, and P. K. Muller (1979): J. Biol. Chem., 254:7016-7023.

62. Yamada, K. M. and K. Olden (1978): Cell Interactions and Development: Molecular Mechanisms. Wiley Interscience, in press.

Morphogenesis and Pattern Formation,
edited by T. G. Connelly et al.,
Raven Press, New York © 1981.

Limb Development: Aspects of Differentiation, Pattern Formation, and Morphogenesis

Stuart A. Newman, *H. L. Frisch, †Mary Ann Perle, and
**James J. Tomasek

*Department of Anatomy, New York Medical College, Valhalla, New York
10595; *Departments of Chemistry and Physics, State University of New York at Albany,
Albany, New York 12222; †Genetics Division, Department of Pediatrics, Children's Hospital,
Medical Center, Boston, Massachusetts 02115; **Department of Anatomy, Harvard Medical
School, Boston, Massachusetts 02115*

During the development or regeneration of all organs at least
three interdependent but distinct processes are brought into play
(44). The process of molecular differentiation involves changes
in gene expression in multipotent progenitor cells resulting in a
characteristic spectrum of terminal cell types. Spatial pattern
formation is a function of the interactions of cells at varying
stages of molecular differentiation and is the means by which
cells are assigned their appropriate relative positions in a
multicellular structure. Morphogenesis depends on movement, shape
change and growth in individual cells and tissues and ultimately
results in the functional form of the organ.

We have been interested in each of these processes as they
relate to the embryonic development of the chick limb. This
structure emerges from the body wall of the embryo as a mound of
mesenchymal cells covered by a thin layer of ectoderm, and takes
on a paddle shape as outgrowth proceeds. The limb skeleton is
laid out as cartilaginous primordia in a proximodistal sequence
between 4 and 7 days of incubation (Fig. 1); only later is the
cartilage replaced by bone.

Several important features of chick limb development will
occupy our attention in this summary:

1. The cell lineage of the muscle component of the limb bud is
distinct from that of the cartilage and soft connective tissue (5,
6, 23). Therefore, the histogenesis of the skeletal elements is a
function of nuclear events in precartilage mesenchymal cells.

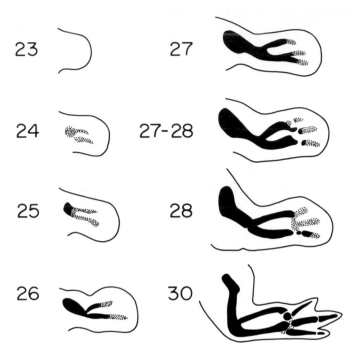

FIG.1. Progress of chondrogenesis in the chick wing bud between 4 and 7 days of incubation. Solid black regions represent definitive cartilage; stippled areas represent early cartilage. Stages are those of Hamburger and Hamilton (13). From Newman and Frisch (26), copyright American Association for the Advancement of Science.

****

2.   The spatial pattern of the developing skeletal elements is prefigured by changes in cellular contacts in those regions of the mesenchyme where cartilage will form (36). If these changes are prevented in culture (23) and conceivably in situ, the precartilage cells differentiate into fibroblasts, or die off (24).

3.   Outgrowth of the limb bud during the patterning process is absolutely dependent on the apical ectodermal ridge (AER) which rims its distal margin (32, 33). The AER provides no limb-type-specific (49), stage-specific (30), or even species-specific (3, 17) information to the mesoderm, but does represent a distinct ectodermal cell type, since other limb or nonlimb ectoderm cannot substitute for it (33).

In what follows we will make use of this background information and summarize some of our recent studies that potentially bear on the mechanisms of these developmental processes.

A Nuclear Protein Involved in Cartilage Differentiation

Programmatic specificity in different cell types of a single organism is thought to be largely determined by the complement of nuclear nonhistone proteins, since the DNA and the main histone protein classes of various somatic cell types are essentially similar (10). Nuclear nonhistone proteins may act at the transcriptional or post-transcriptional levels by, for example, recognizing specific DNA sequences, modifying histones (31), DNA (15) or the conformation of the chromatin subunit (47) on the one hand, or influencing the survival or transport into the cytoplasm of a subset of RNA transcripts (8), on the other.

We have examined by several techniques, the nuclear nonhistone proteins of limb bud precartilage cells and those of cartilage cells. To do this it was necessary to prepare an essentially pure population of cartilage progenitor cells. (Cartilage itself is relatively easy to obtain in a pure form.) Here we made use of an observation that the distal tip of the chick wing bud at five days of incubation is free of myogenic cells (27, 23). This tissue, consisting of cells that are not yet chondrocytes (27, 23, 24), can nonetheless differentiate homogeneously into cartilage when grown in culture under aggregated conditions (27, 23). It can thus be considered operationally a population of cartilage stem cells.

When nuclear proteins of these precartilage cells are compared on one-dimensional gels with those of cartilage cells derived from them in tissue culture the complements of nonhistones appear similar, with the prominent exception of an abundant protein with a molecular weight of 125,000. This protein is present in the precartilage cell nucleus, but absent from the cartilage cell nucleus (25). When precartilage nuclei are compared with nuclei from limb and vertebral cartilages obtained from more developed embryos other differences in the nuclear protein complement are evident, but the most striking change is still the loss during differentiation of the abundant 125,000 M_r component (29).

The 125,000 M_r precartilage chromatin protein, which we term PCP, is not detected in myogenic progenitor cells, definitive muscle cells (16), or fibroblasts (23) and thus, within the mesodermal lineages relevant to limb development, appears to be cell-type-specific.

To determine the relationship of PCP to other components of the precartilage cell nucleus, we have treated these nuclei with various nucleases and monitored protein release. A mixture of ribonucleases does not release PCP, suggesting that it is not among those protein components binding nascent RNA chains during and after transcription (M. A. Perle and S. Newman, in preparation). Transcriptionally active regions of chromatin DNA are highly sensitive to attack by the deoxyribonuclease DNAase I (46, 11). While this enzyme releases a specific subset of proteins from precartilage cell nuclei along with the 55% of the chromatin DNA which is rapidly attacked in this cell type, it does not release PCP (M. A. Perle and S. Newman, in preparation). This further suggests that not only is PCP not part of transcriptional complexes in these cells, but that it is also not among those proteins specifically maintaining the "active" chromatin conformation in precartilage cells (47) (though it may be contiguous to the active regions (28)). The elution characteristics of PCP from chromatin that has been bound to hydroxyapatite is consistent with a DNA-binding role for this protein in precartilage chromatin (28).

The fact that PCP is the major chromatin protein distinguishing precartilage from cartilage cells suggested that it may play a role in the reprogramming event. We subsequently examined the nuclear proteins of precartilage and cartilage cells of the chick mutant talpid² (29). This recessive embryonic lethal exhibits severe skeletal abnormalities in the homozygous state (1). The embryos develop for about 10 days during which time the limbs show a perturbed pattern of chondrogenesis, but apparently normal cartilage at the histological level (Fig. 2). A main target of talpid² gene action is the limb mesoderm, but not its ectoderm (12). We have found that the talpid² precartilage cell nuclei contain a version of PCP that is reduced in molecular weight to 120,000 M_r (Fig. 3a). This protein, like its normal counterpart, is lost during chondrogenesis. Heterozygotes carrying the talpid² gene have only the normal version of PCP in their nuclei. Cartilage nuclei carrying one or two copies of the talpid² gene exhibit no detectable abnormalities in their complement of proteins (Fig. 3b).

Apart from the electrophoretic difference in PCP, homozygous talpid² precartilage nuclei exhibit a "precocious" cartilage-like pattern in the 35-37,000 M_r complement of proteins, which may represent a perturbation in the timing of a normal nuclear event in chondrogenesis. However, because of developmental time course studies we have done (28), we are confident that talpid² precartilage chromatin is not uniformly advanced along the cartilage pathway. In particular, PCP disappears gradually during normal development without changing its molecular weight.

We do not know the role of PCP in normal cartilage differentiation, or whether the alteration in this protein observed in talpid² precartilage cells represents a primary genetic lesion or the abnormal processing of a normal gene product. However, the presence of this developmentally significant nuclear protein in an aberrant form in a cell population that exhibits a disturbance in the spatial pattern of cell differentiation suggests that it may indirectly help regulate cellular interactions during skeletal development.

The Possible Role of Chemical Waves in Skeletal Pattern Formation

Since precartilage mesenchymal cells undergo changed cellular contacts prior to overt chondrogenesis (36), it is reasonable to suggest that a molecule that encourages cell-to-cell contacts could be responsible for the initiation of chondrogenic foci in tissue capable of forming cartilage. One such molecule, the

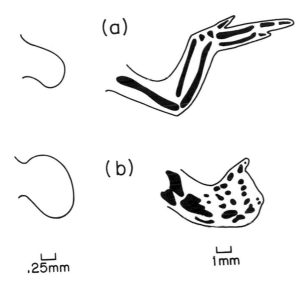

FIG.2. Shapes of 5-day wing buds (left) and skeletal patterns of
9-day wings (right) of (a) normal and (b) <u>talpid</u>[2] embryos.
Drawings of 5-day wing buds are based on <u>camera lucida</u> sketches.
Drawings of 9-day embryonic wing skeletons are based on whole
mount photographs in Goetinck and Abbott (12).

ᛉᛁᛕᛝ ᚨᛩ᚛ᚸᚸᚸᚸᚸᚸᚸᚸᚸᚸᚸᚸᚸᚸᚸᚸᚸᚸᚸᚸᛣ

widely distributed matrix glycoprotein fibronectin (42) has been
found in precartilage mesenchyme, though it is not produced by
mature cartilage cells (21).

    We have undertaken a mathematical analysis of the biosynthesis
and diffusion through the mesenchymal matrix of a glycoprotein
such as fibronectin (26). Soluble fibronectin is presumed to be
produced by the mesenchyme cells and to freely diffuse between the
cells in their hyaluronate-rich extracellular matrix. The
dynamical law governing such processes is known as the reaction-
diffusion equation; its possible role in development was first
suggested by Turing (41) and has been elaborated on by Kaufman et
al. (18).

    In our case the reaction-diffusion equation for a diffusion
chamber of fixed dimensions takes the form:

$$D \nabla^2 c + rc = 0$$

Here c represents the displacement of the concentration of
"fibronectin" from a spatially homogeneous basal value; r is its
biosynthetic rate constant; D is its diffusion coefficient; and ∇^2
is a generalized second derivative along the three spatial

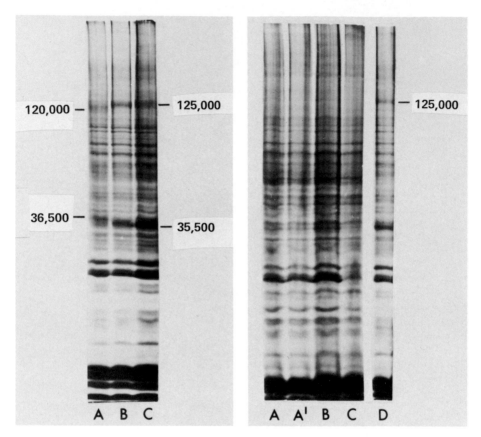

FIG.3(a) Gels (12.5% polyacrylamide-SDS) displaying precartilage
chromatin proteins. A, proteins from talpid² homozygous embryos;
B, proteins from phenotypically normal embryos from the talpid²
flock; C, proteins from embryos from a commercial flock.
(b) Gels displaying cartilage chromatin proteins. A,A', proteins
from talpid² homozygous embryos (two samples); B, proteins from
phenotypically normal embryos from the talpid² flock; C, proteins
from embryos from a commerical flock; D, precartilage chromatin
proteins from normal embryos, presented for comparison. From
Perle and Newman (29), copyright National Academy of Sciences.

****

coordinates inside the developing limb.
    With a source or high point of the putative morphogen, perhaps
fibronectin, at the limb tip (corresponding to the special status
of the apex in development) and its absorption at the periphery,
the concentration of the diffusing molecule becomes non-uniform
throughout the matrix. This can be visualized by imagining a

glass of water with a drop of ink in the center. Diffusion will tend to make the ink spread out uniformly. However, if the ink concentration is kept constant at the top of the glass by constant addition, and is absorbed by the glass itself, the ink will tend to mount up at the center of the glass and form a denser "core." This is the basic principle of the model. The constancy of the values of r, D and the anteroposterior and dorsoventral widths of the limb bud during the pattern forming phase of development, contribute to a constant we have called the "Saunders' Number." Consequently, the number and distribution of dense regions of the morphogen are sensitive to the proximodistal length of the mesenchymal chamber (i.e., the predifferentiated limb tip) in which biosynthesis and diffusion occur (26).

Fig. 4 shows the successive distributions of the hypothetical morphogen (or "chemical waves") on cross-sections of a parallelepiped representing the limb tip as it undergoes a stepwise reduction in its proximodistal length during limb outgrowth.

We have used realistic dimensions (34) for an idealized version of the wing bud, a realistic diffusion constant for a morphogen of the size of the fibronectin dimer in a hyaluronate matrix, and a realistic rate constant for the biosynthetic process.

We have also used the measurements of Summerbell (35) to determine the size of the predifferentiated limb tip at various stages of development. The above factors, taken together with the appropriate solutions to the reaction-diffusion equation, along with a stipulation on the distribution of cells competent to respond to fibronectin (26) govern a process giving the proper number of cartilage elements, emerging in the appropriate proximodistal sequence over a realistic time course as the limb grows out from the body wall (Fig. 5).

We are far from having demonstrated that fibronectin or any similar matrix glycoprotein actually provides a "prepattern" for the developing vertebrate limb skeleton. What we have shown is that well-established mesenchyme cell biochemistry, realistic limb bud dimensions, and the straightforward physics of reaction and diffusion almost inevitably lead to the emergence of a rough skeletal prepattern that could subsequently have been fine-tuned by the evolutionary process.

Morphological and Biochemical Correlates of AER Action

Recent ideas about the basis of morphogenetic epithelial-mesenchymal interactions have centered on the basal lamina, the epithelial-derived matrix that provides an interface between the two tissue types, as a potential locus of such interactions (14, 2 and this volume). Basal laminae, which correspond in part to epithelial basement membranes visualized by the light microscope, consist of collagenous and noncollagenous glycoproteins, glycosaminoglycans and possibly proteoglycans (19). In embryonic systems these structures have been found to exhibit regional and stage-dependent differences in composition (45, 9) and turnover

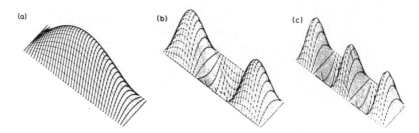

FIG.4. Representation of distribution of "fibronectin" on cross-sections of schematic predifferentiated limb tip at three successive stages of development. Distance above or below rectangular plane represents displacement of fibronectin from a spatially homogenous basal value. From Newman and Frisch (26), copyright American Association for the Advancement of Science.

****

(2) correlating with various morphogenetic activities.

We have examined the ultrastructure and composition of the inductive (AER) and noninductive (dorsal and ventral) ectoderms in developing chick, duck and turtle limb buds by a variety of techniques. Our goal here has been to determine whether the special role of the AER in limb outgrowth can be associated with, and potentially accounted for, by structural or compositional differences between its basal lamina and that of the noninductive ectoderms.

Our studies at the ultrastructural level have made use of recently described methods of fixation using ruthenium red (14, 40) and tannic acid (7) to preserve basal laminae. One interesting observation we have made is that there appears to be a morphological differentiation of the chick limb bud basal lamina that corresponds to the functional differentiation of its ectoderm. The noninductive dorsal or ventral ectoderms of the limb bud when stained with ruthenium red show a very regular basal lamina structure similar to that described in other embryonic epithelia (14, 40). In particular, there is a highly periodic array of ruthenium red-staining, hyaluronidase-sensitive granules on both the ectodermal and mesodermal faces of a continuous and sharply defined lamina densa. The cells of the noninductive ectoderm appear well-spread on their substratum and contain many bundles of microfilaments parallel to their basal surfaces (Fig. 6a).

In contrast, the basal lamina under the AER shows reduced periodicity in the ruthenium red-staining granules and an attenuated lamina densa that is diffuse on its two outer surfaces. The overlying ridge cells show a pseudostratified high columnar cell shape which may be a result of the poor spreading of these cells on their basal lamina substratum (20). These cells do not

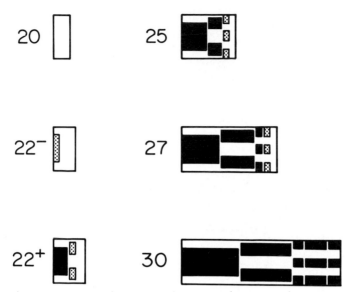

FIG.5. Patterns of chondrogenesis predicted by the model described in text at successive stages of development. Solid black represents cartilage or precartilage condensation; stippling represents hypothetical distribution of fibronectin in competent tissue preceding overt chondrogenesis. Hamburger-Hamilton stages (13) to which model stages correspond are indicated by numbers. From Newman and Frisch (26), copyright American Association for the Advancement of Science.

****

show organized bundles of microfilaments parallel to their basal surfaces; rather microfilaments and microtubules are generally aligned along the long axis of the cell (Fig. 6b). A similar contrast in the organization of lateral ectoderm and AER basal laminae is seen with tannic acid-containing fixatives in the chick (Fig. 6c, d), and with conventional glutaraldehyde-osmium fixation in the turtle (J. Tomasek and S. Newman, in preparation).

We have also examined chick and duck limb buds for the distribution of fibronectin, since this is a known component of some embryonic basement membranes (43, 45). Our collaborator in this effort has been Dr. J. Mazurkiewicz, of Albany (N.Y.) Medical College.

To localize fibronectin we have used an indirect immunofluorescence procedure that involves binding anti-fibronectin antibody raised in rabbits to avian limb sections. This is followed by treatment of the sections with fluorescein-conjugated goat anti-rabbit IgG. The AER basement membrane in both chick and duck was shown by this technique to be highly enriched in fibronectin relative to the non-inductive limb

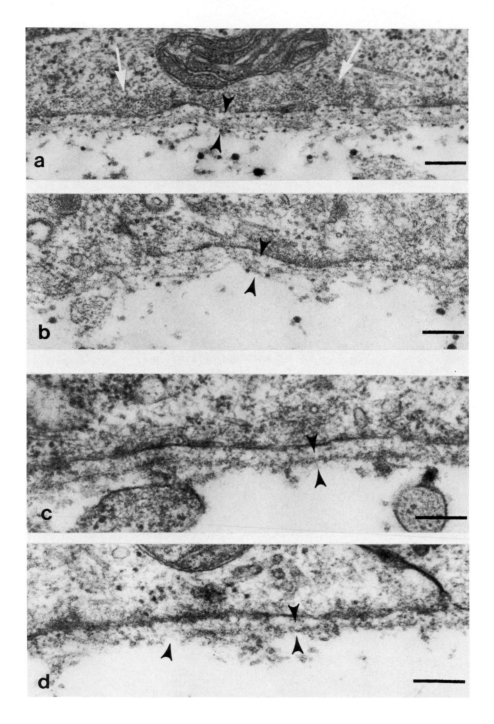

FIG.6. Electron micrographs of the base of an ectodermal cell (top of each panel) and the underlying basal lamina (arrowheads), showing differences in organization of the basal lamina of lateral ectoderm and AER as seen with two different fixatives. a) Chick wingbud lateral ectoderm, stage 21, fixed with Karnovsky's fixative containing 0.2% ruthenium red; postfixed with OsO and 0.05% ruthenium red. Stained with uranyl acetate and lead citrate. Bundles of microfilaments cut in cross-section are evident running along the plasma membrane of the ectodermal cell (white arrows). b) Chick wing bud AER, stage 21; fixation as in (a). c) Chick wing bud lateral ectoderm, stage 23, fixed with glutaraldehyde containing 1% tannic acid, followed by 1% OsO_4 in phosphate buffer. Stained with uranyl acetate and lead citrate. d) Chick wing bud, stage 23; fixation as in (c). All magnification bars represent 200nm.

****

ectoderms.   This is evident in the 5-day chick limb montage shown in Fig. 7.

At the light microscopic level it is not possible to determine whether the subridge accumulation of fibronectin is localized in the basal lamina proper, or in the sublaminar matrix. A relevant point here is our observation(37) of extensive arrays of stacked fibers 3-5nm in diameter localized exclusively in the AER sublaminar space which resemble those identified as fibronectin by Chen et al. (4) in the extracellular matrices of fibroblasts grown in vitro.

Based on these findings our current working hypothesis is that the AER exerts its inductive role in part by elaborating a basement membrane that differs from that of noninductive ectoderm. The basal lamina proper is thought to be less able to assemble into the regular lattice seen in the latter ectoderm and, therefore, to provide a poorer substrate for ectodermal adhesion and spreading. The AER cells would thus minimize their surface contact with the lamina, forming a ridge as a consequence. The attenuated basal lamina could constitute a region of low mechanical resistance to expansion of the mesenchyme. The latter would also tend to migrate along the fibronectin-rich components of the subridge basement membrane. Finally, the acellular space formed beneath the AER and the underlying mesenchyme as a consequence of the incomplete adhesion differences postulated to give rise to the ridge could conceivably provide a reservoir for hyaluronate produced in the ectoderm or mesenchyme, and thus encourage a directional invasiveness of the latter tissue (22, 39). Some or all of these factors could act coordinately to produce inductive outgrowth in the limb bud.

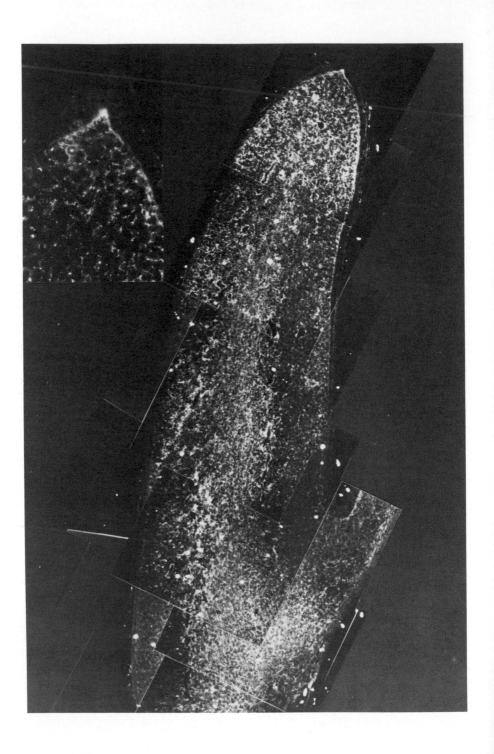

FIG.7. Montage of light micrographic fields of stage 25 chick wing bud photographed under ultraviolet illumination after treatment with antibody against human CIG (fibronectin) raised in rabbit (obtained from L. B. Chen) and staining with fluorescein-conjugated goat anti-rabbit IgG (Miles Laboratories). Cross-section, 37X. Inset, apical tip of a similarly the prepared stage 25 wing tip, 95X.

****

Conclusions: An Integrated Picture of Limb Development

Based on the foregoing discussion we would like to sketch the outlines of a scheme for limb skeletal development that takes into account the cytodifferentiative, pattern forming and morphogenetic components of this process. For most of what follows we can we can only claim plausibility, since few of the assumptions have been put to definitive tests. However, a positive feature of the scheme is that it is testable in detail; in addition to the general ideas which can eventually be proved true or false, predictions are made as to the roles played by specific molecules.

The first step in limb formation is proposed to be the creation on the flank ectoderm, in each limb field, of a line of ectodermal cells having the capacity to make a changed basal lamina, as detailed above. This event, AER initiation, is a problem in cytodifferentiation and pattern formation on a two-dimensional plane whose basis we have not considered.

As the mesenchyme pushes out from the body wall, possibly by overcoming the mechanical restraint normally provided by an organized basal lamina, and possibly under the encouragement of materials accumulated in the subridge space, the paddle shape of the outgrowth arises as a consequence of the anisotropic expansion determined by the original distribution of AER cells.

When the growing limb bud reaches a critical size, and then at subsequent specific times during outgrowth, hyaluronidase is presumed to be induced (38) at the proximal end of the predifferentiated mesenchyme, rendering a portion of its precartilage component susceptible to condensation under the influence of the sequential standing waves of fibronectin entailed by our dynamical model (26; Fig. 4). The cellular interactions promote chondrogenesis and by the time ridge activity has died down, the final pattern in Fig. 1 has been laid out.

Since fibronectin is apparently not found in mature embryonic cartilage (21), it has been suggested that accumulation of fibronectin may act as a __negative__ control element for chondrogenesis during pattern formation (48). However, the montage in Fig. 7 clearly shows a high concentration of this glycoprotein, not only in the predifferentiated distal tip, but also in the chondrogenic core, which at stage 25 consists of precartilage condensation distally, and early definitive cartilage proximally. Therefore, the evidence clearly favors a two-stage process in which fibronectin is involved in the early stages of chondrogenesis, and is only later lost upon maturation of the cartilage cell type (21, 26) (J. Tomasek, J. Mazurkiewicz and S. Newman, in preparation).

Finally, we note the unexpected connection between the abundant precartilage chromatin protein, PCP, and the pattern forming process, as evidenced by the association of an aberrant PCP with abnormal pattern formation in talpid² precartilage mesenchyme. It is premature to speculate on the part played by PCP other than to point out that talpid² precartilage mesenchyme is hyperplastic relative to that of normal limb buds (Fig. 2). Perhaps PCP is involved in the regulation of some component of the mesenchymal matrix (hyaluronate? "ridge maintenance factor" (50)?) that is overproduced when PCP is in an altered state. Now the AER would be discouraged from subsiding pre- and post-axially, and the mesenchyme would expand anomalously in an anteroposterior direction. Our dynamical model, when applied to an expanded diffusion chamber, predicts the polydactyly that characterizes the talpid² limb skeleton (26). Here, molecular differentiation, pattern formation and morphogenesis may interact and converge in the generation of both the normal and abnormal biological structures.

ACKNOWLEDGEMENTS

The authors thank Dr. John Cairns of the Roswell Park Memorial Institute, Buffalo, for fertile eggs from his talpid² flock, Dr. Lan Bo Chen of the Sidney Farber Cancer Institute, Boston, for antibody against cold insoluble globulin, and Mr. Ryland Loos for the line drawings. This work was supported in part by NIH Grants GM26198 and GM27674 to S.N. and NSF Grant CHE76-82583A01 to H.L.F.

REFERENCES

1. Abbott, U. K., L. W. Taylor and H. Abplanalp (1960): J. Hered., 51:195-202.
2. Bernfield, M. R. and S. D. Banerjee (1978): Biology and Chemistry of Basement Membranes, edited by N. A. Kefalides, pp. 137-148. Academic Press, New York.
3. Cairns, J. M. (1965): Develop. Biol., 12:36-52.
4. Chen, L. B., A. Murray, R. A. Segal, A. Bushnell and M. L. Walsch (1978): Cell, 14:377-391.
5. Chevallier, A., M. Kieny and A. Mauger (1977): J. Embryol. Exp. Morphol., 41:245-258.
6. Christ, B., H. J. Jacob and M. Jacob (1977): Anat. Embryol., 150:171-186.
7. Cohn, R. H., S. D. Banerjee and M. R. Bernfield (1977): J. Cell Biol., 73:464-478.

8. Davidson, E. H. and R. J. Britten (1979): <u>Science</u>, 204:1052-1059.
9. Ekblom, P., K. Alitalo, A. Vaheri, R. Timpl and L. Saxen (1980): <u>Proc. Nat. Acad. Sci. USA</u>, 77:485-489.
10. Elgin, S. C. R. and H. Weintraub (1975): <u>Ann. Rev. Biochem.</u>, 44:725-774.
11. Garel, A. and R. Axel (1976): <u>Proc. Nat. Acad. Sci. USA</u>, 73:3966-3970.
12. Goetinck, P. F. and U. K. Abbott (1964): <u>J. Exp. Zool.</u>, 155:161-170.
13. Hamburger, V. and H. L. Hamilton (1951): <u>J. Morphol.</u>, 88:49-92.
14. Hay, E. D. (1978): <u>Growth</u>, 42:399-423.
15. Holliday, R. and J. E. Pugh (1975): <u>Science</u>, 187:226-232.
16. Holtzer, H., N. Rubinstein, S. Fellini, G. Yeoh, J. Chi, J. Birnbaum and M. Okayama (1975): <u>Q. Rev. Biophys.</u>, 8:523-557.
17. Jorquera, B. and E. Pugin (1971): <u>Comptes rendus de l'Acad. des Science, Paris</u>, 272:1522-1525.
18. Kauffman, S. A., R. M. Shymko and K. Trabert (1978): <u>Science</u>, 199:259-270.
19. Kefalides, N. A. (1978): In: <u>Biology and Chemistry of Basement Membranes</u>, edited by N. A. Kefalides, pp. 215-228, Academic Press, New York.
20. Kelley, R. O. and J. G. Bluemink (1974): <u>Develop. Biol.</u>, 37:1-17.
21. Lewis, R. D., R. M. Pratt, J. P. Pennypacker and J. R. Hassell (1978): <u>Develop. Biol.</u>, 64:31-47.
22. Manasek, R. J. (1975): <u>Curr. Top. Dev. Biol.</u>, 10:35-102.
23. Newman, S. A. (1977): In: <u>Vertebrate Limb and Somite Morphogenesis</u>, edited by D. A. Ede, J. R. Hinchliffe and M. Balls, pp. 181-197, Cambridge University Press, Cambridge.
24. Newman, S. A. (1980): <u>J. Embryol. Exp. Morphol.</u> (in press).
25. Newman, S. A., J. Birnbaum and G. C. T. Yeoh (1976): <u>Nature</u>, 259:417-418.
26. Newman, S. A. and H. L. Frisch (1979): <u>Science</u>, 205:662-668.
27. Newman, S. A. and R. Mayne (1974): <u>J. Cell Biol.</u>, 63:245a.
28. Perle, M. A. (1979): Ph.D Thesis. State University of New York at Albany.
29. Perle, M. A. and S. A. Newman (1980): <u>Proc. Nat. Acad. Sci. USA</u>, 77:4828-4830.
30. Rubin, L. and J. W. Saunders, Jr. (1972): <u>Develop. Biol.</u>, 28:94-112.
31. Ruiz-Carrillo, A., L. J. Wangh and V. G. Allfrey (1975): <u>Science</u>, 190:117-128.
32. Saunders, J. W., Jr. (1948): <u>J. Exp. Zool.</u>, 108:363-404.
33. Saunders, J. W., Jr. (1977): In: <u>Vertebrate Limb and Somite Morphogenesis</u>, edited by D. A. Ede, J. R. Hinchliffe and M. Balls, pp. 1-24, Cambridge University Press, Cambridge.
34. Stark, R. J. and R. L. Searls (1973): <u>Develop. Biol.</u>, 33:138-153.
35. Summerbell, D. (1976): <u>J. Embryol. Exp. Morphol.</u>,

35:241-260.

36. Thorogood, P.V. and J. R. Hinchliffe (1975): J. Embryol. Exp. Morphol., 33:581-606.

37. Tomasek, J. and S. A. Newman (1978): J. Cell Biol., 153a.

38. Toole, B. P. (1972): Develop. Biol., 29:321-329.

39. Toole, B. P., C. Biswas and J. Gross (1979): Proc. Nat. Acad. Sci. USA, 76:6299-6203.

40. Trelstad, R. L., K. Hayashi and B. P. Toole (1974): J. Cell Biol., 62:815-830.

41. Turing, A. M. (1952): Philos. Trans. R. Soc. Lond. Ser. B., 237:37-72.

42. Vaheri, A., E. Ruoslahti and D. Mosher, editors (1978): Fibroblast Surface Protein New York Academy of Sciences, New York.

43. Wartiovaara, J., S. Stenman and A. Vaheri (1976): Differentiation, 5:85-89.

44. Waddington, C. H. (1962): New Patterns in Genetics and Development. Columbia University Press, New York.

45. Wakely, J. and M. A. England (1979): Proc. R. Soc. Lond. B., 206:329-352.

46. Weintraub, H. and M. Groudine (1976): Science, 193:848-856.

47. Weissbrod, S., M. Groudine and H. Weintraub (1980): Cell, 19:289-301.

48. West, C. M., R. Lanza, J. Rosenbloom, M. Lowe, H. Holtzer and N. Avdalovic (1979): Cell, 17:491-501.

49. Zwilling, E. (1955): J. Exp. Zool., 128:423-441.

50. Zwilling, E. and L. Hansborough (1956): J. Exp. Zool., 132:219-239.

Morphogenesis and Pattern Formation,
edited by T. G. Connelly et al.,
Raven Press, New York © 1981.

The Adhesive Specification of Tissue Self-Organization

Malcolm S. Steinberg

Department of Biology, Princeton University, Princeton, New Jersey 08544

My concern here will be to describe and in some measure dissect what is perhaps the most awesome feature of embryonic morphogenesis: its goal-directedness. I refer not to the regularity or predictability of normal development but rather to the ability of many systems undergoing morphogenesis to compensate after perturbation and restore themselves to normal form. A simple example is seen in epithelial wound-healing. The wound borders are mobilized and migrate in, ceasing their movement precisely when the gap has been closed. Rand (29) embodied this phenomenon in the dictum "an epithelium will not tolerate a free edge."

Lewis Wolpert has discussed (this volume) under the rubric of "positional information" a form of regulation in which the proper organization of a system's components is achieved by controls which cause originally pluripotential parts to differentiate in the correct location. I am addressing my attention to that mechanism's exact counterpart: that form of regulation in which the proper organization of the parts is achieved by controls which cause already-differentiated but mislocated elements to move to the correct location.

Tissue Affinities: Liquid Properties of Certain Tissues

Our studies in this area grew out of Holtfreter's discovery of "tissue affinities" (13 and 14). Holtfreter observed that embryonic tissue fragments of various kinds when combined in vitro would spread, one over another, to adopt particular geometrical relationships. When the tissues so combined were ones that normally were neighbors in the embryo, the configuration adopted bore a striking resemblance to that normally adopted in the

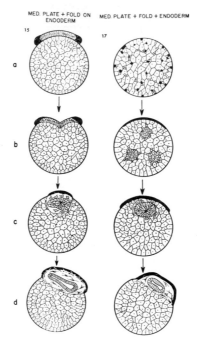

FIG. 1. <u>Left side</u>: a graft of amphibian neural plate with associated neural fold and epidermis is fused with a mass of endoderm. The entire tissue complex spontaneously rearranges itself, more or less as in the embryo, to simulate the organization of a late neurula quite closely. <u>Right side</u>: the same tissues are dispersed into single cells which are mixed together and allowed to reaggregate. By a procedure of cell sorting, quite different from the procedure followed at the left or in normal development, the same ultimate organization is achieved (From Townes and Holtfreter, 1955).

****

embryo. For example, gastrula mesoderm tended to interpose itself between an internally-segregating mass of endoderm and an externally-segregating mass of ectoderm. These "tissue affinities" were found to reside in properties intrinsic to the individual cells, for when the tissues were dissociated and their cells mixed together, the latter unscrambled themselves, moving inward or outward within the aggregates and exchanging partners until the organization characteristic of the particular cell combination was achieved. It is noteworthy that these reorganizations could proceed along totally abnormal morphogenetic pathways (Fig. 1). Holtfreter struggled with several possible explanations of these phenomena, including variations in cellular surface tensions, adhesiveness and chemotactic properties, but did

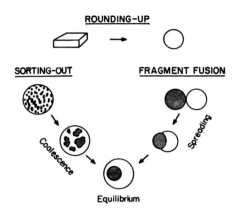

HIERARCHY

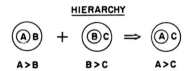

FIG. 2. Syndrome of behaviors shared by certain embryonic cell populations and ordinary liquids or immiscible liquid pairs. Above: a mass of arbitrary shape rounds up, minimizing its surface area. Middle: intermixed phases sort out by a process of coalescence, forming a continuous externalizing phase which envelopes, to greater or lesser degree, a discontinuous, internalizing phase. The same two phases when touched together as separate masses spread, one over the other, to approach the same (equilibrium) configuration approached by sorting-out. Below: in a set of mutually immiscible phases, the property of spreading over another phase is transitive. If b tends to spread over a and c tends to spread over b, c will tend to spread over a. (From Phillips, 1969; cited in Steinberg, 1978b.)

****

not devise experimental tests to distinguish among the various possibilities. The issue came to rest, in his hands, with the suggestion that chemotaxis ("directed migration") guided cells inward or outward within a tissue mass while "selective adhesion" (which was envisioned as including instances of actual repulsion as well as attraction between cells) governed their final assembly into the correct architectural groupings (47).

It occurred to the writer that studies of the pathways of cell rearrangement during "tissue reconstruction" could allow discrimination between alternative directive mechanisms. For

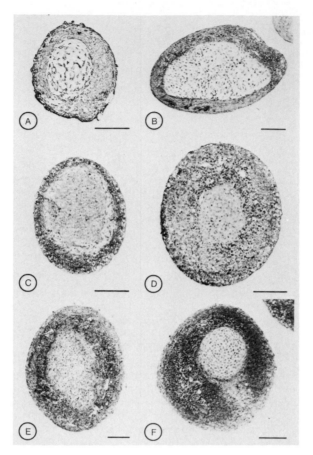

FIG. 3. Equilibrium configurations adopted by chick embryonic cell and tissue combinations through the sorting-out of intermixed cells (A, C, E) and the spreading of apposed, intact tissue fragments (B, D, F). Heart ventricle totally envelops limb bud precartilage (A, B), liver totally envelops heart ventricle (C, D), and liver totally envelops limb bud precartilage (E, F), illustrating the transitivity of inside-outside positioning. According to the differential adhesion hypothesis, a cell population of lesser cohesiveness (sigma) should tend to envelop one of higher sigma. Thus the sigma values of the three tissues represented here should decline in the sequence sigma(limb bud)> sigma(heart) > sigma(liver). (From Steinberg, 1964.)

****

example, the pathways of cells migrating in a chemotactic field differ from those of cells exchanging neighbors on the basis of differences in mutual adhesiveness. In a series of such studies, it was shown that the behavior of cells and tissues in the process of "tissue reconstruction" from experimentally contrived abnormal initial arrangements corresponded in detail with that to be expected if differentials in intercellular adhesive intensities were the sole guiding influence (32-37). Appreciation of these expectations was greatly aided by comparison with the known and well-understood behavior of multi-phase liquid systems, whose rearrangements arise from precisely comparable interactions. Just as certain tissues are collections of mobile, cohering cells, an ordinary liquid consists of a substantial number of mobile, cohering molecules. (If they were not mobile it would be a solid; if they did not cohere it would be a gas; and if there were not substantial numbers of them, they could not be characterized as having any particular phase state.) Because the molecules are free to move, cohesion forces them toward a configuration of minimal interfacial (adhesive) free energy. If molecules of more than one kind are present, the relative intensities of their mutual attractions will determine whether they intermix like water and alcohol or segregate like water and oil. In the latter case, the positions adopted by the phases are likewise determined, a less cohesive phase tending to envelop a more cohesive one. Even the degree of this envelopment, as expressed by the contact angle between two phases, is determined by the relative values of cohesive and adhesive intensities. If disturbed by an external force, the equilibrium configuration will tend to be restored when the force is removed. This will occur by rearrangements which propel the various constituents of the liquid body along whatever pathways lead most directly toward the "desired" configuration. Liquids thus display precisely those behaviors (Figs. 2, 3) which when observed in collectives of living cells, have inspired not only awe but also despair at the possibility of understanding how each cell "knows" where it belongs and can mobilize itself to find and adopt its proper position in the overall structure.

Confirming the Differential Adhesion Hypothesis

The "Differential Adhesion Hypothesis" (34-39) explains these morphogenetic "recognition" properties of cell groups by identifying such populations as liquid bodies whose subunits are not single molecules but entire motile cells. The cells' adhesive properties are held to generate the interfacial free energies or tensions (sigmas) which guide their movements and stabilize the population's ultimate configuration. Testing this theory requires measuring tissues' mutual envelopment tendencies: Any cell population that tends to envelop another must have a lower sigma than the latter. This has been done in two independent sets of experiments (22, 23) and in each case the expected relationship between tissue sigmas and mutual envelopment tendencies has been confirmed (Figs. 4 and 5). In the second set of experiments it was shown in addition that the cohesiveness (sigma) of a cell population can be experimentally either increased or decreased, and that this manipulation not only modulates spreading tendency in the expected manner, but also causes cells so altered to become immiscible with others with which they were initially identical.

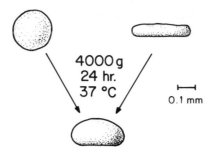

FIG. 4. Like liquid droplets, initially round and initially flat aggregates of chick embryonic cells adopt the same equilibrium shape when cultured in a centrifuge. The profiles shown were traced from photographs of heart aggregates centrifuged in culture medium at 37 C for 24 h. To achieve the equilibrium shape, the initially flat aggregates must round up against the centrifugal force. (After Phillips and Steinberg, 1969.)

****

The adhesive relationships predicted by the Differential Adhesion Hypothesis have thus been confirmed by direct experimental measurement.

The morphogenetic determinants dealt with by the Differential Adhesion Hypothesis are tissue sigmas, sigma representing the <u>reversible</u> work (ergs) required to expand the surface area of a liquid body by a unit amount (cm²) in the course of going from one equilibrium configuration to another in response to a change in the external force field. Such expansions of liquid surfaces are achieved not by stretching surface units (molecules; cells) but by bringing additional units from the interior into the surface. Because this process entails the net breaking of inter-subunit bonds (depicted in Fig. 6), tissue sigmas reflect the intensities of adhesion of internal cells to one another and to extracellular materials to which they may have been adhering.

Is the Differential Adhesion Hypothesis Relevant to Normal Development?

As already noted, the differential Adhesion Hypothesis arose from our experiments designed to clarify the causes of the "self-organizing" behavior of tissues and cells revealed by the work of Holtfreter (13, 47). The design of our experiments required a search for patterns and rules of cell population behavior, and this necessitated combining cells and tissues of a given kind with many others. Other requirements of these experiments imposed additional restrictions upon our choice of experimental cell populations. The result was that the rules we were seeking were indeed clearly revealed, but the cell and tissue combinations

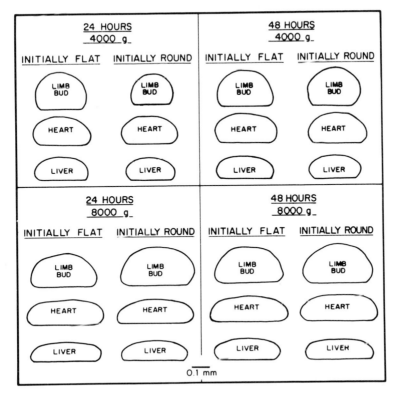

FIG. 5. Profiles of centrifuged aggregates traced from photographs. Each pair was derived from the same kind of primordium. The left-hand member of each pair was initially flat, while the right-hand member was initially round. Upper left: three aggregates spun at 4,000 g for 24h. Upper right: aggregates spun at 4,000 g for 48h. Lower left: aggregates spun at 8,000 g for 24h. Lower right: aggregates spun at 8,000 g for 48h. At the end of each run, the aggregates were fixed in the centrifuge before the speed of the rotor was reduced. (From Phillips and Steinberg, 1969.)

****

employed to reveal them were unavoidably "unnatural." It is not uncommon for the writer to be asked: "What can possibly be the significance of the behavior of heart cells with regard to retina cells?". Or : "What can possibly be revealed about normal morphogenesis by studies of the artificial and unnatural process of sorting-out of contrived cell mixtures?". The answer simply is that all experimentation involves perturbation of a system in order to observe its responses and thereby deduce the rules, and from them the mechanisms, governing its behavior. Holtfreter, together with his student Townes, documented the self-organizing

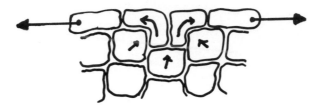

FIG. 6. Illustration of the manner in which applied tension
increases the surface area of a liquid cell aggregate. Cells may
at first be stretched, but originally-subsurface cells continue to
come to the aggregate's surface until the aggregate is again at
shape equilibrium with the forces acting upon it. Because the
surface of a liquid is exposed to anisotropic forces, surface
cells may have a different shape than subsurface cells. (From
Steinberg, 1978b.)

****

behavior in vitro of many "normal" cell and tissue combinations
but fell short of perceiving the rules that were followed and,
therefore, the mechanisms underlying tissue self-organization.
Figure 1, taken from the milestone paper of Townes and Holtfreter
(47), actually depicts cell sorting as proceeding by coalescence
of islands of one cell type in a sea of cells of another kind
(rather than by directed migration toward the aggregate's center)
and the achievement of the same (equilibrium) configuration by
cell sorting and by tissue spreading. Moreover, the tissues used
having been neurula endoderm, neural plate and neural crest
together with some epidermis, the equilibrium configuration
depicted is remarkably embryo-like, with a neural tube surrounded
by neurectodermal mesenchyme and covered by ectoderm; the whole of
this surmounting a belly-like mass of endoderm. This should allay
doubt as to the biological significance of the processes revealed
by such studies, even though these features were not singled out
and interpreted as suggesting any particular mechanism at the
time.

Specific Cell Junctions and Adhesive Specificity

Figure 7 traces the ontogeny of form-regulation by tissue
sigmas from its ultimate structural expression downwards through
two strata of physics to its roots in the chemistry of cell
surface adhesion molecules and their interactions. (The still-
deeper levels descending to the genes await excavation.) Here we
encounter qualitative distinctions for the first time; for the
greater or lesser sigmas of thermodynamics must be resolved into
interactions between molecules at or apposed to cell interfaces;
and these molecules may differ both quantitatively and
qualitatively from cell to cell. They may also differ from region
to region on the surface of a given cell, and it seems a certainty
that they do. Evidence that this is so has been before us for a
long time but has generally been overlooked by investigators of

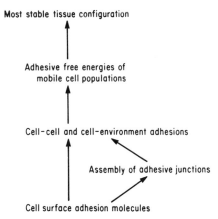

FIG. 7. Causal flow-chart tracing regulation of form by tissue sigmas from the interactions of cell surface adhesion molecules.

****

intercellular adhesion. I am referring to the ultrastructurally differentiated domains characteristic of cell interfaces of so many kinds. There are belt and spot desmosomes, less well organized ahderens junctions, tight junctions, gap junctions, ultrastructurally unexceptional regions of cell apposition and regions that do not support adhesion at all. Except for the last, all of these specialized cell junctions are mirror-symetric structures. Except in early formative stages, one never encounters half-junctions, and mismatched junctions -- for instance, a half-desmosome apposed to a half-gap junction -- have never been reported. (The hemidesmosomes which insert into basal laminae probably have their opposite numbers in the basal lamina itself.) If structure is an expression of chemistry, as of course it must be, this can only mean that the bridging components of each type of association are junction-selective. The number of different kinds of adhesion mechanisms present on a cell must then equal or exceed the number of junctional types that the cell possesses.

Whereas junctional regions of different kinds appear to be exclusive in their associations, comparable junctional regions on cells of different types and even from different vertebrate classes have been shown in certain cases to be capable of interacting [adherens-junctions or desmosomes (1, 2, 18, 19); gap junctions (10)]. In other cases, cells of different types having structurally similar (adherens) junctions seem unable to form these junctions cooperatively (18). A long-extant notion to explain cell sorting has been that adhesions are tissue-specific; that cells recognize "self" through adhesions of a kind unique to each cell type. To bring this concept (17) into accord with the observation that tissues as different as retina, heart, liver and epidermis can all adhere to and spread over one another (e.g., 37) it would be necessary at the very least to postulate that another class of adhesion sites is generally distributed among cells of many kinds. Our view (38, 39) is that the concept of adhesive specificity is generally applicable not at the level of tissues or cells but rather at the level of specific junctions. Cells of different kinds may share certain junctional types but not others and the numbers of junctions of a given type may also differ greatly both among cell types and as a function of the cell's developmental state (e.g., 19, 20). The opportunity therefore exists for precisely the kind of adhesive variation required to produce both the mutual adhesiveness that is so widespread among cells from different vertebrate tissues (and even taxonomic classes) and the adhesive differentials required to cause cells of like construction to group together even as these groups retain their association with groups of another kind. Experiments that support the above view have been reported from two laboratories. Overton (19) coaggregated chick embryonic corneal epithelial and mouse epidermal cells. Desmosome formation by both cell types is developmentally regulated, being faster in older tissue. Desmosomes also form cooperatively between the two cell types. By mixing older corneal cells with younger epidermal cells, mixed aggregates could be produced in which the corneal cells possessed the greater numbers of desmosomes; and by mixing older epidermal cells with younger corneal cells, aggregates were obtained in which the epidermal cells possessed desmosomes in greater abundance. In each case, that cell type with the greater number of desmosomes, whether cornea or epidermis, segregated internally to the other: precisely the behavior expected of the cell type with the greater cohesiveness. Why did the two types of cells, sharing a common adhesion mechanism, not remain randomly intermixed? An answer is suggested by the relative numbers of desmosomes at the three types of intercellular boundary. As we have pointed out earlier (34, 35, 36), two liquid phases become immiscible when heterologous adhesion (a-b) is weaker than the mean of the two kinds of homologous adhesions (a-a and b-b). Overton's counts revealed that in each case the areal frequency of desmosomes joining the heterologous cells was less than the mean of the areal frequencies of desmosomes joining the two kinds of homologous cells. Thus the morphogenetic behavior of the cells in Overton's experiments was exactly that to be expected if the relative intensities of intercellular adhesion at the various intercellular boundaries paralleled the numbers of desmosomes present in each.

This interpretation is strongly supported by experiments of Strickler and Wiseman. These investigators prepared chick embryonic heart cell aggregates and fragments by four different procedures previously shown (23, 50) to increase or decrease both their spreading tendency and their cohesiveness to four different levels. When the areal frequency of desmosomes at the intercellular boundaries was determined, it was found to vary in direct relation to each cell population's spreading tendency [rank in a spreading hierarchy; see (37)] and cohesiveness (40).

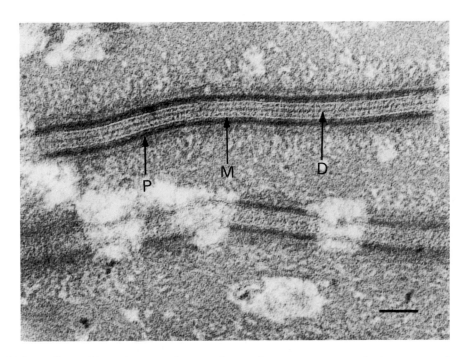

FIG. 8. Structure of <u>macula</u> <u>adherens</u> or spot desmosome in <u>stratum</u> <u>spinosum</u> of bovine muzzle epidermis as seen in transmission electron microscope. <u>D</u>: central lamina of "desmoglea." <u>M</u> (lucent zone): plasma membrane. <u>P</u>: tonofilament-associated plaque on cytoplasmic surface of plasma membrane. X 100,000. Bar = 0.1 m. (From Gorbsky and Steinberg, in preparation.)

****

The Adhesion Components of Spot Desmosomes

The study of intercellular junctions and the search for the molecules mediating intercellular adhesions have until now been separate areas of investigation. Because of the importance of desmosomes as intercellular junctions specialized for adhesion of a particular kind, and in consideration of the earlier isolation of epidermal desmosomes in great quantities (30), we have undertaken to isolate such desmosomes, identify their components and purify the cell-bridging constituents (11). With the latter in hand, we could then investigate their chemical properties, the manner of their assembly, their homologies among desmosomes from various sources and their interactions which produce desmosomally-mediated intercellular adhesion. The structure of desmosomes of the bovine muzzle epidermis is shown in Figure 8. Bundles of tonofilaments containing prekeratins insert into electron-dense cytoplasmic plaques applied to the inner surface of the plasma membrane. Identical plaques are situated directly opposite each

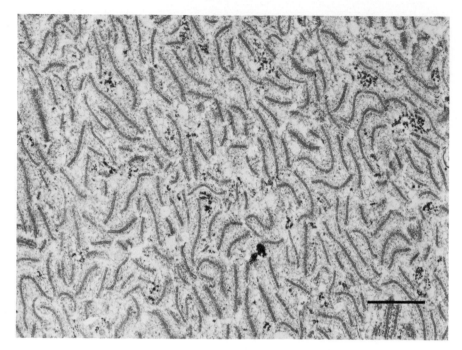

FIG. 9. Desmosomes isolated from bovine muzzle <u>stratum</u> <u>spinosum</u>
by differential centrifugation. Plaques are frayed but intact. X
15,000. bar = 1.0 m. (From Gorbsky and Steinberg,in preparation.)

****

other in adjoining plasma membranes between which is sandwiched an
intercellular material of characteristic appearance. Agitation of
live cell layers of the bovine muzzle <u>stratum</u> <u>spinosum</u> at low pH
in the presence of low concentrations of a detergent dissolves the
tonofilaments and, coupled with sonication, separates the
desmosomes from other constituents and from one another.
Differential centrifugation of the resulting crude homogenate
permits isolation of large numbers of desmosomes with frayed but
apparently intact intracellular plaques and with little
contamination by other materials (Fig. 9). Isopycnic
centrifugation on metrizamide gradients removes most of the plaque
material, leaving purified desmosomal "cores" consisting of the
cell-bridging components and the areas of plasma membrane into
which they insert, together with some residual cytoplasmic
filamentous material (Fig. 10). From twenty muzzles (12-15 grams
of <u>stratum</u> <u>spinosum</u>), about 15-20 mg of such purified desmosomal
cores are obtained. SDS-polyacrylamide gel electrophoresis of
whole desmosomes reveals at least 15 prominent protein bands
(Fig. 11; see also 31). Purified desmosomal cores are greatly
enriched in three closely spaced protein bands of MW ca 155,000,

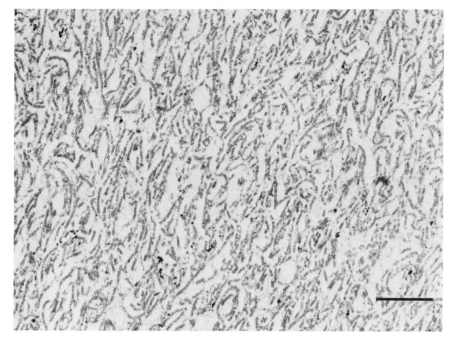

FIG. 10. Purified desmosomal "cores" isolated by isopycnic centrifugation on a metrizamide gradient. Plaque material is largely removed, leaving mainly cell-bridging components and the areas of plasma membrane into which they insert. X 15,000. Bar = 1.0 m. (From Gorbsky and Steinberg, in preparation.)

****

in two broad bands at 115,000 and 100,000, and in a 22,000 MW component, all of which we have called "desmogleins" for their probable function as the principle constituents of the "desmoglea" or intercellular "glue" of the desmosomes. Treatment of gels with periodic acid-dansyl hydrazine, which renders glycoproteins fluorescent (8), labels only the desmogleins and not the other proteins present in whole desmosomes (Fig. 11). These non-glycosylated bands are significantly reduced in gels of desmosomal cores. The desmogleins probably form the intercellular cross-bridges observed in desmosomes by several authors. Their isolation in milligram quantities and the preparation of specific affinity probes directed against them (in preparation, in collaboration with my students and associates Gary Gorbsky, Hisato Shida, Mariko Shida and Stephen Cohen), represent the first steps in our investigation of their contribution to both desmosomal and multicellular assembly.

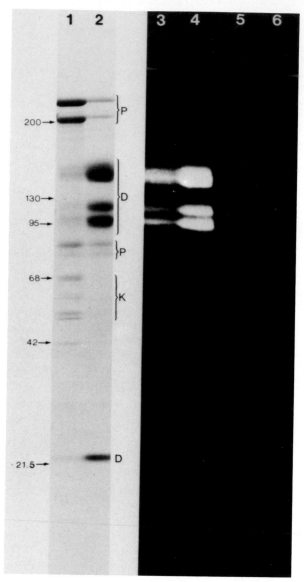

FIG. 11. Lanes 1 and 2: Coomassie Blue stained desmosome preparations in 5-20% polyacrylamide gradient gels loaded with 25 μg of protein per well. Lane 1: whole desmosomes, lane 2: desmosomal cores. (P) plaque-associated bands, (D) desmogleins, (K) prekeratins. Lanes 3-6: periodic acid-dansyl hydrazine staining for carbohydrate in 5-17% polyacrylamide gradient gels. Only the desmogleins are labelled. In lanes 5 and 6, periodate treatment was omitted. Lanes 3 and 5: whole desmosomes; lanes 4 and 6: desmosomal cores. (From Gorbsky and Steinberg, in preparation.)

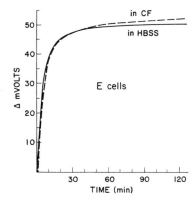

FIG. 12. Aggregometer tracings showing aggregation of 7-day chick embryonic neural retina cells dissociated in EGTA (E cells). <u>HBSS</u>: Hanks' balanced salt solution; <u>CF</u>: calcium-free Hanks' solution. E cell aggregation is Ca^{++}-independent. (From Magnani et <u>al</u>., in press.)

****

<u>Dual Adhesion Mechanisms Shared by Neural Retinal and Optic Tectal Cells</u>

Reference has already been made to the great likelihood that cells of many kinds possess multiple adhesion mechanisms. Multiple adhesion mechanisms have been demonstrated in <u>Dictyostelium</u> <u>discoideum</u> amoebae (4), in vertebrate cells of several kinds (41, 48, 49) and chick embryonic neural retina cells (15, 16, 42, 43, 44, 46). In the latter case it has been possible to dissect the cell surface enzymatically to remove either of the individual adhesion mechanisms, permitting investigation of the behavior and interaction of cells possessing the two mechanisms in various combinations.

The aggregative behavior of neural retina cells dissociated mechanically after treatment with the Ca^{++} - chelator EGTA is shown in Fig. 12. Aggregation is here monitored through the use of our 12-channel, automatic-recording aggregometer (45), which records the decrease in small-angle light scattering that accompanies the aggregation of cells in as many as twelve stirred suspensions simultaneously. Aggregation proceeds at the same rate in the presence or absence of Ca^{++}, indicating the activity of an adhesion mechanism that is Ca^{++} - independent. When retinas are dissociated by trypsin in the presence of Ca^{++}, their subsequent aggregation is very different. It now depends entirely upon the presence of Ca^{++} (Fig. 13), the cells being unable to adhere in the absence of this ion until new Ca^{++} - independent adhesion molecules are synthesized and exported to the cell surface, starting at about 30 minutes of incubation (15; Magnani, Thomas and Steinberg ,in preparation).

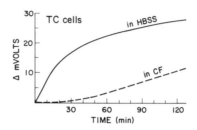

FIG. 13. As in Fig. 12, but cells dissociated with trypsin + Ca⁺⁺ (TC cells). TC cell aggregation is Ca⁺⁺-dependent until the second, Ca⁺⁺-independent adhesion system begins to be restored to the cell surfaces after 20-40 minutes of incubation at 37 C. (From Magnani et al., in press.)

****

The Ca⁺⁺ - independent (CI) and Ca⁺⁺ - dependent (CD) aggregation properties of retinal cells prepared in these two ways are shown to be due to immunologically distinct components by experiments in which antibodies were raised against neural retina cells prepared either with or without the use of trypsin. IgG's from the various antisera were cleaved to make univalent Fab fragments and these were tested for their ability to inhibit the CI and CD adhesion systems. One Fab was obtained which inhibited CI but not CD adhesion, while a different Fab acted in precisely the opposite manner (43, 46). Immunoabsorption and other experiments show that cell trypsinization in the presence of Ca⁺⁺ removes the CI adhesion system and simultaneously activates the CD adhesion system, the latter being present but inefficient until it is proteolytically activated (46). The functional specificity of these two adhesion systems has been demonstrated in reciprocal combinations of retinal cells from which one or the other system has been removed (42, 44). The two cell populations showed a limited ability to cross-adhere in the former experiments (42), but almost no cross-adhesion in the latter ones (44;Fig. 14), probably due to more complete removal of one or the other adhesion mechanism in the second instance. Thus the CI and CD adhesion mechanisms of neural retina cells do not "recognize" one another.

What is the significance of the presence of multiple adhesion mechanisms in a single cell? Why would not a single adhesion mechanism suffice? To a certain extent, multiple adhesion systems may be an unavoidable consequence of the presence of surface molecules with a different primary function. Gap junctions, for example, are widely considered to function in the transmission of small molecules from cell to cell. In order to prevent ion leakage and consequent cell death, the channels must be sealed

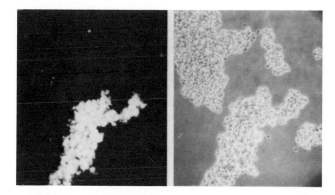

FIG. 14. Paired fluorescence and phase contrast photographs of aggregates formed from a mixture of retinal cells prepared in two ways. The Ca^{++}-independent adhesion system was removed from one subpopulation of cells (FITC-labelled), while the Ca^{++}-dependent adhesion system was removed from the other subpopulation (unlabelled). Both photographs show the same microscopic field. The retinal cells prepared in these two ways aggregate separately, showing the lack of "recognition" of one adhesion system by the other. (From Thomas et al., in press.)

****

against the extracellular medium. This means that gap junctions must constitute a tight physical structure connecting plasma membranes, and this in turn necessitates that gap junctions be regions of intercellular adhesion. Since the function of gap junctions requires that junctional components on one cell "match up" with those on its neighbors, the association between them is certain to be preferential or selective at the molecular level. And since most vertebrate cells can form communicating (presumably gap) junctions with most others, adhesion due to gap junctions is equally certain to be non-selective at the tissue or cell level. In cells with many, large gap junctions, such as lens fiber cells, it is likely that they make a major contribution to intercellular adhesion. In general, however, the fraction of intercellular adhesive energy that is due to gap junctions or indeed to any particular mechanism of adhesion is unknown.

A second reason for the existence of multiple adhesion mechanisms in a single cell must be to produce specific cell orientation. An exocrine cell, for example, must be so oriented that its secretory surface faces the space into which its product must pass. Muscle cells must be properly aligned to transmit tensions. Ciliated cells must not only direct their ciliated surfaces "outward" but must be so oriented that they beat in the correct direction; and so forth. It seems reasonable to suggest that these orientations are achieved, at least in part, through the utilization of different adhesion systems at different points

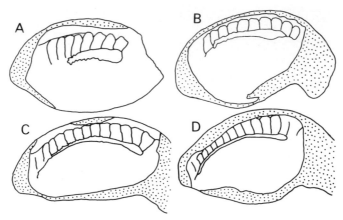

FIG. 15. Tracings of scanning electron micrographs of four
<u>Ambysoma mexicanum</u> embryos from which the epidermis on the right
side was removed after fixation, showing the tailwards extension
of the pronephric duct just ventral to the developing somites.
(From Poole and Steinberg, 1977.)

****

-- for example one system for adhesion to a basal lamina, another
for lateral adhesion to neighboring cells and perhaps a non-
adhesive surface to abut (or even to determine) cell-free space
(36).

A third reason for multiple adhesion mechanisms in a single
cell may be particularly cogent in cells of the nervous system,
such as retinal cells, for here more than anywhere else it is
necessary to arrange cells and to specify their contacts with
precision. The retina must be mapped precisely upon the optic
tectum of the brain. It has been suggested that systems of graded
adhesiveness of retina to optic tectum may provide or at least
contribute to the coordinate systems that orient one to the other
(3, 5). To map one plane onto another in this manner, at least
two independent coordinate systems or axes must be specified. It
is, therefore, interesting that two non-interacting adhesion
systems have been found in the chick retina. If they should play
a role in the matching of retina to tectum, the tectum would have
to share these adhesion mechanisms. We have, therefore,
investigated this question and found that these two retinal
adhesion mechanisms are indeed shared by the optic tectum but not
by certain other embryonic tissues (Thomas, Edelman and Steinberg,
in preparation). The actual significance of this finding remains
to be explored.

Adhesive Guidance of Pronephric Duct Migration

The goal of our studies has always been to understand how cell
and tissue rearrangements are controlled in normal development.

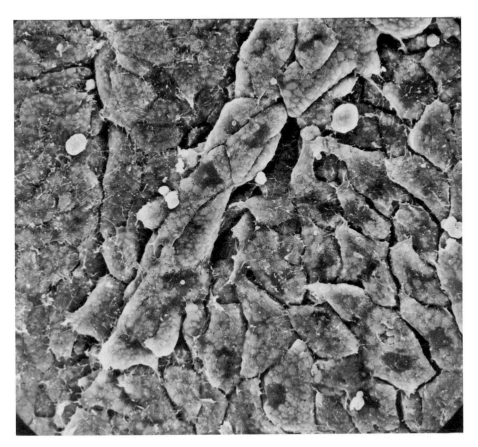

FIG. 16. Posterior quarter of Schreckenberg and Jacobson stage 29
A. mexicanum pronephric duct, showing craniocaudally elongated
cells of the migrating duct tip adhering to both somites (above)
and lateral mesoderm (below) by cell processes. (Courtesy of
Thomas Poole.)

****

This has been a difficult matter to confront because of a variety
of technical obstacles to progress. In the last few years,
however, we (24, 25, 26, 27, 28) have been investigating the
extension of the vertebrate pronephric duct and have found this to
be not only amenable to experimental approaches but a rich source
of clues to morphogenetic control mechanisms.
    The Ambystoma pronephric duct rudiment segregates from the
lateral mesoderm just ventral to the anterior somites and then
extends caudally along the ventrolateral margins of the segmenting
somites, eventually fusing with the cloacal wall (24, 26, 27;
Fig. 15). During all this time it is readily accessible both to
observation by scanning electron microscopy and to surgical

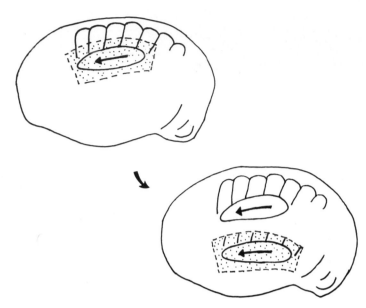

FIG. 17. Operation diagram showing the transplantation of a second pronephric duct primordium from a donor embryo to the right flank of a host of the same stage. The transplant is here placed in normal orientation ventral to but at the same craniocaudal level as the host duct primordium. (From Poole and Steinberg, in preparation.)

✳✳✳✳✳✳✳✳✳✳✳✳✳✳✳✳✳✳✳✳✳✳✳✳

manipulation. The thinning of the duct as it elongates, the reduction in the number of cells across its diameter, the shapes of cells in its different regions, and the spreading and caudal extension of vital dye marks placed within it all make it apparent that the <u>Ambystoma</u> duct extends tailward by the active locomotion of cells near its tip (26, 27; Fig. 16). The more proximal (anterior) cells rearrange by cell slippage (rather than cell stretching) to accommodate this increase in the duct's length.

Since the duct tip in its caudad excursion keeps strictly to the boundary between the lateral mesoderm and the forming somites, one might have supposed that zone to be uniquely able to support duct migration. Earlier observations of Holtfreter (14) and transplantations of extra duct tips to a more ventral position on the flank (26, 28) have eliminated this possibility. Following the operation sketched in Fig. 17, the tip of the transplanted duct migrates dorsocaudally across the foreign mesodermal terrain. In doing so, it is not "contact-guided" by the edges of the elongated somatic mesoderm cells that constitute its substratum. (It hardly adheres to the overlying ectoderm.) Rahter, it migrates at an angle to the mesoderm's "grain." Nor is the duct attracted by some distant summons from dorsal or caudal tissues,

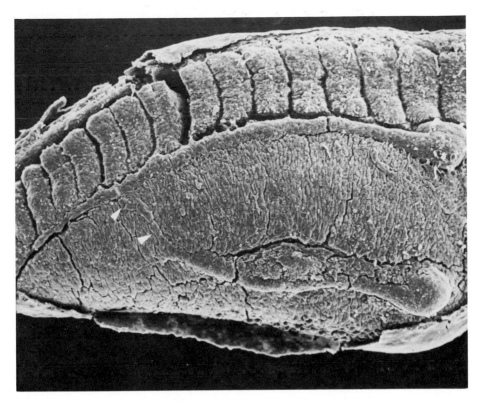

FIG. 18. Consequences of the operation diagrammed in Fig. 17. The tip of the secondary pronephric duct primordium has streamed dorsocaudally (arrows) across the host's flank mesoderm to merge with the host's migrating pronephric duct.

****

for its migration proceeds even after these have been removed (26, 28). The information guiding the duct's migration must, therefore, be local. When the tip of a transplanted duct encounters the primary duct, the two merge in the manner of two streams converging to form a river and flow toward the cloaca as one (Fig. 18). This demonstrates the miscibility of duct with duct in contrast with the immiscibility of duct with somatic mesoderm or somite, clearly indicating the relevance of tissue miscibility/immiscibility relationships in specifying tissue boundaries within the embryo. If the primary duct has been blocked, however, a new point emerges. When the transplanted duct's tip encounters the absent primary duct's path, it turns sharply caudad -- never cephalad -- and proceeds in the normal manner toward the cloaca. This is the case even when the duct tip strikes the duct path at an angle of 90°. Moreover, duct tips transplanted to aim cephalad rather than caudad will not migrate, nor will they migrate ventrad except to skirt a mechanical barrier or hug a protruding tissue edge. Thus the information guiding the pronephric duct's migration must be not only local and oriented; it must be polarized as well.

It is noteworthy that normal duct extension proceeds in precise synchrony with the separating-off of new somites, the duct tip pursuing the last-formed intersomitic furrow at a distance of about two somite lengths. In the transplants which gave good migration, like that depicted in Figure 18, the primary and secondary duct tips were always aligned at the same transverse level. When the graft was shifted a distance of some four somite lengths anterior to the primary duct tip, little migration occurred. By varying the stages of host and donor and the anteroposterior level of graft implantation, it was discovered that the capacity of the flank mesoderm to support pronephric duct tip migration itself moves caudad as a wave. This wave is exactly coordinated with the anteroposterior wave of differentiation as expressed in somite formation.

These and other grafting results involving flank mesoderm grafts, rotations, etc. have led us to conclude that the Ambystoma pronephric duct tip proceeds caudad following the slope of a developmentally regulated adhesion gradient. This gradient -- the posterior end being of higher and the anterior end of lower adhesiveness -- itself progresses caudad as a wave travelling at the rate of developmental advance. At any given moment, filopodial extensions of the cells of the duct's tip, which must constantly make and break adhesions to the substratum, will be more apt to break the weaker (more anterior) adhesions and establish stronger (more posterior) ones. As the wave progresses, these stronger adhesions themselves weaken, and the exchange process is repeated. In embryos transected while the the wave is in the anterior half, it appears on schedule (as do somites) in the posterior half. The wave is, therefore, not propagated caudad like a wave in water, but is rather kinematic, representing the expression of a series of intracellular clocks or timers set earlier to "go off" in anteroposterior succession. Migration of cells up an artificial adhesion gradient has earlier been demonstrated in vitro (termed haptotaxis by Carter, 6; see also 12).

It is interesting to consider our results in connection with recent work on the mechanisms of somite formation, with which pronephric duct extension is so closely linked. Cooke and Zeeman (7) have proposed a clock and wavefront model for the control of somite formation. According to this model: "The wavefront is a front of rapid cell change moving slowly down the long axis of the embryo; cells enter a phase of rapid alteration in locomotory and/ or adhesive properties at successively later times according to anterior-posterior body position". Elsdale et al. (9, 21) demonstrated, by serial administration of heat shocks, the existence of precisely such a wave involved in predetermining somite formation and established that this earlier wave is not propagated but kinematic. Thier conclusions and ours, even though they are based upon entirely different bodies of experimental data, agree completely.

In summary, there exists a substantial and growing body of evidence that developmentally regulated adhesion mechanisms play a central role in the control of multicellular assembly during development. In particular, the kinds of adhesion systems present, the quantities in which these molecules are produced and the domains of the cell surfaces in which they are displayed will act as a set of morphogenetic determinants -- a morphogenetic code (36). When cells come together in groups, their spontaneous locomotory activity -- the counterpart of Brownian motion in an ordinary liquid -- provides constant adhesive alternatives which are chosen between on a simple thermodynamic basis. Thus the kinds of cells that are present determine the structure that will emerge. A striking feature of this mode of structure-determination is that the rules of construction specify the end-structure itself and not any particular pathway of morphogenesis by which it is to be achieved. It is through appreciation of this fact that the goal-directedness referred to at the outset -- the ability of organized, multicellular systems to compensate after perturbation and restore themselves to normal organization -- can be understood.

ACKNOWLEDGEMENTS

The research from my laboratory discussed in this article has been carried out with the excellent technical assistance of Mr. Edward Kennedy, Mrs. Doris White and Ms. Dorothy Spero. Our recent studies have been supported by research grants nos. CA 13605 and GM 26047 and training grants nos. CA 09167 and GM 07312 from the National Cancer Institute and the National Institute of General Medical Sciences, DHEW. We have also benefitted from the central equipment facilities in the Biology Department, Princeton University, supported by the Whitehall Foundation. Gary Gorbsky was the recipient of a predoctoral fellowship from the National Science Foundation.

REFERENCES

1. Armstrong, P. B. (1970): J. Cell Biol., 47:197-210.
2. Armstrong, P. B. (1971): Wilh. Roux Arch., 168:125-141.
3. Barbera, A. J., R. B. Marchase, and S. Roth (1973): Proc. Nat. Acad. Sci. U.S., 70:2482-2486.
4. Beug, H., F. E. Katz ,and G. Gerisch (1973): J. Cell Biol., 56:647-658.
5. Cafferata, R., J. Panosian ,and G. Bordley (1979): Devel. Biol., 69:108-117.
6. Carter, S. B. (1967): Nature, 213:256-264.
7. Cooke, J. and E. C. Zeeman (1976): J. Theor. Biol., 58:455-476.

8,   Eckhardt, A. E., C. E. Hayes,and I. J. Goldstein (1976):
     Anal. Biochem., 73:192-197.
9.   Elsdale, T., M. Pearson,and M. Whitehead (1976): J. Embryol.
     Exp. Morph., 35:625-635.
10. Epstein, M. C. and N. B. Gilula (1977):   J. Cell Biol.,
     75:769-787.
11. Gorbsky, G. and M. S. Steinberg , in preparation.
12. Harris, A. (1973): Exp. Cell Res., 77:285-297.
13. Holtfreter, J. (1939):   Arch. fur Exp. Zellforsch.,
     23:169-209.
14. Holtfreter, J. (1944): Rev. Can. Biol., 3:220-250.
15. Magnani, J. L. (1979): Ph.D. thesis, Princetan University.
16. Magnani, J. L., W. A. Thomas ,and M. S. Steinberg (1980):
     Devel. Biol., (in press).
17. Moscona, A. A. (1968): Devel. Biol., 18:250-277.
18. Overton, J. (1974): Prog. Surf. Sci., 8:161-208.
19. Overton, J. (1977a): J. Theor. Biol., 65:787-790.
20. Overton, J. (1977b): Devel. Biol., 55:103-116.
21. Pearson, M. and T. Elsdale (1979): J. Embryol. Exp. Morph.,
     51:27-50.
22. Phillips, H. M. and M. S. Steinberg (1969): Proc. Nat. Acad.
     Sci. U.S.A., 64:121-127.
23. Phillips, H. M., L. L. Wiseman,and M. S. Steinberg (1977):
     Devel. Biol., 59:150-159.
24. Poole, T. J. and M. S. Steinberg (1977): In: Scanning
     Electron Microscopy/1977 Vol. II, edited by O. Johari,
     pp. 43-52, ITT Research Institute, Chicago.
25. Poole, T. J. and M. S. Steinberg (1978): J. Cell Biol.,
     79:337a.
26. Poole, T. J. (1980): Ph.D. dissertation, Princeton
     University, Princeton, N.J.
27. Poole, T. J. and M. S. Steinberg (1980a): J. Embryol. Exp.
     Morph., (submitted for publication).
28. Poole, T. J. and M. S. Steinberg (1980b): Devel. Biol.,
     (submitted for publication).
29. Rand, H. W. (1915): Wilh. Roux Arch., 41:159-214.
30. Skerrow, C. J. and A. G. Matoltsy (1974a): J. Cell Biol.,
     63:515-523.
31. Skerrow, C. J. and A. G. Matoltsy (1974b): J. Cell Biol.,
     63:524-530.
32. Steinberg, M. S. (1962a): Proc. Nat. Acad. Sci. U.S.,
     48:1577-1582.
33. Steinberg, M. S. (1962b): Science, 137:762-763.
34. Steinberg, M. S. (1962c): Proc. Nat. Acad. Sci. U.S.,
     48:1769-1776.
35. Steinberg, M. S. (1963): Science, 141:401-408.
36. Steinberg, M. S. (1964): In: Cellular Membranes in
     Development, edited by M. Locke, pp. 321-366. Academic Press,
     New York.
37. Steinberg, M. S. (1970): J. Exp. Zool., 173:395-343.

38. Steinberg, M. S. (1978a): In: Specificity of Embryological Interactions, edited by D. R. Garrod, pp. 97-130. John Wiley and Sons, New York.
39. Steinberg, M. S. (1978b): In: Cell-Cell Recognition, edited by A. S. G. Curtis, pp. 25-49. Cambridge University Press, New York.
40. Strickler, J. and L. L. Wiseman (1978): J. Cell Biol., 79:39a.
41. Takeichi, M. (1977): J. Cell Biol., 75:464-474.
42. Takeichi, M., H. S. Ozaki, K. Tokumaga ,and T. S. Okada (1979): Devel. Biol., 70:195-205.
43. Thomas, W. A. (1979): Ph.D. thesis, Princeton University.
44. Thomas, W. A., J. Thomson, J. L. Magnani, and M. S. Steinberg: Devel. Biol., (in press).
45. Thomas, W. A. and M. S. Steinberg (1980a): J. Cell Sci., 41:1-18.
46. Thomas, W. A. and M. S. Steinberg (1980b): Devel. Biol., (in press).
47. Townes, P. L. and J. Holtfreter (1955): J. Exp. Zool., 128:53-120.
48. Ueda, M. J. and M. Takeichi (1976): Cell Struct. Funct., 1:377-388.
49. Underhill, C. and A. Dorfman (1978): Exp. Cell Res., 117:155-164.
50. Wiseman, L. L., M. S. Steinberg, and H. M. Phillips (1972): Devel. Biol., 28:498-517.

Morphogenesis and Pattern Formation,
edited by T. G. Connelly et al.,
Raven Press, New York © 1981

The Genetic Basis of Pattern Formation: Systems of Genetically Caused Abnormal Morphogenesis

Salome Gluecksohn-Waelsch

Department of Genetics, Albert Einstein College of Medicine, Bronx, New York 10461

The program of this afternoon's session poses two questions: one refers to the contributions which the understanding of normal morphogenesis may make to an analysis of abnormal development. The second question, the converse of the first, inquires about clues to normal developmental mechanisms that may be obtained from analytical studies of abnormal development. It is my belief that in general the latter approach has proven to be particularly productive, as evidenced, for example, by the many contributions which studies of pathology have made to knowledge of physiology. Even closer to my own concerns are the insights obtained through the study of mutant gene effects which have helped the identification of normal metabolic pathways. This is exemplified particularly well in the work of Ephrussi, Beadle and Tatum, who used an "aggressive pursuit of mutations as tools for the dissection of biochemical pathways and their genetic control" in the words of Lederberg (13).

In the causal analysis of mechanisms of morphogenesis and their genetic control, developmental abnormalities due to the action of abnormal genomes have played a decisive role ever since Boveri's ingenious work provided definitive proof that in the sea urchin normal development depended on the qualitatively distinct action of each individual chromosome. In his experimental system Boveri made use of polyspermy and the resulting dispermic eggs with developmental abnormalities which he interpreted by subjecting them to causal analysis.

In higher vertebrates, the most outstanding characteristics of causal mechanisms of development are interactions and interdependencies of cells, tissues and organs. These were revealed by the exciting transplantation experiments and their interpretations on the part of experimental embryologists in the

first third of this century. The picture of a well defined
pattern of epigenetic development unfolding in sequential order
emerged but the role played by genes in the responsible
developmental mechanisms remained largely unknown. Potential
clues in this direction may be derived from analytical studies of
gene mutations which interfere with the orderly normal patterns of
vertebrate development and differentiation. In this way, specific
sequences of developmental pathways as well as interactions and
interrelations of developmental processes may be exposed, making
possible the identification of cellular and molecular processes
operative in embryogeny, as well as the analysis of the relevant
genetic control. Some examples will serve to illustrate this
point.

Pleiotropic Patterns of Gene Action

In vertebrates, as in other high eukaryotes, a characteristic
phenomenon of gene action is its pleiotropic nature. This term
refers to the fact that multiple targets appear to be under the
control of a single gene inherited in simple Mendelian fashion.
Examples for pleiotropic gene action are manifold; I shall cite
several from the literature of developmental genetics of the
mouse, my favorite experimental object. Various mutations have
been shown to affect differentiation of red blood cells. Two
allelic series in particular were studied in great detail (15),
that of the W-alleles and that of the Steel-alleles, the two of
them mapping on different chromosomes. In both cases, the
differentiation of germ cells and of pigment cells was regularly
affected in addition to that of the red blood cells. From the
developmental point of view, this indicated that the three tissue
systems - blood cells, germ cells, pigment cells - might have a
common developmental denominator which in turn was under the
control of the particular mutant alleles under study. Thus, the
pattern of genetically caused abnormalities demonstrated a normal
developmental interrelationship between three quite different
tissue systems, and exposed it to further analysis. The
literature of mouse developmental genetics includes many examples
where mutational analysis revealed a connection between developing
systems previously thought to be distinct.

Gene Effects on Specific Differentiation Patterns

In many cases abnormalities caused by mutational systems in the
mouse serve to reflect the respective normal patterns of
morphogenesis. An illustration of this is provided by a recessive
mutation (mdg) which affects differentiation of striated voluntary
muscle only. Whereas all striated skeletal muscle cells of
homozygous mutants are affected early in embryogenesis and fail to
differentiate, heart muscle cells and those of involuntary muscle
differentiate perfectly normally. Thus, the unique character of
the striated skeletal muscle cell and of its pattern of

differentiation is underscored by the specificity and the pattern of the mutational effect.

The genetic control of pattern formation during development was studied and discussed extensively many years ago by Stern (17) who focussed his attention on the pattern of bristles in Drosophila. In the mouse, abnormalities of the extremities caused by a recessive mutation, phocomelic, were traced back to a consistently abnormal pattern of mesenchymal cell aggregation in earliest stages of limb bud differentiation in the embryo. It seems that this mutation interferes with the aggregation pattern of mesenchymal cells, possibly by affecting cell surface properties (5).

Temporal Patterns of Development

Abnormal patterns of development involve dimensions not only of space but also of time. A developmental analysis carried out many years ago of a semi-dominant mutation in the mouse causing the congenital absence of kidneys in mutant homozygotes suggested that the observed failure of nephrogenesis was due to a shift in the temporal pattern of differentiation of the two kidney components, i.e., the ureteric bud and the metanephrogenic mesenchyme. In normal development, these two primordia grow until they are close together and able to interact in order to induce each other's differentiation. In the mutants, there is a failure of the essential synchronization of growth of the two elements to provide the basis for mutual inductive interaction; subsequently, tubular and glomerular differentiation fails to occur. An experimental system in which the two elements, i.e., ureteric bud and nephrogenic mesenchyme, were brought together and grown under organ culture conditions, overcame the disturbances of temporal relationships and resulted in normal differentiation of kidney tubules and secretory elements (7). The experimental analysis of this model system thus revealed the essential role of a specific temporal pattern in differentiation and its genetic control.

The T-complex in the Mouse

Cell interactions, their genetic control, and the mechanisms by which these operate, have been the focus of studies of developmental genetics for many years. Among the most famous and intriguing systems in this connection is the T-complex in the mouse. As long as about 50 years ago mutations at this locus seemed to offer a potential for the demonstration of inductive interactions and their role in the development of the mammalian nervous system. Chesley (2) interpreted the observed deficiency of the notochord-mesoderm material in homozygous mutant T/T embryos as being responsible for the failure of neural induction of the overlying undifferentiated ectoderm and consequently for the abnormal nervous system in these mutant embryos. This reasoning was based on an analogy with the results of experimentally produced lesions in amphibian systems as described in the work of Spemann and his school (16).

In the years since, the puzzle of the interference of mutations within the T-complex with differentiation has been pursued by various laboratories, including our own.   Mechanisms of effects have been proposed and discounted, and to this day the modes of action of mutant or wild type genes in the T-complex still remain to be identified. There is no doubt that this complex represents an outstanding example of a genetic system exerting regulatory control on differentiation.   About 10 years ago, Erickson and I (8) proposed that the abnormalities of development in embryos homozygous for lethal mutations at and near the T-locus involved defects in processes including cell to cell recognition and interaction as well as morphogenetic movements, all of them essential and significant events in the development of higher vertebrates.   This resulted in our suggestion that T-locus products might be located at the cell surface, interfering when mutant, with normal mechanisms of cell interactions. Since that time different laboratories have devoted much work to attempts of achieving identification of such cell surface molecules, but considerable controversy continues to surround the results and their interpretations. On the basis of immunological studies, it was postulated that antigens specific for the recessive mutations at the T-locus were present on the surfaces of sperm, testicular cells and embryos (19). However, convincing evidence was recently presented that argues against the existence of t-allele determined antigens on spermatozoa (4, 10) and there are experimental indications of possible metabolic abnormalities expressed by t- carrying sperm (12). At this time it appears that in spite of strong theoretical arguments indicating the possible existence of T-complex coded or controlled cell surface molecules, their actual identification has not been achieved. Without question, the T- complex is a prime example of a genetic system intimately involved in the regulation and control of a pattern of early morphogenesis. This pattern concerns the notochord-mesoderm cells of the early embryo and their specific and essential inductive interaction with the overlying ectoderm in the course of differentiation of the nervous system. Identification of possibly abnormal gene products would contribute to the analysis of normal, i.e., wild type gene products in the T-complex region possibly located at the cell surface and instrumental in the pattern of normal morphogenesis.

Regulation of Tissue Specific Patterns of Differentiation

The final system of genetically caused abnormal morphogenesis that I would like to discuss in this symposium is that of lethal deletions at and around the albino locus in the mouse which appear to reveal the existence of regulatory genes concerned with specific patterns of differentiation. Work on this system began about 13 years ago when Erickson and I puzzled over the cause of death of certain homozygous albino newborns (3).   The relevant lethal albino mutations were products of studies of X-ray mutagenesis at Oak Ridge in this country and Harwell in England; later they turned out to be not point mutations but overlapping chromosomal deletions at and around the albino locus in chromosome 7 of the mouse (11, 14). At the time, Erickson was impressed by the similarity of clinical symptoms between these lethal albino newborn mice and hypoglycaemic newborn babies, an observation responsible for much of the subsequent experimental analysis of this system. The effects of lethal albino deletions on morphogenesis and biochemical differentiation have been the object of an extensive recent review (6), and I shall restrict myself here to the discussion of those aspects of this genetic system which I consider to have particular relevance to the main topics of this symposium.

In the course of the past 13 years a plethora of biochemical and morphogenetic abnormalities has been described in feLuses and newborns homozygous for certain of the lethal albino deletions. The pattern of these abnormalities appears strictly determined: on the biochemical level, deficiencies of five enzymes pertain exclusively to those specific for liver and kidney, primarily glucose-6-phosphatase, tyrosine aminotransferase and serine dehydratase. However, the majority of liver specific enzymes have perfectly normal activities. Synthesis of certain liver proteins is affected also, but deficiencies are restricted to particular proteins, i.e., albumin, α-fetoprotein and transferrin, while the general protein synthesizing machinery remains normal. Thus, 3 specific plasma proteins are added to the list of 5 specific liver enzymes as targets of the biochemical effects of the lethal albino deletions.

This pattern of biochemical defect is reflected on the level of morphogenesis. Electron microscope studies revealed ultrastructural defects of specific subcellular compartments, i.e., the microsomal membranes, the Golgi apparatus and the nuclear membrane. Thus, within a particular liver cell, these subcellular structures are severly affected only in the homozygous mutants whereas all other cellular membranes remain perfectly normal. These latter include mitochondia, peroxisomes and the plasma membrane (18). In addition to this specific pattern of intracellular effects, the lethal albino deletions cause an equally distinct intercellular pattern of abnormalities. Only liver and kidney cells show ultrastructural defects whereas all other cell types have perfectly normal rough endoplasmic reticulum, Golgi apparatus and nuclear membranes. These include intestinal cells, islets of Langerhans, exocrine cells of the pancreas, adrenal cortical cells and thymus. Therefore, it appears that subcellular structures, e.g., microsomal membranes, Golgi apparatus and nuclear membrane, which might be assumed to be analogous in different cell types, are actually not identical. Their specific susceptibility to mutant effects in liver or kidney cells of homozygotes suggests that similar appearing membranous structures of cells of different cell types may differ on the

molecular level and that a Golgi apparatus of a pancreatic cell is
an entity different from that of a liver cell. The specific
pattern of ultrastructural abnormalities in the lethal albino
homozygotes brings to light a new aspect of ultrastructural cell
differentiation, i.e., that of molecularly distinct species of
subcellular membranes which might be assumed to play a causal role
in cellular differentiation.

An interesting feature of the ultrastructural differentiation
of liver cells of lethal albino homozygotes is the pattern of
appearance of subcellular abnormalities in successive fetal
stages. At 18 days of fetal life only a few scattered abnormal
liver cells among a majority of normal cells are found in the
mutants. Within an abnormal cell the abnormalities are identical
in quality and extent to those of newborn mutant liver cells. At
19 days, a striking increase in the number of abnormal cells is
observed, and at birth all liver parenchymal cells of mutants
express the abnormality (18). During fetal development of mutant
homozygotes the progressive increase in numbers of abnormal cells
rather than degree of abnormalities within a cell, is paralleled
by the developmental pattern of glucose-6-phosphatase activity in
the normal fetal liver. Here also, an increasing number of cells
expressing glucose-6-phosphatase activity rather than an increase
of enzyme activity per cell accompanies differentiation of the
liver specific enzyme (13a). This parallelism raises the question
of the possible causal role of glucose-6-phosphatase in
subcellular membrane differentiation of the normal liver.

In the context of the present discussion of problems of pattern
formation and its genetic control in morphogenesis one particular
experiment carried out with the lethal albino deletions appears to
be relevant. As mentioned before, several of the albino deletions
cause perinatal death of homozygotes. It proved possible to
rescue such homozygotes and render them viable by a process of
chromosomal engineering which makes use of a chemically induced
insertion translocation between chromosome 7, on which the albino
locus maps, and the X-chromosome. This insertion includes the
wild type alleles of genes deleted in the lethal albinos and known
to be essential for survival. A female can be "constructed" with
homozygous deletions of the relevant genome at and around the
albino locus in chromosome 7 but with a stretch of 21 cM, derived
from chromosome 7 and including the respective wild type alleles,
inserted in one of its X-chromosomes. Such females turned out to
be viable in the case of four perinatal lethals tested (9). Their
chromosomal types include three instead of the normal two
representative regions at and around the albino locus, i.e., they
are trisomic for this region. Genotypically, they carry one dose
of wild type alleles inserted into one of their X-chromosomes and
two doses of deletions in their chromosomes 7. The one dose of
wild type alleles complements the homozygous deletions and is
responsible for the females' survival.

The mechanism of survival raises interesting questions since it
is known that in any one cell of a female mammal one X-chromosome

only is active, the other having been inactivated in the course of development. Thus, any female heterozygous for a mutation mapping on the X-chromosome includes a mosaic of cells in which either one or the other X-chromosome was inactivated at random, leaving only one functional X-chromosome expressing either the mutant or the wild type allele. In the case of the females carrying Cattanach's translocation, the mosaic pattern is made up of those cells in which the ordinary X-chromosome is active and those in which the translocation carrying X-chromosome, including the wild type alleles of the deletions, is active. Only in the latter cell type are the deletions complemented; the former cell type is homozygous mutant and deficient. Nevertheless, all such females survive, as evidenced by breeding data, and liver enzyme activities are perfectly normal and uniform throughout the liver. Thus, the newborn liver of these females fails to express the mosaic pattern of liver cells expected on the basis of X-inactivation.

There exist two possibilities to account for this: cell selection at the time of differentiation in fetal stages might favor growth of those cells in which a translocation carrying X-chromosome, complementing the deletions, is active. Alternatively, interactions between the two types of cells might induce those homozygous mutant cells with an active ordinary X-chromosome, which one expects to be deficient, to express normal enzyme function as the result of normal regulatory signals coming from the complemented cells.

Such an interpretation assumes that the deletions include not the structural genes for the relevant enzymes but rather controlling and regulatory genes required for inducibility and expression of enzymes. The pattern of enzyme activity as observed in the differentiated organism is the result, of course, of a highly complex system of interactions between structural genes, which determine the amino acid sequence of an enzyme, and controlling and regulatory genes which are involved in temporal, e.g., time of expression and spatial, e.g., subcellular localization, aspects of enzyme differentiation. In the case of the lethal albino deletions, the relevant structural enzyme genes map most likely outside the deletions, perhaps even on other chromosomes, whereas regulatory factors responsible for the pattern of enzyme differentiation are products of genes inside the deleted regions.

PROSPECTS

Several foci of particular interest for possible future studies of mammalian developmental genetics emerge from the brief review presented here. There seems to be a shift of attention towards an analysis of the role of regulatory genes in morphogenesis and pattern formation. Obviously, neither a short nor a direct route leads from the structural gene that codes for the amino acid sequence of a peptide to a morphogenetic phenomenon or to the execution of a cellular differentiation pattern. An enormous complexity of interacting factors and processes underlies differentiation, and genes play a paramount role in guiding the essential pathways from transcription of structural genes to their expression. Among the genes involved, those which regulate and control gene expression are of paramount importance. However, at this time, next to nothing is known of their nature nor of their mode of action.

The identification and genetic analysis of cell surface substances instrumental in differentiation is another area of considerable current interest. Even though much circumstantial evidence supports their very existence and genetic control, their actual demonstration awaits further experimental proof. This would no doubt add significantly to the understanding of morphogenetic movements, so essential not only to the understanding of morphogenetic movements, and in cell and tissue differentiation, but also to that of the responsible genetic mechanisms.

The possible correlation of patterns of biochemical and of morphological differentiation remains another unexplored problem area at this time. Genetic systems which affect both may offer the chance of exploring possible causal connections between patterns of morphological and of biochemical genesis.

Decisive progress in the elucidation of these and numerous additional problems of morphogenesis will be achieved by the study of mammalian mutant systems. In this way it may be possible to disentangle the maze of processes instrumental in normal and abnormal morphogenesis and pattern formation.

ACKNOWLEDGEMENTS

Work carried out in the author's laboratory was supported by grants from the National Institutes of Health, the American Cancer Society and the National Science Foundation.

REFERENCES

1. Boveri, T. (1902): In: Foundations of _ Experimental Embryology, edited by B. W. Willier and J. M. Oppenheimer, pp. 74-97. Prentice Hall, Englewood Cliffs, N. J.
2. Chesley, P. (1935): J. Exp. Zool., 70:429-459.
3. Erickson, R. P., S. Gluecksohn-Waelsch and C. F. Cori (1968): Proc. Nat. Acad. Sci., USA 59:437-444.
4. Gable, R. J., J. R. Levinson, H. O. McDevitt and P. N. Goodfellow (1979): Tiss. Ag., 13:177-185.
5. Gluecksohn-Waelsch, S. (1964): In: Genetics _ Today, Proc. of XI International Congr. of _ Genetics, pp. 209-219. Pergamon Press, N. Y.
6. Gluecksohn-Waelsch, S. (1979): Cell, 16:225-237.
7. Gluecksohn-Waelsch, S. and T. R. Rota (1963): Dev. Biol., 7:432-444.
8. Gluecksohn-Waelsch, S. and R. P. Erickson (1970): In:

Curr. Topics Dev. Biol., edited by   A. A. Moscona and A. Monroy, pp. 281-316.   Academic Press, N. Y.

9. Gluecksohn-Waelsch, S., L. S. Teicher and   C. F. Cori (1980): Submitted to Developmental   Genetics.

10. Goodfellow, P. N., J. R. Levinson, R. J. Gable and H. O. McDevitt (1979):   J. Reprod. Immunol.,   1:11-21.

11. Jagiello, G., J. S. Fang, H. A. Turchin,   S. E. Lewis and S. Gluecksohn-Waelsch (1976):   Chromosoma, 58:377-386.

12. Katz, D. F., R. P. Erickson and M. Nathanson   (1979): J. Exp. Zool., 210:529-535.

13. Lederberg, J. (1979): In: Ann. Rev. Genet., 13,   pp. 1-5. Palo Alto, Calif.

13a. Leskes, A., P. Siekevitz and G. E. Palade (1971):   J. Cell Biol., 49:264-287.

14. Miller, D. A., V. G. Dev, R. Tantravahi,   O. J. Miller, M. B. Schiffman, R. A. Yates and   S. Gluecksohn-Waelsch (1974): Genetics,   78:905-910.

15. Russell, E. S. (1979):   In: Adv. in Genetics, 20,   pp. 357-459. Academic Press, N. Y.

16. Spemann, H. (1938): Embryonic Development and   Induction. Yale University Press, New Haven,   Conn.

17. Stern, C.   (1956):   Cold Spring Harbor Symp. on Quant. Biol., 21:375-382.

18. Trigg, M. J. and S. Gluecksohn-Waelsch (1973):   J. Cell Biol., 58:549-563.

19. Yanagisawa, K., D. R. Pollard, D. Bennett,   L. C. Dunn and E. A. Boyse (1974):   Immunogenetics, 1:68-73.

Morphogenesis and Pattern Formation,
edited by T. G. Connelly et al.,
Raven Press, New York © 1981

Mechanical Forces and Patterns of Deformation

David W. Smith

*Dysmorphology Unit, Department of Pediatrics, Child Development and Mental Retardation
Center, and the Center for Inherited Diseases, University of Washington, School of Medicine,
Seattle, Washington 98195*

Mechanical forces are integral to morphogenesis and unusual mechanical forces tend to yield unusual form in developing tissues. The consequences are termed a deformation or deformation sequence. The latter term refers to the manifold consequences of a single deforming cause, such as the oligohydramnios deformation sequence. These types of defects are to be distinguished from malformation, in which there has been an intrinsic problem in the development of one or more tissues, and from disruptions in which there has been a breakdown of a previously normal tissue.

Given a structural defect which is presumed to be caused by aberrant mechanical forces, it is prudent to strive to determine whether the unusual forces were of extrinsic origin affecting an otherwise normal fetus, or of intrinsic origin resulting from a fetal problem such as a malformation. The distinction is based on a number of historical and physical findings. The major emphasis of this presentation is on extrinsic deformations which are due to in utero constraint.

Extrinsic Deformations Due to Uterine Constraint

The presumption in this category is that there is no primary problem within the fetus, but that the deformations are secondary to extrinsic forces which have deformed an otherwise normal fetus. The most common cause for extrinsic deformation is uterine constraint. About 2 percent of babies are born with an extrinsic deformation; hence these are relatively common problems (1, 2).

There is usually an adequate amount of amniotic fluid to cushion the fetus and allow for full growth and mobility prior to 36 to 37 weeks of gestation (from conception). Thus, as Harrison and Malpas (3) indicated, one of the functions of the amniotic fluid is to distend the uterus and enable the fetus to move freely, to develop and to grow with equal pressure in all regions and no excessive or localized constraint. As the fetus becomes crowded in its uterine "sac" during late gestation it will usually settle into a position in which the largest mobile fetal parts, the relatively bulky legs, have ample room. Thus, the fetus tends to assume the vertex presentation. The implication that many of the extrinsic deformations are produced during late fetal life is supported by the observations of Nishimura (4), who found that dislocation of the hip and club foot are both rare features in abortuses prior to 20 weeks of gestation.

After about 35 to 38 weeks of gestation the human fetus tends to grow out of proportion to the uterine cavity. During this time the fetus is growing rapidly while the relative proportion of amniotic fluid is decreasing. The fetus thus usually becomes increasingly constrained. Uterine constraint of the rapidly growing malleable fetal tissues may result in mechanically-induced deformations.

Since the cause of one deformation may often have lead to other problems of constraint in the pliable fetus, there is a nonrandom occurrence of more than one deformation in the same child (2). Dunn found that 30 percent of newborn infants with a deformation problem had more than a single deformation. A number of deformations due to consequence of the same extrinsic cause are referred to as a deformation sequence.

Uterine constraint also tends to reduce the rate of fetal growth and is one cause for prenatal growth deficiency. Such newborn babies frequently show deformational evidence of uterine constraint other than growth deficiency alone.

Any situation which tends to overdistend the uterus may be associated with early onset of labor, with prematurity. This is a major concern for twins who simply distend the uterus prematurely and for a woman with a bicornuate uterus of the type which tends to become overdistended before term.

If the diagnosis is not clear at the time of birth the early postnatal course may provide valuable clues as to whether the deformations noted at birth are extrinsic in causation or not. The otherwise normal infant who has been constrained in late fetal life tends to show progressive improvement in growth and form after being released from the deforming situation at birth. If growth has been slowed by constraint in late fetal life the infant tends to show catchup growth toward his or her genetic potential in early infancy, usually within the first 2 months. If growth of particular parts has been restrained, they tend to show catchup growth toward normal form. This was dramatically evident for nasal growth in an example of prolonged face presentation. Joints which have been externally constrained tend to show progressive increase in their range of mobility after birth.

Historical Perspective

During recent times there has been less recognition of mechanical constraint factors as a cause for problems of prenatal morphogenesis than was true during some periods in past history. As far back as Hippocrates it was noted that uterine constraint could cause fetal deformation (1). Aristotle carried out experiments which showed that crowding of developing chicks caused limb deformation (5). However, there was little written about constraint deformations from then until the renaissance era. In 1573 Ambrossio Paré of France wrote that "narrowness of the uterus produces monsters by the same manner that the Dame of Paris carried the little dogs in a small basket to the end that they didn't grow." A little over a half century ago the text on Diseases of the Newborn by von Reuss (6) contained an entire chapter on postural deformations, whereas present day texts about the newborn have scanty coverage of this subject. One reason for the limited recognition of the more common mechanical factors in morphogenesis during the recent era may be the relative preoccupation with biochemical and physiological factors in morphogenesis. Though the latter are of obvious importance, so are the mechanical factors. This understanding is certainly important for the clinician dealing with problems of morphogenesis.

A number of investigators have made major contributions to our knowledge and understanding of extrinsic deformation during this century. A few brief summations and quotations from representative individuals will serve to emphasize some of their important observations and interpretations.

Thompson (7). "We are ruled by gravity." "There is freedom of movement in the plane perpendicular to gravitational force." "Gravity affects stature and leads to sagging of tissues and drooping of the mouth."

von Reuss (8). This early Viennese neonatologist made the following statement about contractural deformities: "...the deformities occur probably most frequently from pressure on the part by the uterine wall; sometimes marks of pressure may be observed on the skin."

Chapple and Davidson (9). Chapple and Davidson noted that the "position of comfort" of the deformed infant soon after birth tends to be that which had existed in utero. Repositioning the baby into the "position of comfort" may allow the clinician to more readily deduce the causative compressive factors which resulted in the deformation.

Browne (11). Dennis Browne, who was an orthopedist at Great Ormond Street Children's Hospital in London, recognized that deformed infants were often the product of an "uncomfortable" pregnancy, implying uterine constraint. He emphasized the need for controlled forces, utilizing functional growth, in the correction of such deformations.

Dunn (1, 2). Peter Dunn, a pediatrician and neonatologist in Bristol, England who has been responsible for resurrection and extension of knowledge about extrinsic deformation, states that: "intra-uterine forces capable of moulding the fetus increase throughout pregnancy as the infant grows, the mother's uterus and abdominal wall are stretched, and the volume of amniotic fluid diminishes. At the same time the ability of the infant to resist deformation also increases as the rate of fetal growth slows, the skeleton ossifies, and leg movements become more powerful. All these factors are, of course, themselves directly or indirectly under the influence of heredity and are involved in a dynamic interplay throughout fetal life. Nature plays her hand to the limit. The price paid for a larger and more mature infant at birth, better able to withstand the stresses of extrauterine life, is a 2% incidence of deformities".

Table 1

Factors which increase the likelihood of fetal constraint in utero

Environment	Variables
Maternal	Primigravida Small Maternal Size Uterine Malformation Uterine Fibromata Small Maternal Pelvis
Fetal	Early Pelvis Engagement of the Fetal Head Unusual Fetal Position Oligohydramnios Large Fetus, Rapid Growth Multiple Fetuses

Factors Which Enhance Fetal Constraint In Utero

Table 1 summarizes some of the factors which increase the likelihood of fetal constraint in utero and these are presented in more detail below.

Primigravida: The first fetus may be liable to experience more constraint than later offspring because he or she is the first to distend the uterus and the mother's abdominal wall. As a consequence, most of the constraint types of deformations are more common in children of primigravidas than those of multigravidas.

This greater magnitude of late fetal constraint in the primigravida is considered a major reason why the first born is normally smaller at birth than are later born offspring. Though the first born tends to be 200 to 300 gm smaller than later offspring, they are of comparable size to subsequent offspring by one year of age (12). Thus the mild, late fetal growth deficiency in the offspring of a primigravida is transient and they tend to rapidly "catch up" to their genetic pace of growth postnatally. Usually this catch up is achieved within the first few months after birth. The first born is also more likely to become constrained in an unusual position such as the breech presentation and to have consequent deformations relating to such a position.

Small Mother: The smaller the mother in relation to fetal size, the greater is the liability of deforming uterine constraint in late fetal life. Thus most deformations are more common for the small woman than for the larger woman. The impact is readily evident in terms of birth size. Maternal size has a much greater impact on birth size than does paternal size. However, by one year of age the length of the infant relates equally to maternal and paternal stature (12). Much of this maternal impact on birth size appears to relate to the transient effect of the smaller mother in restraining late fetal growth via uterine constraint. Postnatally the infant moves into his or her own genetic pace of growth, which is usually evident by one year of age.

Uterine Malformation: Limitation in the capacity of the uterus to accommodate a fetus may result in early miscarriage, stillbirth, prematurity and/or an offspring who survives to be born with sufficient constraint to give rise to deformation(s). Such reproductive problems are particularly liable to occur with uterine malformations such as a bicornuate or unicornuate uterus (13). It is estimated that about one to two percent of women have a uterine malformation. The likelihood of a deformation problem in the fetus reared in a bicornuate uterus has been crudely estimated to be about 30 percent (13). The recognition that a malformation of the uterus has caused a fetal problem may lead to corrective surgery of the uterus, thus providing a better opportunity for the next fetus to grow without as much constraint.

Uterine Fibromata: A large fibroid of the uterus may limit intrauterine space and therefore have gestational impact similar to that of a bicornuate uterus. The possibility of surgical removal of the tumor, allowing for better fetal space, merits consideration in such cases. Fortunately most uterine fibromata either develop late in reproductive life or after reproduction and are an infrequent cause of fetal deformation.

Small Maternal Pelvis: Vaginal delivery through a small pelvic outlet in relationship to the size of the fetus may result in appreciable molding of the craniofacies. This is usually quite transient. However, if there has been prolonged engagement of the fetal head in a small pelvis the degree of molding can be severe and there may be a rather slow resolution towards normal form postnatally.

Early Pelvic Engagement of the Fetal Head: Early descent of the fetal head into the maternal pelvis is often accompanied by maternal symptoms of pelvic pressure and discomfort that sometimes include pains radiating down the legs with walking. It is very unusual for the fetal head to descend more than six weeks before term and it seldom does so more than one month prior to delivery. Early fetal head descent is more common in the primigravida. When the symptoms are severe it may be difficult for the mother to walk during the later period of gestation. The fetal consequences are predominantly craniofacial deformation. One potential result is vertex craniotabes (4), secondary to prolonged compression of the top of the calvarium, resulting in poorly mineralized, malleable bone in the region of compression. Another potential consequence is constraint of fetal head growth in one dimension, resulting in a lack of growth stretch across one or more of the sutures. If there is a lack of growth stretch across a given suture, then that suture is more liable to become ossified and result in a problem of craniosynostosis (15).

Fetal Position: Prior to 36 to 37 weeks from conception, when the fetus usually has adequate room for movement in its aquatic environment, it is not unusual for the fetus to be in varying positions in utero, including the breech presentation. As the fetus becomes more crowded, he or she will tend to shift into the vertex presentation, there being more ample room in the fundal portion of the uterus for the bulkier legs. The more common reason for aberrant fetal position is in utero constraint which has limited the capacity of the fetus to move into the vertex presentation. Abnormal fetal position during late fetal life may result in unusual constraint forces on fetal morphogenesis. Examples include breech presentation, face presentation, brow presentation and transverse lie. Breech presentation, though only occurring in about 4 percent of pregnancies, is associated with about 32 percent of the overall frequency of extrinsic deformations (16).

Large Fetus, Rapid Growth: The fetus manifests a rapid rate of growth. For example, it doubles in weight during the 6 week period from 28 to 34 weeks in utero. The faster the growth rate and the larger the fetus, the greater is the liability toward external constraint types of deformation. The male is normally larger and grows more rapidly in late fetal life than does the female. Therefore, most extrinsic deformations are more common in the male than in the female, except for dislocation of the hip and other deformations which appear to relate to greater connective tissue laxity in females.

Multiple Fetuses: Multiple fetuses fill out the uterine cavity sooner than average. The average uterus is capable of handling about 4 kg of fetal mass. For twins this combined size is usually achieved by about 34 weeks gestation, and thereafter there tends to be a slowing in growth as the uterine cavity becomes filled (11). Other deformations besides transient growth deficiency also tend to be more common in twins, especially malpositioning of feet and molding of the craniofacies. This is one reason why monozygotic twins may not appear to be identical at the time of birth. One of the twins may have been constrained in a different manner and to a different degree than the other twin. Some of this may relate to aberrant fetal positioning, especially breech presentation in one of the twins.

Oligohydraminios: A deficit of amniotic fluid in late fetal life may be due to a variety of causes such as early rupture of the amnion with chronic leakage of amniotic fluid, lack of urine flow into the amniotic space, or maternal hypertension. However, regardless of the cause, a lack of amniotic fluid tends to give rise to an unusual degree of uterine constraint which affects fetal growth, including thoracic and lung growth, and may also cause a number of craniofacial and limb deformations (17). The consequences are referred to as the oligohydramnios deformation sequence.

Prognosis, Management and Counsel

When a deformation is due to external constraint in late fetal life in an otherwise normal individual, the prognosis for a return towards normal form is usually excellent. The management for extrinsic deformations may vary with the cause. Sometimes it is simply worthwhile to observe the spontaneous changes for several days to several weeks after birth before making a decision as to whether any therapy is indicated. The mode of treatment may simply utilize corrective mechanical forces, similar to those which gave rise to the deformation, striving to <u>force</u> the deformed tissues into a more normal form. When possible, this mechanical therapy should take advantage of normal growth. However, there should be caution in attempting to treat one deformation with a mode of management which may produce additional deformations.

The actual mode of management for reforming constraint deformations may vary appreciably and yet accomplish the same purpose. Simple manual manipulation with molding and stretching toward normal form may be all that is needed. This is a common and ancient practice in India, where "massage women" are employed to mold and shape the baby. They come to the home daily for two to three months, or as long as indicated. By massage with oil and stretching, they form the baby into a normal shape and remove any extrinsic deformations which may have been present at birth. In a similar fashion, parents can be instructed to accomplish such molding or stetching at home. More consistent forces may be applied to foot deformities by frequent adhesive taping, with gradual improvement in the form. When such benign measures do not result in improvement, more rigorous means of molding and stretching, such as casting of the limbs or helmet molding of the head, may be utilized. When a joint is seriously dislocated or malpositioned and conservative measures have not been successful in accomplishing a repositioning to normal form, surgical intervention may be indicated. Ideally, this should be done as soon as it is established that conservative measures are not working. The tendency is toward earlier surgery for such defects. This is especially important for severe equinovarus club foot in which the calcaneous and talus are at least partially dislocated. Proper bony alignment is necessary to foster normal subsequent joint development.

The counsel given to parents of a baby with an extrinsic deformation problem can usually be quite favorable. With rare exception the parents may be counseled in the following manner: "I believe your baby is normal. He (or she) became crowded in the uterus before birth and this resulted in the somewhat unusual features at birth. Having been released from this constraint, the baby's features will return toward normal with no after effects. It is for this reason that I say your baby is normal". If any treatment is merited this is then explained to the parents along with the recurrence risk. The recurrence risk depends on the cause of the extrinsic deformation. For most deformations it is a low recurrence risk. However, the risk may be quite high if the cause is a persisting one such as a uterine malformation.

Obviously, it is important to distinguish between an extrinsic deformation and an intrinsic deformation problem secondary to a malformation, since this distinction has major impact on the prognosis and management for the child and the recurrence risk for the parents.

REFERENCES

1. Dunn, P. M. (1969): The influence of the intrauterine environment in the causation of congenital postural deformities, with special reference to congenital dislocation of the hip. Thesis for MD degree, University of Cambridge, Cambridge.
2. Dunn, P. M. (1976): Br. Med. Bull, 32:71.
3. Harrison, R. G. and P. Malpas (1953): J. Obstet. Gynaec. Brit. Emp., 60:632.
4. Nishimura, H. (1970): In: Congenital Malformations, edited by F. C. Fraser and V. A. Mokusick, p. 275. Excerpta Medica, Amsterdam and London.
5. Tarruffi, C. (1881): Storia della teratologia (History of Teratology), 8:Bologna:Regia Tipografia.
6. von Reuss, A. R. (1921): The Diseases of the Newborn. William Wood and Co.
7. Thompson, D'Arcy Wentworth (1942): On Growth and Form. The University Press, Cambridge.
8. Chapple, C. C. and D. T. (1941): J. Pediatr., 18:483.
9. Browne, D. (1934): Lancet, 2:969.
10. Browne, D. (1935-6): Proc. Roy. Soc. Med., 29:1409.
11. Browne, D. (1955): Arch. Dis. Child., 30:37.
12. Smith, D. W. (1975): Growth and its Disorders. W. B. Saunders Co., Philadelphia.
13. Miller, M. E., P. M. Dunn and D. W. Smith (1979): J. Pediatr., 94:387-390.
14. Graham, J. M. and D. W. Smith (1979): J. Pediatr., 95:114-116.
15. Graham, J. M., M. de Saxe and D. W. Smith (1979):

     J. Pediatr., 95:747-750.
16. Dunn, P. M. (1976): 5th Europ. Cong. Perinatal Med., 76.
17. Thomas, I. T. and D. W. Smith (1974): J. Pediatr., 84:811-814.

Morphogenesis and Pattern Formation,
edited by T. G. Connelly et al.,
Raven Press, New York © 1981.

Discussion of Sections III and IV

WAELSCH: I would like to ask Dr. Newman about the non-histone chromosomal proteins which he says are different in the talpid homozygote. Now, first of all, if you consider them to be direct gene products, then I fail to understand why the heterozygote does not have some of the 120 K chromosomal protein. Secondly, what role do you ascribe to them, the chromosomal proteins, a gene-controlling role or what? I would not expect to find any differences in the cartilage material proper if, indeed, there is a difference in chromosomal proteins that play a controlling role.

NEWMAN: The first thing I want to emphasize, is that I was looking at the proteins in the nuclei so I wasn't looking at whole cellular proteins. What I suggested is that if this is a direct gene product, whatever is made in the cytoplasm might be in the heterozygote in both a normal and an abnormal version. I'm suggesting that once it gets to the nuclear level the abnormal version gets assembled into the chromatin, but the normal version fails to get assembled. Since the spectrum of proteins are so complex in the whole cell, I just haven't searched for the aberrant version in the whole cell. Now, as far as the possible role ascribed to this, we've probed the chromatin of the precartilage cells with nucleases to try to distinguish putatively active from putatively inactive regions of the template material; i.e., template active and template inactive. This particular protein seems to be associated with DNA which is contiguous with but not part of, the transcribing units in the DNA, but that's as far as I can say. I know it's a DNA-binding protein. And I agree, I wouldn't expect any differences in the cartilage per se, and in fact we don't see any nuclear differences in the cartilage of the homozygote versus the normal. What we do see is differences in this particular protein in the precartilage, and the precartilage seems to be the target tissue for the action of the mutation.

RIZKI: Have you tried to get antibodies against this protein so you could see the distribution of it along the axis of the limb bud?

NEWMAN: No, each of those gel slots that you saw is the result of the nuclei taken from about 50 limbs, and particularly in the case of talpid it is very difficult for us to get enough material to even characterize the proteins biochemically any more than we have. Furthermore, in the normal limb the protein is present in only microgram amounts in about 25 animals worth of limbs. We'd need several thousand embryos to get enough protein for even one shot at making an antibody. We have thought of it but since it is so scarce we haven't attempted to make antibodies.

RIZKI: In Drosophila, Sue Elgin has been able to take the band from one of the salivary gland proteins and hybridize them by indirect methods to localize them. If you can do that, then you can find out the distribution of active and inactive nuclei.

NEWMAN: Right, I agree.

SMITH: This question isn't directly down the line of what you gave, but I'd like to get your interpretation again in terms of the muscle. Are you implying from your work that the precartilage is setting the stage for everything that's going to happen in terms of where the muscle location will be and where the tendon locations will be?

NEWMAN: Not in my own work, but I think that's pretty well established by work from Kieny's lab and other labs that it doesn't matter where the somites come from; the muscle coming in follows that pattern that the cartilage has laid out. So I think that the muscle is pretty non-specific.

KOLLAR: My question for Mert Bernfield is on the mammary cultures. Have you lifted the collagen gels, in the way Emerman, Pitelka and Shannon do?

BERNFIELD: You don't have to lift the collagen to get a basal lamina. We have lifted the collagen gel.

KOLLAR: Are the cells in better shape; do they do different things?

BERNFIELD: If you lift the collagen gels, you see a change in cell shape, you see organization of actin filaments somewhat different than if you don't, and you see a slightly thicker basal lamina; but we see no difference in the rate of proteoglycan degradation, whether you chase on a lifted collagen gel or nonlifted collagen gel. Also, when we do the incorporation, and assess the amount of proteoglycan which is present, there is about the same.

KOLLAR: Well the question really is two-pronged because they are using primary cultures, and I wonder whether your refrigerated cells acted differently from, say, primary cells, when they are lifted.

BERNFIELD: Yes, they do.

DAVIS: This pertains to the retino-tectal stuff you were talking about earlier. Have you been able to distinguish between different retinal cell types in your retinal cell aggregates, i.e. can you distinguish which cell types are participating in the adhesion phenomenon in general, and in particular, can you localize the two "processes", calcium-dependent and calcium-independent, to particular cell types? The reason I'm asking is because if one is attempting to draw some physiological significance from the *in vitro* data (and since it is only the retinal ganglion cells which project to the tectum *in vivo*) one would like to be able to demonstrate that the ganglion cells themselves are, in fact, partaking in aggregate formation and be able to localize the calcium dependent or independent systems on the ganglion cells.

STEINBERG: OK, the answer has to have several parts. I'll try to make them as brief as I can. First, all of the cells in the retina, within our ability to demonstrate this, contain both systems. It's not that the ganglion cells do and the prospective photoreceptor cells don't, or anything of the sort, and this goes for the tectum as well. It's not easy to show because what you can do is remove one or the other adhesion system or inhibit it with the appropriate univalent antibody (Fab) then you allow the remaining cells to aggregate. Only the ones that have the other system can aggregate. You can then remove them and see whether the ones that are left are missing. If they are, one of two things must be true, either they lack that adhesion system, or they haven't happened to get together yet. It's easy then to show that they simply haven't happened to get together yet. When you collect the ones still remaining and resuspend them at the original concentration, the aggregate at the same rate as the original population. So all the cells have both of the adhesion systems. Now the second thing, we, and the "we" is really Bill Thomas in my lab, have been trying to determine is whether one or the other of the two adhesion systems has some role in retino-tectal connectiveness. First of all, we're using the technique that Marchase and others have used of making instant monolayers of cells, either dorsal or ventral in origin, and then using labelled cells. In our case we use fluorescently labeled cells instead of radioactively labeled cells from dorsal or ventral retina, and we put them on and see if there is a preference of one for the other. This is an instant cell pickup assay and no one has yet demonstrated whether or not this assay, which demonstrates graded preferences across the retina, correlates or has anything to do with the projection of the retina onto the tectum, which has putative gradients. We don't yet know whether this is going to be relevant to the actual projection process, but at the moment, it's the best we can do. We've shown that the calcium-dependent system does have dorso-ventral polarity to it. There is a dorsal-ventral gradient, and at this moment the calcim-independent system is under investigation.

CONNELLY: In the cases where the entire calvarium is removed, and
the skull reforms normally, is this an example of morphogenetic
memory?

SMITH: I'd rephrase it and say that it's an example of allowing
the skull to form under normal principles in the wake of the
disturbing situation in utero. And in the examples where we've
done total calvariectomy, in at least one example, the calvarium
reformed   under   normal   principles and had normal sutural
positioning and all.   Interestingly, it was a little thinner
calvarium than average. That child is now 4 years of age, and no
further procedure is needed to be done. These have all been
functional sutures that have reformed at the time, so I think the
earlier one can move in on that kind of thing, the more one can
take advantage of normal morphogenesis in the reformational
process.

BRINKLEY: How long, developmentally, will the dura respond in
terms of forming bone in the overlying connective tissue when the
calvarium is removed?

SMITH: The answer there is that if you remove the calvarium
within the first four months, usually you can throw away the bone
and from the underlying calvarium new bone will form. If you do
it after four months, the procedure is basically the same, you
remove the dura but you put back islands of bone onto the dura
interlaced as a mosaic to serve as niduses (foci) for
mineralization.   But I think the best results are obtained the
earlier it is done.

BURDI: I can see where you had a filling out of these negative
contours of the skull, in terms of the brain catching up and
giving a nice shape. But what about where you had a positive
outgrowth with a suspected encephalocoele; where did all that
material go to give you a normally shaped head?

SMITH: The one case which others interpreted as encephalocoele we
did nothing to. Because there was no synostosis or anything to
impair the molding we just let the normal brain molding take its
course.   We have had cases of plagiocephaly in which the head is
grossly oblique in shape and one area is particularly prominent.
In those cases we use the helmet to prevent any further outgrowth
from the prominence and then the only other place where the brain
can mold out is where the skull is shallow and uninhibited by the
helmet.   This has worked out beautifully.

QUESTION: Elaborate on the evidence that the t-locus alleles do
not specify abnormal cell surface antigens.

WAELSCH: Dr. Erickson, who has had a lot more direct contact with this work and is himself involved in it, might agree to answer that question.

ERICKSON: I guess the very brief answer is two references from Hugh Mc Devitt's group, one of which appeared in Tissue Antigens (13:177, 1979) with Gable as the senior author, the other in J. Reprod. Immunol. (1:11, 1979), with Goodfellow as the senior author. One has a massive amount of data but did not use precisely the same system, the other did use precisely the same system as the positive data which has all emanated from one laboratory, that of Dorothea Bennett. In a slightly wider sense, there's the problem that t alleles suppress crossing over and "lock-in" H-2 haplotypes. Craig Hammerberg and a number of workers have elucidated this. Most t alleles carry a private H-2 in cis. This means that it's very difficult to study t antigens because you've got that H-2 carried along, pari passu. There is also the very recent work of Alena Lengerova, who passed away last year, and her collaborators, who have shown that within the t region is a locus, (which they call Hye for "histocompatibility Y expression") which changes the amount of the Y antigen (J. Immunogen.,6: 429, 1979). So here again we have something in the t region that affects the amount of an antigen, but doesn't change the antigen, and is "locked-in" cis again by t alleles. I think that besides those two references with a lot of negative data, there's the complexity of the proximal portion of chromosome 17 and, therefore, a large number of controls, etc. that have to be used before there can be clear evidence for t antigens.

CONNELLY: Would you expect there to be an increase in fibronectin in the basement membrane of ectoderm induced to thicken by grafts of ZPA into the anterior region of the anterior limb?

NEWMAN: I would insofar as ZPA grafts apparently just bring out the capacity of marginal ectoderm to make ridge. As far as I'm aware, ZPA grafts don't make dorsal or ventral ectoderms into apical ectodermal ridge, but they might essentially stimulate a ridge that is becoming quiescent at it's antero-posterior margins. I think that since the buildup of fibronectin in the basement membrane is probably associated with the functional state of the ridge, I would expect a local buildup if the ridge were stimulated in those regions:

CONNELLY: What sort of connective tissue framework does one find in the mutants described by Dr. Waelsch in which there is no striated muscle. Particularly in view of the possibility that connective tissue might act as a mold for muscle morphogenesis?

WOLPERT: The answer is, one doesn't know. The prediction would be that the connective tissue would be there just as the tendons are there. You can make a limb without muscle simply by irradiating the somites as Madeleine Kieny and Chevalier have done. If you look early enough you find the tendons in the right places, but afterwards they disappear.

Can I take this opportunity to ask a question? It's really of Dr. Steinberg. I'm left slightly uneasy. I believe in the liquid model of cells, but cells also actively move, as for example, in the pronephros. What about the role of active cell movement, or are the cells behaving simply as liquid drops? In general it would be very nice to know what role active cell movement plays in all the processes that you've been describing.

STEINBERG: Yes, in the case of the pronephric duct it's very clear, and I should say it's Tom Poole who has done this work. In the case of the pronephric duct, it's very clearly a creeping of the posterior lead cells. The others show following behavior. The lead cell never gets out ahead of the others, but they all creep along behind. It gives the appearance that the active creeping is restricted to cells nearest the tip. In the case of cell sorting movements, it's even hard to know how one would find this out. But, our supposition is that the cells jostle about a bit and relax tensions that one imposes upon them. There's no hard evidence that the cells are using metabolic energy to produce some of these movements. The closest thing to that is Peter Armstrong's demonstration 7-8 years ago that when certain cell mixtures in artificial aggregates, are put in cytochalasin the sorting is stopped, but with others it's not stopped. It goes up to a certain point until the clusters are far enough apart. There's apparently no random probing about of cells in the interior of those mixtures in the presence of the cytochalasin (which inhibits active cell motion). With cytochalasin, the cells already in contact evidently can exchange adhesions just on the basis of zipping up one and those forces breaking the other. However, they can't seek out any new ones, and so the sorting out bogs down at an earlier stage. . If you then wash out the cytochalasin they pick up and go the rest of the way. So, It seems that both passive and active cell movements play a role in cell sorting. Of course, the cell sorting itself is just a sort of model way of getting at the question of what determines the rearrangement of cells and tissues in embryos.

BRINKLEY: Just a point of information. Is the posterior extension of the pronephric duct sensitive to cytochalasin?

STEINBERG: We haven't asked.

QUESTION: Can you relate your work to the studies of Dr. Elizabeth Newfeld on the mucopolysaccharidoses?

BERNFIELD: I think the question refers to the "capture-recapture" hypothesis that Dr. Newfeld has had in which it has been thought that lysosomal enzymes are first secreted before they can be taken up into the lysosomes. I have recently spoken with her and understand that she no longer holds the recapture hypothesis. She now feels that the phosphomannosyl group which is the "address" on many lysosomal enzymes is indeed an intracellular address rather than an extracellular one. I hope that was an adequate answer.

LILLIE: Can your observations on the mouse salivary gland be extended to differentiated adult tissues, or are they in fact characteristic of embryonic systems only?

BERNFIELD: We have no direct evidence on this point, but I would like to comment and introduce some ideas of Vracko who is at the University of Washington. He has done a number of studies demonstrating that in adult tissues the basal lamina acts as a scaffold for preserving tissue boundaries. The studies have included inducing experimental necrosis, killing the cells: the parenchymal tissues die, cells die and the basal lamina remains. It appears to be resistant to the necrotic process even over large areas. In addition, other work I'd like to mention, which bears on this argument, indicates that in an adult, the basal lamina turns over really very slowly. So these two pieces of evidence, together with our work indicating that in embryonic tissue the basal lamina turns over rapidly, specifically at certain sites, suggest that the embryonic morphogenetic systems might be unique. I should point out in this regard that the differing distribution of histochemically identifiable GAG at epithelial surfaces has also been found by Morris and Solursh and by Dr. Cunha, who is with us here at the meeting.

LILLIE: Can you distinguish between cell surface matrix and the basal lamina? Does this lamina contain hydroxyproline and type IV collagen?

BERNFIELD: Let me put those together in the following way. I've attempted to define the cell surface matrix as the material which is on the cell surface and associated with it, and which contains materials which we would normally ascribe to the matrix. In the instance of the submandibular salivary gland we have not been able to label this with radioactive proline . That includes the basal lamina by the way. That work has been published and I can give you the reference if you like. Immunological studies to determine whether type IV collagen in fact exists are currently in progress.

LILLIE: Does this lamina have any specializations, such as hemidesmosomes?

BERNFIELD: We find very, very few of these specializations.
I just want to say one thing, which is that I was extraordinarily impressed with the mechanical influence on development that Dr. Smith has clearly shown. The more I thought about them, the more I realized that many aspects of development

are mechanical, including those which we have looked at in the morphogenesis of glandular organs. Indeed, this is an area which has not been pursued as well at the basic biological level as he seems to have done clinically, and I just wanted to thank him.

Morphogenesis and Pattern Formation,
edited by T. G. Connelly et al.,
Raven Press, New York © 1981.

Morphogenesis of the Neural Plate and Tube

Antone G. Jacobson

Department of Zoology, University of Texas at Austin, Austin, Texas 78712

Early morphogenesis of the central nervous system consists of distortions of a sheet of cells, the neuroepithelium. A neural plate shapes itself out of the embryonic ectoderm, rolls into a tube, then expands at the brain end and forms bulges and furrows. In embryos of mammals, birds and many amphibia, the neuroepithelium remains but one cell thick throughout these transformations.

Many efforts have been made to identify the mechanisms of neurulation. Fate maps and analyses of cell movements have been made in early neural plates in amphibia (43, 44, 12, 33, 32, 57, 86, 22), and in bird embryos (71, 77, 87, 89). Early stages of plate formation in mammals, including human embryos (63, 64), have been described, but not mapped. The mammal appears to have a neural plate quite similar to that of the bird, but with a very wide brain area.

Neural tube formation has attracted attention for over 100 years. Roux (72) held that changes in the neural plate itself were responsible for tube formation. Some investigators invoked pushing forces in the epidermis that surrounds the neural plate (35, 75, 76, 18). However, slits made in the epidermis always gape immediately, suggesting that the epidermis is under tension, not pushing (30, 42, 52).

Rhumbler (69) and others have proposed a model in which cells become wedge-shaped to create curving of the sheet of cells. Glaset (20) proposed that such a change in cell shape resulted from the imbibing of water into the basal ends of the cells which in turn caused the sheet to fold. This notion was later refuted by Glaset (21) and by Brown et al. (9) who found that the density of neural plate cells changes very little during neural tube formation. Measurements that show that the amphibian nervous system has a constant volume throughout neurulation (19, 30, 28) are also evidence against this mechanism.

Increasing adhesion among the neural plate cells has been invoked as a driving force of neurulation (9, 25). The idea was that neural cells would get taller because they would tend to adhere more to one another. Bellairs, et al. (5) claim to have measured adhesiveness of various tissues of the chick embryo and report the neural cells are less adhesive than the cells of the epidermis. Both tissues double in adhesiveness during neurulation, but only neural tube thickens and rolls up. They say their evidence refutes a role of adhesiveness in neural tube formation.

Lewis (52) proposed a physical model in which tension in the top surface of the plate was responsible for rolling the plate into a tube. His physical model was unrealistic in that the sides of the adherent units (representing plate cells) were rigid and of invariable length.

Some investigators have suggested that underlying somites or mesenchyme and matrix may help push up the neural folds (75, 61). However, the amphibian neural plate will roll into a tube when isolated with no other tissue than the underlying notochord (30).

There have been many studies using electron microscopy of neurulation in amphibian embryos (56, 70, 60, 54, 10, 40, 79, 75, 45, 1, 2), in bird embryos (62, 13, 68, 74, 3, 41, 27, 24, 4), and in mammalian embryos (91, 73, 88, 17).

Many chemical and physical treatments have been found that halt neural tube formation. These include UV irradiation (15), the lectins concanavalin A (48) and wheat germ agglutinin (50), Cytochalasin-B (53, 58, others), colchicine (41, 11, 55), 2,4-dinitrophenol (8), actinomycin-D (51, 7), 5-bromodeoxyuridine (49), heavy water (40), and beta-mercaptoethanol (34).

While a great amount of information about neurulation has accumulated, and many possible mechanisms have been proposed, most possibilities have been disproved or are still unproven. There have been several reviews in recent years (82, 42, 83).

I will now review the attempts of myself and my colleagues to analyse and model the processes of neurulation using observations, experiments, computer simulation and mathematical analysis. New interpretations and results are included.

Our early studies of neural morphogenesis were done in salamander embryos (West Coast newt, Taricha torosa) in which cells are large enough to follow individually, and whose nervous system does not grow at all during the time studied (28, 30, 19); so growth does not obscure the morphogenetic processes mainly responsible for these early changes of shape in the nervous system. Neural tube shaping is also examined in the chick embryo. Both amphibian and chick neurogenesis are, at these early stages, quite similar to that of the mammal, but much easier to study.

Three phases of development of the central nervous systems of vertebrate embryos will be considered. The morphological stages of development that include these three phases are shown in Figure

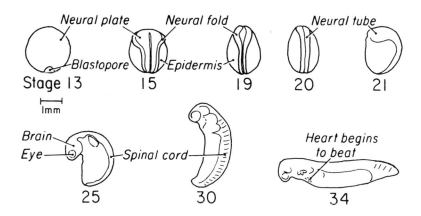

FIG. 1. Morphological stages of development of the embryo of the West coast newt, *Taricha torosa* (as defined by Twitty and Bodenstein (84)) during neural plate shaping (stages 13-15), neural tube formation (stages 15 to 19-20), and brain expansion and shaping (stages 21 to 34 and beyond). All stages are drawn to the same scale.

****

1 for the newt embryo.

In the first of the three phases, the newly induced neural plate thickens and shrinks from a hemisphere to a disc then into a keyhole or pear shape (newt stages 13 to 15, Fig. 1). By the end of this phase the flat keyhole-shaped plate is just about to roll into a tube and the various parts of brain and spinal cord have been ·determined (32, 33). The whole plate is by then composed of about 14,000 cells (30, 19).

In the second phase, the neural plate suddenly elongates and rolls into a tube (newt stages 15 to 19-20, Fig. 1).

In the third phase, the closed neural tube expands at the brain end and bulges and furrows appear (85), some of which become major divisions of the brain (newt stages 21 to 34 and beyond, Fig. 1). At newt stage 34, the heart begins to beat and for the first time growth of the nervous system begins· (at the expense of gut wall tissue (28). During neurulation, cell division occurs at a slow pace, but daughter cells remain half the size of their progenitor cell so this is not growth.

ANALYSIS OF THE SHAPING OF THE NEURAL PLATE

In the newt embryo, by late gastrula stage 13 (small yolk plug stage, Fig. 1), the neural plate has been induced from the dorsal hemisphere of ectoderm, and the hemisphere has begun to flatten into a disc. To convert from a hemisphere to a disc of the same diameter, the surface of the plate must shrink by 50%. The disc elongates along the midline of the embryo and distorts into a keyhole shape by stage 15. The plate surface shrinks 40% during the conversion from disc to keyhole shape (30).

Mapping cell positions in the forming neural plate

The changes of cell position between stages 13 and 15 were mapped with time-lapse cinematography (12). Cells could be identified by variegations in pigmentation. The cells followed were at intersections of a coordinate grid (a D'Arcy Thompson grid (81)). The grid was superimposed on the projected images of the movies of neurulation and frame-by-frame analysis was made to determine the new positions of cells and the resulting distorted grid (Fig. 2).

Two sorts of information were obtained: cell pathways (at the grid intersections) and local changes of area (changes of area of the original squares of the grid as they are distorted). We noted an inverse correlation between cell height and changes of local area (12), as had others (33). We also noted that cells generally moved toward the midline and anteriorly along the midline (Fig. 3).

Changes in cell shape in the neural plate

Changes of cell shape were measured between stages 13 and 15 in this mapped system (10). For example, cell heights and apical surface areas were measured at stage 13 when cells were at "A" in Figure 3, then cells at "B" were measured at stage 15 at the site where "A" cells would be displaced by then. This was one of the first studies that described changes of the shape of cells in a mapped system, so the cells measured at the beginning of the study, and as displaced at the end of the study, were known to be the same cells. Others have described changes of the shape of cells in typical sections of embryos, but the "changes" they described were not in the same cells through time (1, 75).

The changes in shape of the cells involves contraction of bundles of microfilaments at the apical surfaces (1, 10, 11), and elongation of microtubules in the long axes of the cells (10, 11). At these stages the activities of microfilaments and microtubules are somehow coordinated so the reduction of apical surface is inversely proportional to the increase in cell height (Fig. 4).

Mapping the regional differences of changes of cell shape in the neural plate

Additional measurements of changes of shape of neural plate cells between stages 13 and 15 (30) were made to construct, on the stage 13 neural plate, the prospective changes of cell shape over

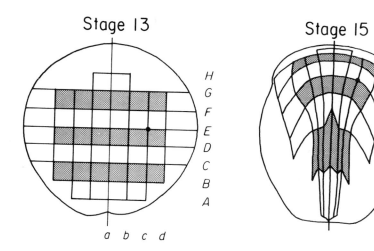

FIG. 2.   Neural plate formation was recorded by time-lapse
cinematography (1 frame per minute, 17 C).   The movies were
analyzed frame by frame.   The 50 points followed   at   the
interactions of the grid superimposed on the projected images were
cells identified by variegations in egg pigmentation. The grid
became distorted due to cell relocations. (Modified from 12.)

****

the whole plate (Fig. 5). Since they are inversely proportional,
the map represents both apical cell surface shrinkage and cell
elongation. Cell elongation was most conveniently measured from
serial cross sections.   The data was grouped into nine natural
categories with regions labeled 9 shrinking apical   surfaces (and
elongating)   most,   and   those   labeled 2 least. Category one was
used to represent contiguous epidermis that flattened and expanded
rather then getting thicker and contracting.

Experiments to show the changes in cell shape in the
neural plate are programmed by stage 13

We (30, 31) did several experiments to demonstrate that the
pattern   of   prospective   cell   surface   shrinkage (and cell
elongation) mapped on the stage 13 neural plate was already
programmed at stage 13.   One such experiment is illustrated in
Figure 6. Cells from an "8-9" region (Fig. 5) at stage 13 were
transplanted to a "2" region.   The cells shrank their apical
surfaces and elongated an amount appropriate for the region from
which they were taken, not for the region into which they were
transplanted. The amount of elongation to be done between stages
13 and 15 was already programmed by stage 13 and not changed by

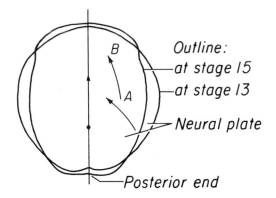

FIG. 3. This diagram of dorsal views of superimposed outlines of stage 13 and 15 embryos shows three typical pathways of cells (of the 50 followed). Rates of movement (at 17 C) ranged from 4 to 95 m/hr and some cells moved almost a millimeter. For example, the cell at A (at stage 13) moved 819 m at an average rate of 64 m/hr to end at B at stage 15 (12.8 hrs later). Cells on the midline moved cranially along the midline. (Modified from 10, 12.)

****

the strange environment.

Epidermis transplanted into the neural plate of a stage 13 embryo expands apical surface, while the reciprocal experiment, plate cells implanted among epidermal cells, shrink apical surfaces and elongate normally (30).

Behavior of the notoplate

We (30, 23) observed that the area of the neural plate that overlies the notochord (the notoplate) behaves differently from the rest of the neural plate. The notoplate is intimately attached to the underlying notochord (see Fig. 9), and makes the same movements as the notochord (36, 30).

In time-lapse color movies of neurulation, the notoplate area can be distinguished from the rest of the plate by its color, by the way light penetrates through it compared to surrounding neural plate, and by its behavior through time. The changing boundary between notoplate and the rest of the neural plate can be followed quantitatively in these movies (30).

At stages 13 to 15, neither isolated notoplate nor isolated notochord will elongate by themselves, but if isolated together (notoplate attached above notochord) they elongate as much as normal through the stage 13 to 15 time period (30). In both notoplate and notochord, the cells converge toward and relocate

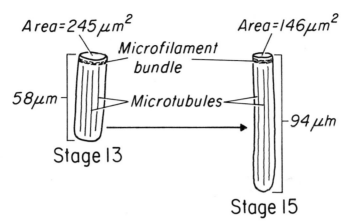

FIG. 4. The change in shape of this cell occurs while moving from position "A" to position "B" in Figure 3. Most microfilaments and microtubules are disposed as shown, and the change of cell shape requires their activities. The cell volume remains constant through these changes. Increase in cell height is inversely proportional to decrease in apical area during this period. (Modified from 11.)

☆☆☆☆☆☆☆☆☆☆☆☆☆☆☆☆☆☆☆☆☆☆☆☆☆☆☆☆

along the midline. At these stages, notochord is still a flat sheet. By stage 15, the notochord begins to rearrange into a rod and to form a sheath. The overlying notoplate cells make the same movements, converting the notoplate area from a broad sheet at stage 13 to a long column of cells stretched along the midline at stage 15 (Fig. 7).

Experiments with isolated neural plate

The neural plate explanted at stage 13 shrinks, but does not elongate along the midline and does not achieve a keyhole shape. If the underlying notochord is left in place, the isolated stage 13 neural plate elongates normally and does achieve a keyhole shape by stage 15 (30).

Computer simulation of neural plate shaping

Gordon and I (30, 23) did a computer simulation to help determine whether the stage 13 pattern of prospective shrinkage of apical cell surfaces (Fig. 5), plus the change in shape of the notoplate region (Fig. 7), were necessary and sufficient mechanisms for changing the shape of the neural plate between

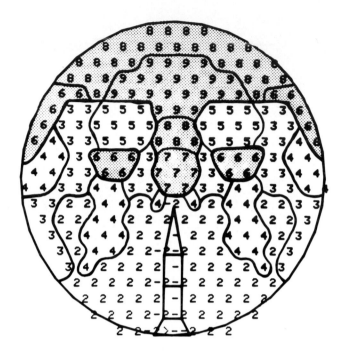

FIG. 5. On this map of a stage 13 neural plate, the numbers in each region indicate the amount of apical area shrinkage of the cells (and inversely, the amount of cell elongation) that will occur between stages 13 and 15. Regions labelled 9 shrink the most, and 2 the least. Areas of greatest shrinkage are shaded. The rocket-shaped region is the <u>notoplate</u>, the area of the neural plate that overlies the notochord. (adapted from 30.)

****

stages 13 and 15.

In the simulation, the shrinkage of cell surfaces was carried out as indicated on the empirical map (Fig. 5). As each shrinkage unit (representing the cell surfaces) shrank, it pulled on its neighbor cells equally in every direction (isotropically)and they pulled on their neighbors, etc. The resulting changes in position of the cells was worked out with a repacking algorithm.

The extension of the notoplate along the midline was also modeled from empirical data. Changes in shape of the perimeter of the notoplate (as observed in time-lapse movies) were made stepwise and the rest of the cells of the neural plate responded to the repositioning of the notoplate by adjustments in their positions worked out by the repacking algorithm. Results of the

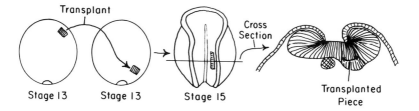

Transplant

Stage 13   Stage 13   Stage 15

Cross Section

Transplanted Piece

FIG. 6. The experiment illustrated here was one of the tests of whether the cells are already programmed at stage 13 to shrink (and elongate) the amounts indicated in Figure 5. A piece of neural plate from an 8-9 region was transplanted into a 2 region of a host embryo (in place of a 2 region previously removed). The embryo was then reared to stage 15 and cross-sectioned through the transplant. Even though surrounded by "2" cells, the transplanted piece elongated (and shrank its apical surfaces) as much as would be expected of "8-9" cells, so they must have been programmed to do so at stage 13. (Modified from 31.)

****

simulations are shown in Figure 8.

The neural plate was modeled as a sheet of viscoelastic material. The units (representing cells) of the plate were held together in a continuous sheet in the simulation by bonds between the centers of the units. The bonds were given the properties of a spring and dashpot in parallel. As units shrank and the notoplate boundary moved, the bonds between units were stretched. The repacking algorithm relieved the stretch by repositioning of the units. This was done in small steps so the simulation kept the system in a quasistatic state. When stretched more than limits observed in stretched apical surfaces of cells of neural plates, the bonds were allowed to break and the units changed neighbors. This models the viscous component of the tissue.

The driving forces for neural plate shaping have two origins. One set of forces comes from the contractions of the apical bundles of microfilaments of the plate cells as they shrink their apical surfaces. (The simultaneous and inversely proportional elongation of the cells, involving microtubules, is necessary if the plate is to remain flat.) We have modeled the global consequences of the operation of these shrinkage forces to cell positions over the whole neural plate.

The other set of forces is the elongation of the notoplate cell group along the midline that results in the extension of the neural plate. We modeled the consequences of these forces by adjusting cell positions to the changing perimeter of the notoplate area. Possibilities for how and why notoplate cells relocate along the midline are discussed below.

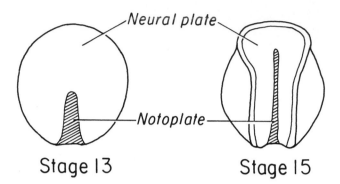

FIG. 7. These outlines of an embryo at stage 13 and at stage 15 are traced from a time-lapse movie of neurulation of the embryo. The notoplate region (the region of neural plate that overlies the notochord) is shown as observed in the movie. (adapted from 30).

****

Extension of the notoplate along the midline is the most important of the two forces leading to the change in shape that forms the keyhole shape, but a normal result comes only when both mechanisms act together (Fig. 8).

Lines of shear in and around the forming neural plate

Both cell surface shrinkage and notoplate extension produced lines of shear (changes of neighbors among cells). The boundary between neural plate and epidermis is a line of shear produced by disparate shrinkage programs in the plate and epidermal cells. Cells change neighbors everywhere within the notoplate area, and immediately adjacent to it. Thus at and near the midline is a line of shear.

We (30) suggest that lines of shear resulting from morphogenetic processes may serve to help isolate adjacent domains of cells embarking on different courses of differentiation. Epidermal-plate domains are separated by one line of shear, and the midline shear line separates right and left symmetrical halves of the nervous system.

An approach to the mathematics of morphogenesis: Morphodynamics

In an appendix to our simulation paper (30), Gordon describes approaches to a mathematics of morphogenesis that we call morphodynamics.

The neural plate may be considered a two-dimensional hydrodynamic system with special properties. These properties include fluid elements (cells) that differ one from another. The sheet of cells has a surface density (mass of protoplasm per unit

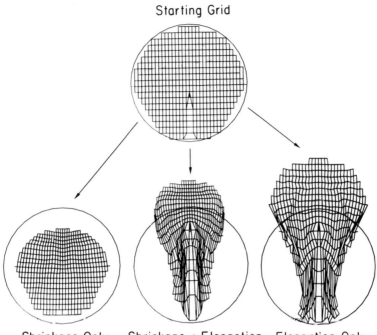

Starting Grid

Shrinkage Only Shrinkage + Elongation Elongation Only

FIG. 8. Results of computer simulations of neural plate shaping are shown with these photographs of a computer graphics terminal . A starting grid represents the stage 13 neural plate. The simulation rearranges cell positions as a result of apical surface shrinkage of cells (map, Fig. 5) and elongation of the notoplate area along the midline (Fig. 7). Shrinkage alone does not achieve a keyhole shape, either simulated or when the stage 13 neural plate is explanted alone. Simulation with elongation alone makes a keyhole shape that is too long and broad. This is an experiment that can be done with the computer, but not with the embryo. Only a simulation where both shrinkage and midline elongation operates gives a normally shaped result. (adapted from 30.)

****

area) that varies from place to place and with time. The sheet of cells acts as if it were a compressible two-dimensional fluid because the surface density may vary. The properties of such a system are best described in Lagrangian, or material, coordinates that move with the fluid elements. Equations are given for isolated neural plates, with and without notochord, and for a three-dimensional growing system whose mass changes with time.

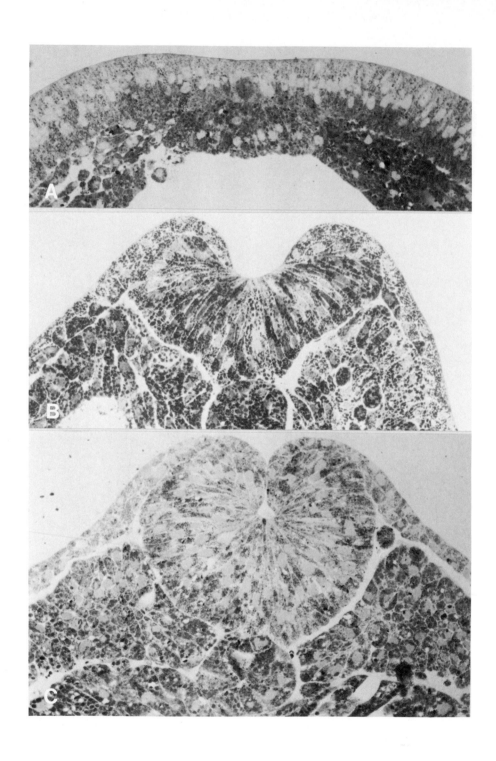

FIG. 9. These light micrographs of plastic cross-sections (1 m thick), of embryos fixed in glutaraldehyde and stained with methylene blue, show the changes in shape of cells of the neural epithelium as the neural tube forms (X 390). (A) Neural plate at stage 15. The notochord is still flat and is intimately attached beneath the midline of the neural plate. (B) By stage 17, tube formation is underway. Cells of the plate have greatly contracted their apical surfaces and increased in height. Notochord beneath the plate at the midline is now a round cylinder. (C) At stage 19 the neural folds appose one another and tube formation is nearly complete. All stages are shown at the same magnification, and all show the region just posterior to hind brain.

****

NEURAL TUBE FORMATION

The neural plate rolls into a tube between stages 15 and 19 in the newt embryo (Fig. 9). The same two mechanisms that acted during plate shaping continue to act through neural tube formation, but each changes rather dramatically during this period.

Cell behavior during tube formation

Apical surfaces of neural plate cells shrink greatly during tube formation (Fig. 10), but elongation of the cells, while continuing, does not keep pace and the basal ends of the cells become broader than the apical ends (Fig. 11).
By actively becoming wedge-shaped, the cells could cause the plate to roll up (Fig. 12). Gordon and I are presently modeling tube formation and we call this the wedging model. Alternatively, if the tube were rolled up by some other mechanism, the cells could be passively constrained to assume the wedge shape.

Midline elongation during tube formation

We (30, 28) found that just during those stages when the plate closes into a tube (stages 15 to 19), notoplate extension along the midline goes 10 times faster than before or after (Fig. 13).
This is an enticing correlation. The newt neural plate rolls into a tube all at once between stages 15 and 19, but in bird and mammal embryos the anterior end of the embryo is neurulating while the posterior end is still gastrulating through the primitive streak. As a result, there are stages when the anterior plate is already a tube, the middle plate is in the process of rolling into a tube, and more posterior plate is still open.
If more rapid elongation of the midline has a role in rolling

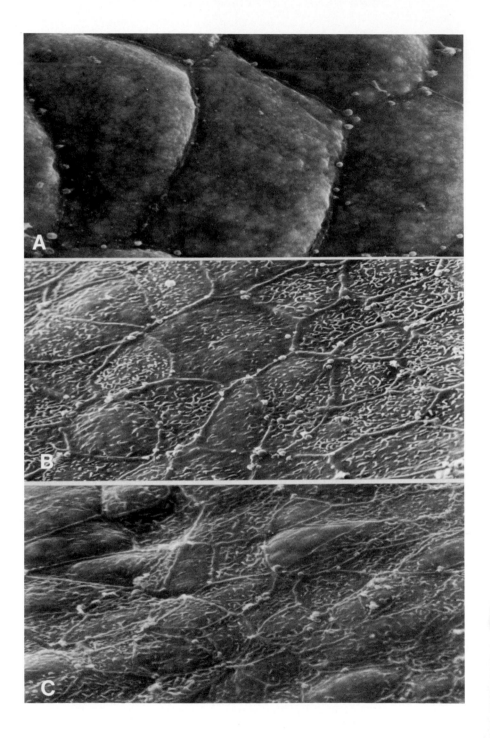

FIG. 10. Scanning electron micrographs (all at 1500 X) of the
surfaces of neural plates in the hind brain region at (A) stage
13, (B) stage 15, (C) stage 19. The apical surfaces of the neural
plate cells progressively shrink during this period.

****

the plate into a tube, then one would expect the part of the plate
that is closing to be elongating faster than either closed tube or
open plate. I have measured elongation of these regions over a
four hour period in a stage 9 chick embryo marked with lines of
nile blue sulfate. The results (Fig. 14) were as predicted.
Closing plate elongates four times as fast as open plate and seven
times as fast as closed tube (29).

  This close correlation between rapid midline elongation and
tube formation suggests a possible causal relationship.   I
suggested (28, 23, 29) that if the plate began to act like an
elastic sheet, then stretching it along a line could roll it into
a tube (Fig. 15). The extension of the midline should buckle the
plate lateral to the midline out of the plane and roll it into a
tube. Gordon and I call this the buckling model. We are making a
computer simulation of tube formation and will test the wedging
and buckling models

Experimental tests of the wedging and
elongation models of tube formation

  As part of my work with Gordon to model tube formation, I have
been doing a series of experiments on newt embryos to test the
models. I will give here preliminary results for two of these
experiments.

  A transverse strip was explanted from the neural plate of a
stage 15 embryo (Fig. 16). If wedging of the plate cells drives
tube formation, then the strip should roll up into a circle,
apical surface innermost. If stretching of the midline drives
tube formation, then the strip might be expected to remain fairly
flat since so little of the notoplate is in the explant.   In all
cases the strip either rolled up in the wrong direction or
remained flat. This result weakens the wedging model, but is not
conclusive since wounded surfaces produce new conditions.

  In another series of experiments, stage 15 embryos were severed
from anterior to posterior end, but off the midline so the left
part contained no notoplate, and the right part contained all of
the notoplate (Fig. 17).   The length of the nervous system was
measured with an ocular micrometer (and thus included some optical
foreshortening). Of twelve cases, initial nervous system length
averaged 2.2 mm. Forty-eight hours later, when controls were at
closed tube stage 21, the length of left and right halves of the

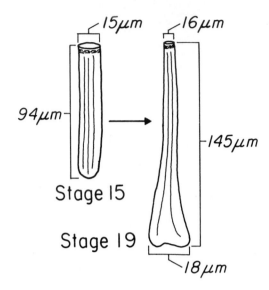

FIG. 11. this diagram shows changes in apical and basal areas, and cell height, of a neural plate cell of the brain region between stages 15 and 19. During this period, increase in cell height does not keep pace with apical surface shrinkage and the cell becomes wedge-shaped. (Modified from 10, 11).

****

experimental embryos were measured again and they were fixed, sectioned and examined in cross-section. The left halves (lacking notoplate) averaged 2.14 mm in length (-3%), and the right halves (containing all the notoplate) had elongated to 2.52 mm (+15%). In each case, the half-plates had partly, or completely, folded into a tube, but right halves most consistently completed tube formation (Fig. 17).

These results suggest a strong role of elongation in tube formation, but do not eliminate other mechanisms. The results also clearly indicate that the notoplate region is responsible for nervous system elongation at these stages.

What are the mechanisms of midline elongation?

The experiment just described implicates the notoplate region in extension of the neural plate midline during tube formation, but does not eliminate a possible role of the underlying notochord. Kitchin (46) had reported that the nervous system elongates and the tube closes as usual if the notochord is

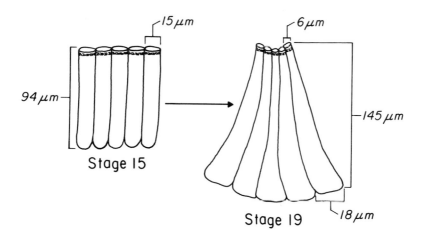

FIG. 12. This diagram shows how several cells undergoing the shape changes shown in Fig. 11 could begin to roll the flat plate into a tube.

****

carefully removed from beneath at keyhole stage 15 in the axolotl embryo. His results thus suggest that after stage 15, the notochord is not essential for elongation of the plate.

I have explanted neural plates at stage 15 with and without underlying notochord to attempt to see what is needed for plate elongation. In a 24 hour period following explantation, neural plates alone average 16.4% increase in length, while neural plates with underlying notochords average 28.9% elongation. Elongation can certainly occur without notochord, but more elongation occurs if notochord is present. This leaves us with the question of how notoplate can elongate itself.

There is no mystery about how the notoplate elongation occurs, only about what drives it. The cells of the notoplate change neighbors and relocate in a line along the midline. Length of neural plate is increased at the expense of cross-sectional area, and the number of cells in cross-sections decreases (28, 29).

One possibility for a driving mechanism is differential adhesion between notoplate cells and cells of the rest of the neural plate. Gordon and I are examining the possibility that these two cell populations meet the criteria for <u>mixing</u> defined by Steinberg (78). That is, if the strengths of adhesions are W_a for neural plate cell to neural plate cell, W_b for notoplate cells to notoplate cells, and W_{ab} for adhesions between the two kinds of cells and $W_{ab} \geq (W_a + W_b)/2$, then mixing will occur. In contrast to the situation in which sorting out occurs and minimal

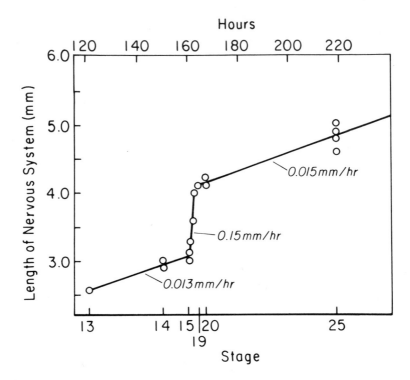

FIG. 13. Neural plates or tubes were excised at the stages
indicated, laid flat on agar and their lengths measured. The rate
of elongation abruptly changes at stage 15 to go ten times faster
between stages 15 and 19 when it returns to the old rate.
(modified from 30, 28.)

****

(spherical) boundaries are established between cell types, in a
mixing situation the boundary tends to maximize. We believe the
neural plate-notoplate situation may fit the criteria for mixing
with one additional constraint.   The plate cells other than
notoplate are bound to one another by many desmosomes connected to
the microfilament bundles (10). This creates an interconnected
microfilament network over the plate surface that may greatly
limit the ability of the cells to change neighbors, and may thus
prevent actual mixing with notoplate cells. The boundary between
notoplate area and the rest of the neural plate is then unstable
and will tend to maximize (as when it extends along the midline).
A bias to extend along the midline rather than in some other
direction may be imposed by association with underlying notochord
and/or may be imposed by contraction of the tongue of highly

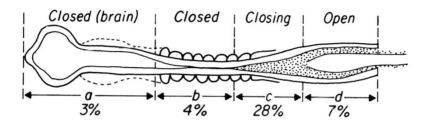

FIG. 14. Chick embryos were marked with lines of vital dye (Nile blue) at the dashed lines to delimit closed portions of the neural tube, closing neural plate, and open plate. Four hours later, when the closing region of the plate was just completing tube formation, the lengths of the regions were measured and the increases in length divided by the original lengths to get the percentage increases in length shown (figures are an average of ten cases). The closing portion of the plate elongated much more rapidly than closed or open regions. (Modified from 29.)

✳✳✳✳✳✳✳✳✳✳✳✳✳✳✳✳✳✳✳✳✳✳✳✳✳

contractile cells in the cranial midline at stage 13 (see hatched areas in the map in Fig. 5).

If notoplate cells contacted neural plate cells, they would stick there. Any tangential forces acting among the cells would tend to hasten the midline extension by making such contacts more frequent. At least two active sources of tangential forces are possible. The observed contractions of the apical microfilaments

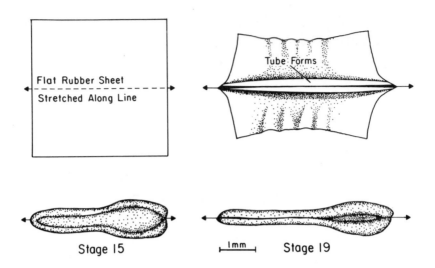

FIG. 15. This figure compares tube formation in a rubber sheet, pulled along a line, with neural tube formation between stages 15 and 19 in a newt embryo. The neural plate and tube are drawn to scale to accurately show the amount of midline elongation during this period of tube formation. (Derived from 28, 29).

****

that decrease apical surface area are tangential forces. Cell processes or filopodia (known to be capable of contractile forces) could extend among the cells and produce tangential forces. we have found such filopodia (and lamellipodia) all over the basal ends of the cells of the neural plate at stages 13 and 15 (Fig. 18).

<u>Does the neural plate change state from a viscoelastic system to an elastic system during neural tube formation?</u>

The notoplate area must behave during tube formation like a viscous fluid with its cells changing neighbors as they relocate along the midline, but the rest of the plate must behave like a solid or elastic system if midline elongation is to buckle the plate out of the plane.

One could imagine that the ten-fold increase in rate of midline elongation could emphasize the elastic properties of the surrounding tissue, but even though relatively faster, the rate of elongation at this time is still slow (0.15 m/hr).

By stage 15, neural plate cells are much longer than earlier, and their apical surfaces have greatly contracted (Figs. 10, 11).

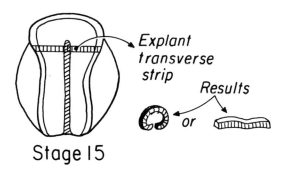

FIG. 16. This drawing illustrates an experiment in which a transverse strip of neural plate (vertical hatch) is explanted onto an agar plate in physiological saline solution. If neural tube formation is driven by change of cell shapes to a wedge form, then the excised strip should roll into a circle with the apical surface inside. In six cases, four rolled up in the wrong direction and two remained flat.

****

With the apical microfilament bundles drawn tight, with many filopodia and lamellipodia linking together the basal ends of the cells, and with long lateral surfaces of the cells adhering to one another, the changing of neighbors among plate cells could be much slowed, or stopped. It is possible that the plate has become, by stage 15, much more elastic and less viscous so the more rapid midline elongation might effectively work on an elastic system.

By limiting mixing with plate cells, increase of boundary between notoplate and neural plate would come from faster midline extension. The change of state of the plate could thus bring on the faster elongation.

We are examining the state of the neural plate after stage 15 with time-lapse cinematography, scanning electron microscopy, and experiments.

Do contracting plate cells pull equally in every direction?

For our simulation of neural plate shaping (30) we assumed that when the microfilament bundles contract the apical surface of a cell, nearby cells are drawn toward the center of shrinkage with equal force in every direction. The shapes of the plate cells at stage 13 make this assumption quite likely (Fig. 19).

By stage 15, apical surfaces of plate cells are stretched in the direction perpendicular to the long axis of the embryo, especially near the neural folds. The most likely causes of this

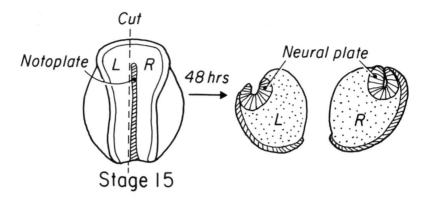

FIG. 17. This drawing illustrates an experiment in which embryos were cut in two just to the left of the notoplate region. The parts were then reared until controls reached closed tube stage 21, then were measured, fixed and sectioned. The part (L) with no notoplate (or notochord) failed to elongate at all, but the plate partially rolls into a tube. The part that contained all the notoplate (R) elongated normally and rolls the plate into a tube. Results were similar in 12 cases.

****

stretching are the tensions produced by the elongating midline and the resistance of the contiguous epidermis. Neural plates, removed from the embryo at stage 15 and later, immediately narrow toward the midline (see Fig. 4 in 28). I judge this to be due to the relaxation of the elastic stretch in these cells.

Jacobson and Gordon (30) searched for cells maximally stretched in the plane of the plate of the stage 15 embryo. Long axes were always in the medio-lateral direction, and cells were most stretched near the neural folds. We calculated the average length to width ratio of ten such maximally stretched cells at 9.6.

One possible consequence of such stretching of plate cells in the plane of the plate is that subsequent contraction of their microfilament bundles to reduce their apical surfaces would produce anisotropic forces in the plane of the plate; the pull in the medio-lateral direction would be much greater than in the anteroposterior direction.

The extension of the midline, which most likely stretched the apical surfaces in the mediolateral direction, would now co-opt most of the shrinkage of those cells to augment plate closure into a tube. This is a kind of transfer of anisotropy.

Other simulations of neurulation

Oster, Odell, Burnside and Alberch (65, and personal communication) are simulating amphioxus gastrulation, insect ventral furrow formation, and vertebrate neural tube formation with a model that describes the mechanical forces of contracting microfilament networks in cells.

The advantage of the model they propose is that the driving force is directly related to mechanical properties of microfilaments in changing cell shape, and the mechanical interactions among cells seem to account for coordinated movements.

So far their simulations have all been done on sections through embryos and have not yet encompassed the global properties and observed behaviors in, for example, the whole neural plate.

We (Gordon and I, Oster and Odell) have been discussing what is necessary to adapt this approach to the whole plate.

The failure of proper tube formation

Defects of the neural tube are the most common congenital malformations in human beings. Anencephaly, which occurs in one per thousand births (59), results from a failure of the cranial ends of the neural plate to complete tube formation. Anencephaly, together with spina bifida cystica and hydrocephalus account for more than 90% of congenital malformatons of the nervous system, and nearly a third of all major congenital malformations recognizable at or shortly after birth (47).

To understand the mechanisms that cause such defects, the mechanisms of normal development must be understood first.

NEURAL TUBE EXPANSION AND BULGE AND FURROW FORMATION

Organized mechanical forces have an important role in further shaping the neural tube once it forms. As neural tube closes, it enfolds within itself a space that becomes the ventricles of the brain and the spinal canal. Some time after tube closure, these cavities greatly enlarge and the expanding brain becomes pinched into bulges and furrows.

During the five hour period between chick embryo stages 11 and 12 (26), little expansion of the brain occurs, but in the five hours between stages 12 and 14 the brain expands greatly, bulges and furrows form, and cranial flexure takes place (Fig. 20).

the key event at stage 12 that brings this on is the occlusion of the spinal canal in the trunk region. The sides of the spinal canal press tightly together, creating a closed fluid compartment in the brain ventricles and anterior spinal canal. Prior to this occurence, cerebrospinal fluid could move down the spinal canal and exit through the open plate at the rear. Once the canal closes, cerebrospinal fluid accumulates in the brain ventricles

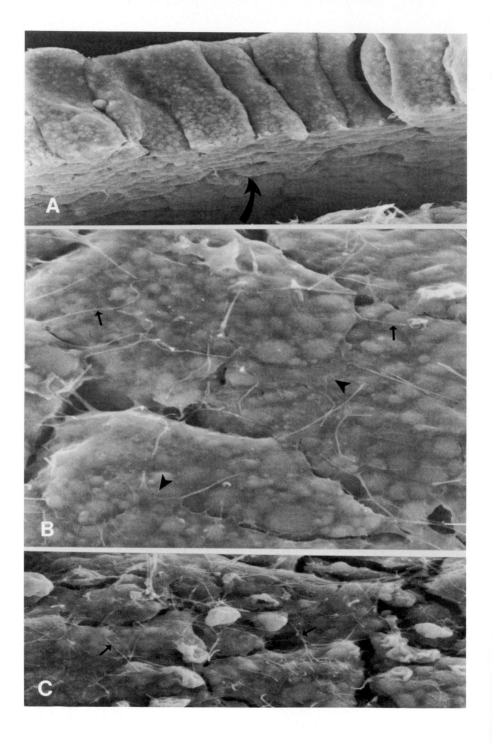

FIG. 18. Scanning electron micrographs show (A) the edge and underside of the neural plate of a newt at stage 13. The mesoderm has separated cleanly from the plate (500 X). (B) the undersurface of the stage 13 neural plate (1500 X) shows numerous filopodia (small arrows) stretching between the basal ends of the plate cells, as well as broad lamellipodia (arrow heads) stretching from cell to cell. (C) the undersurface of the stage 15 neural plate is similarly covered with filopodia passing between the basal ends of the cells (small arrows) (1500 X).

****

and produces an internal pressure that blows the brain up like a balloon (16, 38, 39, 67, 14).

The role of cerebrospinal fluid pressure can be demonstrated by putting a capillary tube into the brain ventricle and releasing the cerebrospinal fluid ("intubated", Fig. 20). The brain ventricles fail to expand and nervous tissue folds into the cavities (16). Early brain expansion requires a positive cerebrospinal fluid pressure.

Brains of intubated chick embryos appear very similar to the malformed brains in aborted human fetuses that Patten (66) attributed to "neural overgrowth." The experimentally produced malformation in chick embryos is definitely an undergrowth of brain tissue (6, 37, 90, 16).

When the ventricle fails to expand due to loss of cerebrospinal fluid pressure, the brain wall continues to grow at a reduced rate and folds into the cavity (16).

The normal ballooning of the brain must follow some interesting rules. for example, the neural tube approximates a closed hollow cylinder with an internal fluid pressure. Such a system must follow the law of Laplace, which for these circumstances could be stated: the forces that tend to expand the walls are proportional to the radius of the cylinder.

Since, during plate shaping, most of the bulk of the neural plate is packed into future brain plate (30), when the neural tube is formed, the brain is already of much greater radius than spinal cord. Thus it is brain that commences expansion when cerebrospinal fluid pressure appears. Once expansion has begun, brain radius becomes even greater and expansion increases. The brain balloons.

The embryo might take advantage of the ballooning to shape itself into bulges and furrows. Differential resistance to expansion in the brain walls, the matrix and mesenchyme surrounding the brain, or the epidermis around that could produce furrows some places and bulges others. This possibility is being systematically investigated.

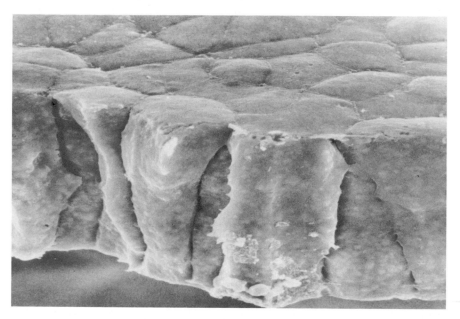

FIG. 19. Scanning electron micrograph (700 X) of the top and edge of a stage 13 neural plate. The apical surfaces are mostly not stretched, so when they contract they pull equally in every direction.

****

After these studies were done in chick embryos, I took a look at similar stages in the newt embryo (28). Brain expansion is evident in the newt embryo between stages 21 and 34 when growth commences (Fig. 1) and the brain has made bulges and furrows and formed a cranial flexure. Assuming that cerebrospinal fluid pressure is responsible for this early brain expansion, then two interesting conclusions emerge. First, there is no heart beat between stages 21 and 34 so any cerebrospinal fluid pressure in these embryos would have to result from secretion pressure since no filtration pressure exists. Secondly, if the brain is to expand as the cavity enlarges, the brain must do so at the expense of wall thickness since no growth is occurring. Measurments show this is exactly what happens. The walls of the various brain vesicles thin (by different amounts) to stage 34 (when growth commences) then they thicken while they continue to expand (28).

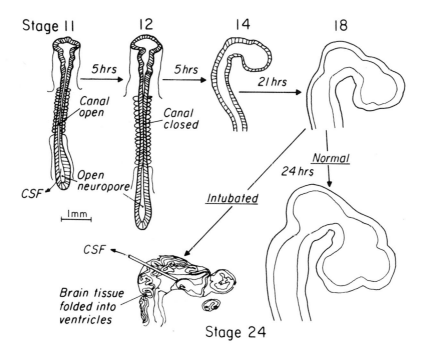

FIG. 20. Drawings of chick embryos and brains, all to the same
scale. At stage 11, any cerebrospinal fluid (CSF) formed in the
brain ventricles would pass down the spinal canal and out the
posterior neuropore where the neural plate is still open. At
stage 12, the walls of the spinal cord become apposed and close
the spinal canal. CSF will now accumulate in the brain ventricles
and anterior spinal canal. The brain immediately begins to
expand, and bulges and furrows form. If a brain is intubated in
the mesencephalic cavity to release the CSF pressure, the cavity
and brain fail to expand, and brain tissue folds into the
ventricles (based on 16).

****

CONCLUSIONS

Some of the mechanisms responsible for shaping the
neuroepithelium into plate, tube and brain with bulges and furrows
have been identified and their relative contributions to shaping
processes assessed.

The forces within and among cells generated by contractions of
microfilament networks and bundles certainly help shape the neural
plate and tube, but cannot account for major aspects of shape

change such as the very prominent midline elongation of the plate and tube.

Midline elongation is largely responsible for plate shaping and may be the dominant factor in buckling the plate out of the plane and folding it into a tube. This enigmatic anisotropic force is localized in the part of the neural plate that overlies the notochord (the notoplate), and possibly in the notochord as well. As the midline elongates, notoplate cells relocate along the midline, reducing plate width and cross-sectional area. This expansion of the boundary between notoplate cells and the cells of the rest of the neural plate may be driven by relative differences in adhesion between notoplate cells and other neural plate cells, together with jostling around by tangential forces generated by apical microfilament bundles and contractile filopodia among basal ends of the plate cells.

Midline elongation stretches plate cells in the mediolateral direction so any subsequent apical contraction they do is anisotropic, augmenting plate closure.

The viscoelastic properties of the neuroepithelium are critical factors in the shaping processes. It seems likely that most of the plate changes state from viscoelastic to elastic just as tube formation begins. This may allow the plate to buckle into a tube as the midline suddenly elongates.

Once the tube is closed, cerebrospinal fluid pressure accumulates within the brain ventricles and spinal canal and is responsible for the initial expansion of the brain. As the early brain blows up like a balloon, there is good opportunity to acquire the observed bulges and furrows by imposition of differential resistance to expansion in or on the walls of the tube.

It will take much more probing of these complicated physico-chemical systems to discover finally all the rules of nervous system shaping. We must be willing to deal with the complexities, to make testable models, to test them, and to discard or change models until they finally conform to what embryos are doing.

ACKNOWLEDGEMENTS

Much of the work described in this chapter was done with my collaborator, Richard Gordon. Some of the brain expansion studies were done with Mary Desmond. My former student, Beth Burnside, mapped the cell movements in the neural plate. Technical assistance for most of these studies was provided by Gertrud Threm. My colleague Stephen Meier assisted with the scanning electron micrographs. The work was supported by grant number HD 03803 from the National Institutes of Health.

REFERENCES

1. Baker, P. C. and T. E. Schroeder (1967): *Develop. Biol.*, 15:432-450.

2. Balinsky, B. I. (1961): Symposium on Germ Cells and Development, pp. 550-563, Inst. Int. d'Embryologie e Fondazione A. Baselli, Pavia.
3. Bancroft, M. and R. Bellairs (1975): Anat. Embryol., 147:309-355.
4. Bellairs, R. (1959): J. Embryol. Exp. Morph., 7:94-116.
5. Bellairs, R., A. S. G. Curtis, and E. J. Sanders (1978): J. Embryol. Exp. Morph., 46:207-213.
6. Berquist, H. (1960): J. Embryol. Exp. Morph., 8:69-72.
7. Billett, F. S., P. Bowman, and D. Pugh (1971): J. Embryol. Exp. Morph., 35:385-403.
8. Bowman, P. (1967): J. Embryol. Exp. Morph., 17:425-431.
9. Brown, M. G., V. Hamburger, and F. O. Schmitt (1941): J. Exp. Zool., 88:353-372.
10. Burnside, B. (1971): Develop. Biol., 26:416-441.
11. Burnside, B. (1973): Amer. Zool., 13:989-1006.
12. Burnside, B. and A. G. Jacobson (1968): Develop. Biol., 18:537-552.
13. Camatini, M. and S. Ranzi (1976): Acta Embryol. Exp., 1:81-113.
14. Coulombre, A. J. and J. L. Coulombre (1958): Anat. Rec., 130:289-290.
15. Davis, J. O. (1944): Biol. Bull., 87:73-95.
16. Desmond, M. E. and A. G. Jacobson (1977): Develop. Biol., 57:188-198.
17. Freeman, B. G. (1972): J. Embryol. Exp. Morph., 28:437-448.
18. Giersberg, H. (1924): Roux. Arch., 103:387-424.
19. Gillette, R. (1944): J. Exp. Zool., 96:201-222.
20. Glaser, O. C. (1914): Anat. Rec., 8:525-551.
21. Glaser, O. C. (1916): Science, 44:505-509.
22. Goerttler, K. (1925): Roux Arch., 106:503-541.
23. Gordon, R. and A. G. Jacobson (1978): Scientific American, 238:106-113.
24. Granholm, N. H. and J. R. Baker (1970): Develop. Biol., 23:563-584.
25. Gustafson, T. and L. Wolpert (1967): Biol. Rev., 42:442-498.
26. Hamburger, V. and H. Hamilton (1951): J. Morphol., 88:49-92.
27. Handel, M. A. and L. E. Roth (1971): Develop. Biol., 25:78-95.
28. Jacobson, A. G. (1978): Zoon, 6:13-21.
29. Jacobson, A. G. (1980): Amer. Zool., (in press).
30. Jacobson, A. G. and R. Gordon (1976): J. Exp. Zool., 197:191-246.
31. Jacobson, A. G. and R. Gordon (1976): J. Supramolecular Structure, 5:371-380.
32. Jacobson, C.-O. (1959): J. Embryol. Exp. Morph., 7:1-21.
33. Jacobson, C.-O. (1962): Zool. Bidrag (Uppsala), 35:433-449.
34. Jacobson, C.-O. (1970): J. Embryol. Exp. Morph., 23:463-471.
35. Jacobson, C.-O. and A. Jacobson (1973): Zoon, 1:17-21.
36. Jacobson, C.-O. and J. Lofberg (1969): Zool. Bidrag (Uppsala), 38:233-239.

37. Jelínek, R. (1961): Cesk. Morfol., 9:151-161.
38. Jelínek, R. and T. Pexieder (1968): Physiol. Bohemoslov., 17:297-305.
39. Jelínek,   R.   and T. Pexieder (1970): Folia Morphol., 18:102-110.
40. Karfunkel, P. (1971): Develop. Biol., 25:30-56.
41. Karfunkel, P. (1972): J. Exp. Zool., 181:289-302.
42. Karfunkel, P. (1974): Int. Rev. Cytol., 38:245-271.
43. Keller, R. (1975): Develop. Biol., 48:222-241.
44. Keller, R. (1975): Develop. Biol., 51:118-137.
45. Kelley, R. O. (1969): J. Exp. Zool., 170:157-180.
46. Kitchin, I. C. (1949): J. Exp. Zool., 112:393-415.
47. Kurtzyke, J. F., I. D. Goldberg, and L. T. Kurland (1973): Neurology, 23:483-496.
48. Lee, H. (1976): Develop. Biol., 48:392-399.
49. Lee, H., A. K. Deshpande, and G. W. Kalmus (1974): J. Embryol. Exp. Morph., 32:835-848.
50. Lee, H., N. Karasanyi, and R. G. Nagele, Jr. (1978): J. Embryol. Exp. Morph., 46:5-20.
51. Lee, H. and W. Poprycz (1970): Growth, 34:437-454.
52. Lewis, W. H. (1947): Anat. Rec., 97:139-156.
53. Linville, P. L. and T. H. Shepard (1972): Nature New Biol., 236:246-247.
54. Lofberg, J. (1974): Develop. Biol., 36:311-329.
55. Lofberg, J. and C.-O. Jacobson (1974): Zoon, 2:85-98.
56. Mak, L. L. (1978): Develop. Biol., 65:435-446.
57. Manchot, E. (1929): Roux Arch., 116:689-708.
58. Messier, P.-E. and C. Auclair (1974): Develop. Biol., 36:218-223.
59. Moore, K. L. (1977): The Developing Human. Clinically Oriented Embryology, Second edition, W. B. Saunders Company, Philadelphia, London, Toronto.
60. Moran, D. J. and R. W. Rice (1975): J. Cell. Biol., 64:172-180.
61. Morriss, G. M. and M. Solursh (1978): J. Embryol. Exp. Morph., 46:37-52.
62. Nagele, R. G. and H. Lee (1979): J. Exp. Zool., 210:89-106.
63. O'Rahilly, R. (1973): Developmental Stages in Human Embryos. Including a Survey of the Carnegie Collection. Part A: Embryos of the First Three Weeks (Stages 1 to 9). Carnegie Institution of Washington Publication 631.
64. O'Rahilly, R. and E. Gardner (1971): Z. Anat. Entwickl.- Gesch., 134:1-12.
65. Oster, G. F., G. Odell, B. Burnside, and P. Alberch (1979): Amer. Zool., 19:1014.
66. Patten, B. (1952): Anat. Rec., 113:381-393.
67. Pexieder, T. and R. Jelinek (1970): Folia Morph., 18:181-192.
68. Revel, J. P. and S. S. Brown (1976): Cold Spring Harbor Symp. Quant. Biol., 40:433-455.
69. Rhumbler, L. (1902): Roux Arch., 14:401-476.

70. Rice, R. W. and D. J. Moran (1977): <u>J. Exp. Zool.</u>, 201:471-478.
71. Rosenquist, G. C. (1966): <u>Contrib. Embryol. Carnegie Inst.</u>, 38:71-123.
72. Roux, W. (1885): <u>Z. Biol.</u>, 21:411-526.
73. Sadler, T. W. (1978): <u>Anat. Rec.</u>, 191:345-350.
74. Santander, R. G. and G. M. Cuadrado (1976): <u>Acta Anat.</u>, 95:368-383.
75. Schroeder, T. E. (1970): <u>J. Embryol. Exp. Morph.</u>, 23:427-462.
76. Selman, G. G. (1955): <u>Proc. R. Phys. Soc. Edinburgh</u>, 24:24-27.
77. Spratt, N. T. (1952): <u>J. Exp. Zool.</u>, 120:109-130.
78. Steinberg, M. S. (1964): In: <u>Cellular Membranes in Development</u>, edited by M. Locke, pp. 321-366. Academic Press, New York.
79. Tarin, D. (1971): <u>J. Anat.</u>, 109:535-547.
80. Tarin, D. (1972): <u>J. Anat.</u>, 111:1-28.
81. Thompson, D. W. (1952): <u>On Growth and Form</u>. Cambridge Univ. Press, Cambridge.
82. Trinkaus, J. P. (1969): <u>Cells Into Organs. The Forces that Shape the Embryo</u>, pp. 159-165. Prentice-Hall, Inc., Englewood Cliffs, New Jersey.
83. Trinkaus, J. P. (1976): In: <u>The Cell Surface in Animal Embryogenesis and Development</u>, edited by G. Poste and G. L. Nicolson. <u>Cell Surface Review</u>, 1:225-329.
84. Twitty, V. C. and D. Bodenstein (1962): In: <u>Experimental Embryology</u>, R. Rugh, p. 90. Burgess, Minneapolis.
85. Vaage, S. (1969): <u>Advan. Anat. Embryol. Cell Biol.</u>, 41:8-87.
86. Vogt, W. (1929): <u>Roux Arch.</u>, 120:385-706.
87. Waddington, C. H. (1932): <u>Phil. Trans. Roy. Soc. London, Ser. B.</u>, 221:179-230.
88. Waterman, R. E. (1976): <u>Am. J. Anat.</u>, 146:151-172.
89. Wetzel, R. (1929): <u>Roux Arch.</u>, 119:118-321.
90. Wilson, D. B. (1974): <u>Brain Res.</u>, 69:41-48.
91. Wilson, D. B. and L. A. Finta (1980): <u>J. Embryol. Exp. Morph.</u>, 55:279-290.

Morphogenesis and Pattern Formation,
edited by T. G. Connelly et al.,
Raven Press, New York © 1981.

Coordinate Systems and Morphogenesis

Fred L. Bookstein

Center for Human Growth and Development, University of Michigan, Ann Arbor, Michigan 48109

In recent years the theoretical framework of morphogenetic studies has undergone a morphogenesis of its own, culminating in a novel structure: positional information. According to this concept, normal, uncommitted cells are presumed to discern their position in a cell mass by interpreting values or gradients of unnamed, hypothetical qualities and to respond by directed differentiation. Certain striking experiments in dysmorphogenesis are shown to be consistent with the existence of such values or gradients. The results of these experiments are often interpreted in terms of coordinate "systems", usually Cartesian or polar, with convenient formal symmetries and order relations. The axiom of positional information has been applied to studies of budding, metamorphosis, regeneration, retinotectal connectivity, and other diverse phenomena.

I do not intend here to survey this literature from my formal, geometric point of view. I hope rather to show, through examples, that the range of meaningful coordinate systems is much broader than biologists generally realize. Coordinate systems can be unearthed which match biological structure rather closely.

Types of Coordinate Systems

Conventional applications of the notion of coordinate systems to morphogenesis are rooted in a fundamental mathematical misunderstanding. Consider, for instance, the familiar Cartesian coordinate system of squared grid paper. The essence of this arrangement is the collection of grid lines themselves. These are loci of points which are quite literally co-ordinated-- which have the same value on abscissa or ordinate, one coordinate or the other. The ordered pairs (x,y) which we use to label individual points are pairs of curves, not pairs of numbers. Of course, we are used to labelling each curve by a very convenient number of its own, the position at which it intersects a fixed axis; and these numbers have an algebra which corresponds to the ordinary geometry of the plane. However, more general coordinate systems, such as I shall display below, do not allow this unambiguous association of number pairs with points. When it is mere points we intend to describe, that is a clear advantage of the Cartesian and polar systems. But when our interest is in gradients, polarities, or boundaries of extended regions, then the coordinate curves themselves must take priority. In such circumstances the formalism of the ordered pair of numbers is highly misleading.

The two systems most familiar to us, Cartesian coordinates and polar coordinates, are unfortunately not typical of coordinate systems likely to be encountered in practice. In these special systems the curves fall into two distinct <u>families</u> (vertical and horizontal lines, or radii and circles) such that each curve of either set intersects each curve of the other set once and only once. If we assume this about the coordinate system "suggested" by an experiment, its particulars naturally become derivable from the data at hand. But an indefinite variety of other coordinate systems can be devised all consonant with any set of experiments. These will lead to quite different schemes of morphogens and predictions and different modes of explanation.

To grasp the differences of the typical coordinate system from the Cartesian or polar, one should set aside questions of how the coordinate curves of a family are spaced and how they curve, and should also ignore such singularities as the origin of the polar system. There still remain to be considered the intersections and interconnections between the curve systems, which may bear unfamiliar intricacies and contingencies. For a formal classification the reader must turn to modern treatises of global differential geometry. In this short pictorial note, I must content myself with four sketches of interesting examples.

<u>Multiple Families of Coordinate Curves.</u> There may be more than two families of coordinate curves necessary for the specification of a two-dimensional system. Consider the set of coordinate curves in Figure 1. The curves labelled "1" clearly compose a systematically varying family perpendicular to all the curves labeled "2" wherever they intersect. The "2" curves are likewise perpendicular to the "3" curves, but these latter, in turn, are perpendicular to the "1" curves. To specify a point, therefore, may require coordinates 1 and 2, 2 and 3, or 3 and 1, depending on the sector of the diagram. The three separate quantities required here are uncorrelated, but their domains of influence are different.

The absence of appropriate literature notwithstanding, it is easy to imagine experimental results suggesting a coordinate system such as this, in which there are more than two morphogens. Suppose that we transplant a patch of tissue from the 1-2 sectors of Fig. 1, NNE or SSW. If we move this patch to the 2-3 sector, its differentiation ought to be guided by values (or reversals or gradients) on coordinate "2"; but if we transplant it to the 1-3 sector its fate would be decided instead by values of coordinate "1". A bit of the 2-3 sector transplanted to the same place would have its fate determined by coordinate "3" instead. Such a

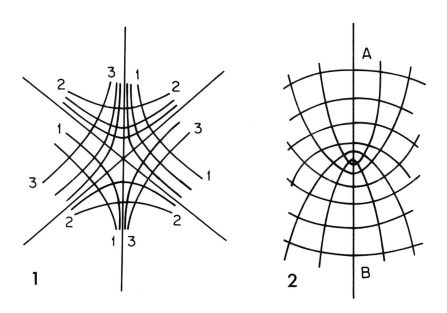

1

2

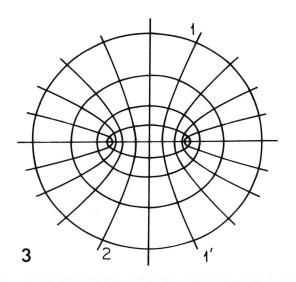

3

"superfluous dimensions model" can usually be arranged to reconcile inconsistencies among the results of diverse manipulations.

Independent Polarities.   Independent polarities, which I will here refer to as "horizontal" and "vertical", may reverse themselves or be interchanged from region to region of an extended structure.   In this regard consider Figure 2.   The patches of coordinate grid near A and B look like perfectly ordinary graph paper;   but the verticals at A are coordinated in fact with the horizontals at B, and vice versa.   Above the middle of interval AB, the grid is aligned with neither end, but rather is halfway in between, rotated by 45 degrees.

It   is   also   possible   for   polarities   to   be   consistently discriminable but individually reversed from end to end of a tissue.   Figure 3, when viewed from a distance, strongly resembles polar   coordinates: it   shows   ovals   and   radii.   However, end 1 is coordinated not with end 2 but with end 1'.   Clockwise may be interchanged with counterclockwise, in other words, across an axis which   appears   at   a   distance to have no special function in the system at all, i.e. which might go   unsuspected.   If we further reverse   vertical   polarity between the middle and both ends there results the system of Fig. 4, two polar schemes conjoined at their radii   while   the   cyclic   families   remain   separate.   Figure 5 displays   yet   another   transformation   of Fig. 3 wherein the left half has been inverted with respect to the   right.   (Notice that another singularity has been forced upon us.)

Only   a   complex   series   of   experiments   is   capable of discriminating among these alternatives to polar coordinates.   In the absence of this more precise geometric analysis the researcher will   seriously   misapprehend   the   form   of the morphogenetic gradients putatively responsible for the phenomenon.

Polar-like Systems.   Coordinates generally "radial" with respect to one   singularity   (center)   can   be   generally   azimuthal   with respect   to   another.   In   Figure   6   we   see an instance of this interlacing of polar-like systems.   Note that, as with   Figure   1, more   than two coordinates are required to specify the position of a point in terms of the coordinate curves--we   need   to   know,   as before,   which   families   of   curves   are   involved   in   the specification.   Figure 7 shows   a   related   example   in   which   the interlacing   involves   non-adjacent   centers.   As in the previous examples, the full record of findings generated   by   this   spatial arrangement   of   gradients   and   polarities   is   perplexing in the context of any simpler model.

Surfaces in Three-Dimensional Space.   The geometry likeliest   to be   directly   relevant   to our experiments is not of ovals on two-dimensional paper, but of   surfaces   in   three-dimensional   space. The nonmathematician expects a three-dimensional coordinate system to   look   like a packing crate: three families of surfaces each of which intersects all surfaces of the other two families in   simple curves.   As   in   the   plane,   these   natural   criteria   admit possibilities fundamentally different from Cartesian or   spherical

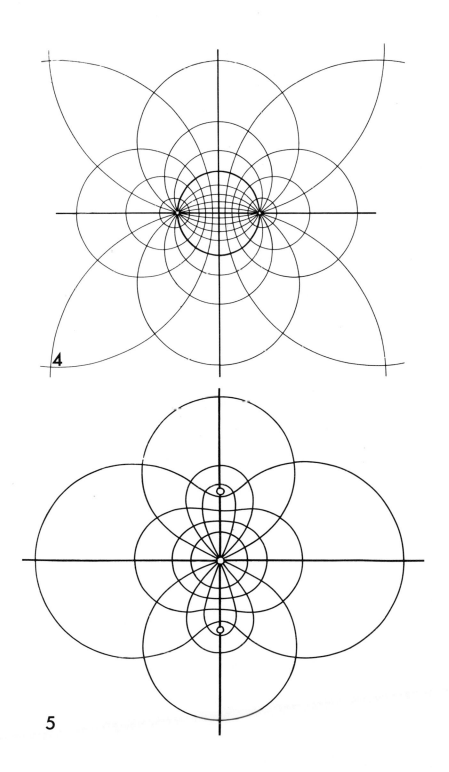

4

5

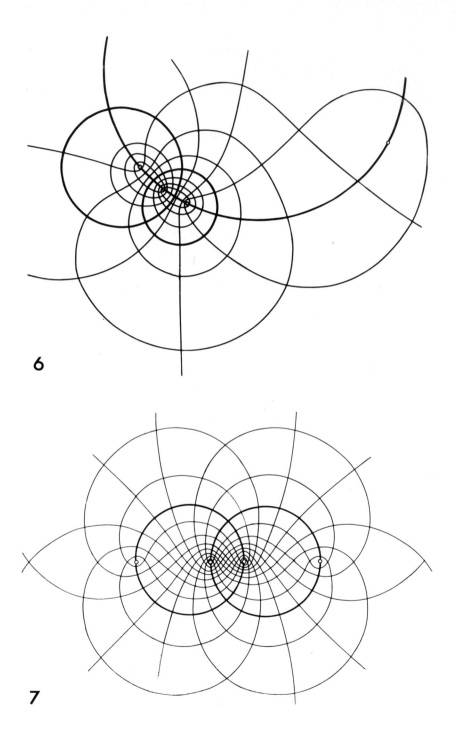

6

7

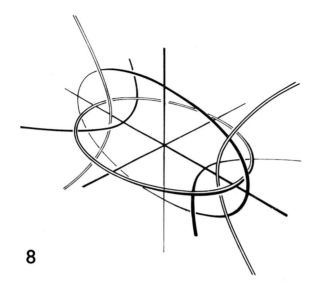

8

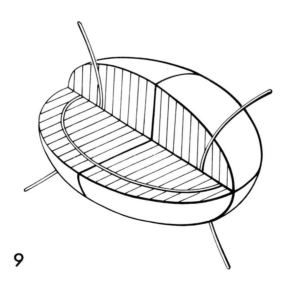

9

coordinates. For instance, consider Figures 8-12, taken from the classic work Geometry and the Imagination of Hilbert and Cohn-Vossen. Figure 8 shows a framework of three curves in space, two ellipses and a hyperbola, about which we hang three families of surfaces. The first family, one member of which is shown in Figure 9, consists of ellipsoids spanning the ellipse of Figure 8. The second family consists of two-piece hyperboloids like that of Figure 10. The third family, the one-piece hyperboloids, is exemplified in Figure 11. Together these surfaces compose the so-called confocal system assembled in Figure 12. (The reader should distinguish between hyperbolas and ellipses, which are flat curves, and hyperboloids and ellipsoids, which are curving surfaces.) For instance, the intersections of any of the ellipsoids with each surface of the other two types yields, for the ellipsoids, a coordinate system sketched in Figure 13. This is just a version of the interlaced system of Figure 16. The coordinate curves are now all overlapping loops, as in Figure 14. Such curves can be distorted to apply to any closed surface, that is, any surface which has an interior.

Figure 15 is from an ongoing project on vertebrate limb regeneration directed by my collaborator, Dr. Thomas Connelly. By reconstruction of serial sections the figure depicts two surfaces, one inside the other. The outer form, drawn in solid lines, is the epithelial-mesenchymal boundary of an Early Digit stage regeneration blastema of the newt. The animal had been injected with labeled thymidine 4-5 hours prior to sacrifice. The inner form, drawn in dashed lines, is the surface of the region within which the thymidine labeling index, derived by automated counts of nuclei in radioautograms, was 25% or greater. The form of this surface, which presumably adumbrates the region of highest mitotic activity, strongly resembles the centric system I have just been sketching. In fact, the centers (foci near the endpoints of the elongated inner surface) correspond closely to the tips of two digits: that most recently formed, and that about to be formed next. There is suggested here a model for digit determination in terms of a sequence of chemical foci rather than standing waves--- but this speculation is beyond the scope of the present essay.

In the confocal coordinate system the curves scribed on the tall hyperboloids (Fig. 11) have the form of horizontal ellipses and vertical hyperbolas: one coordinate linear, one angular. But these hyperboloids could have been just as well assigned the coordinate system shown in two views in Figure 16. Just as with two-dimensional Cartesian coordinates, we have two systems of straight lines such that each line of either system intersects each line of the other system just once. Now, however, the coordinates of the lines themselves are values on a single shared elliptical curve such as the equator. Unlike closed surfaces, tubular structures may have a left "angle" and a right "angle", two coordinates of opposite sense of spiraling, with no length coordinate at all.

These algebraically simple coordinate systems may be reflected

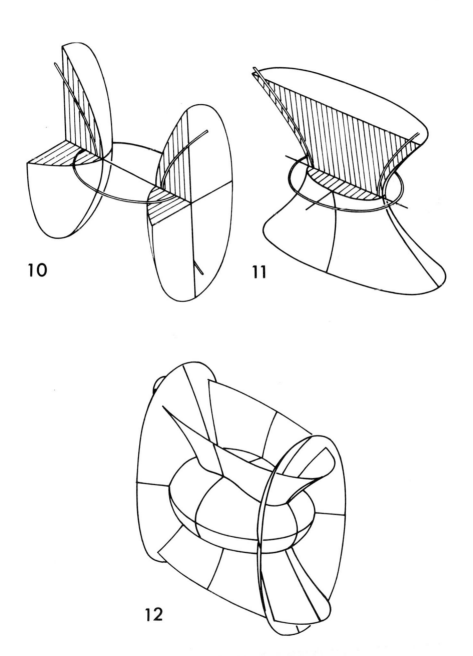

10

11

12

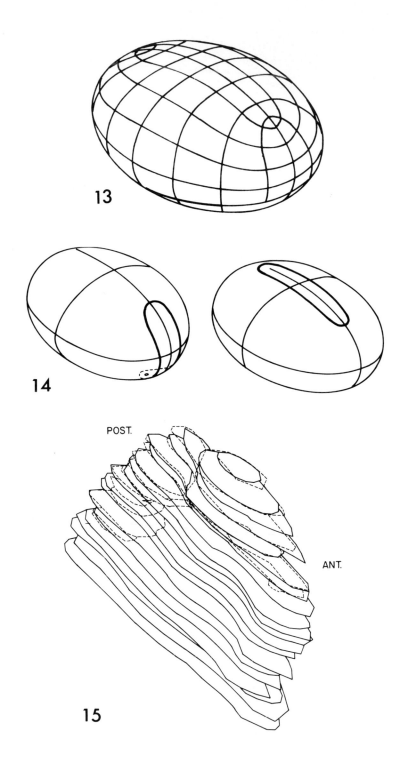

13

14

POST.

ANT.

15

in lines or planes, by halves of their ranges, to yield more oddly polarized versions analogous to Figures 4 and 5. Or the axes of Figure 8 may be bent around into more general position. Then the surfaces become quite a bit more organic-looking, as in Figures 17 and 18 (which each show a single family of surfaces to which two others are orthogonal).

By this point it should be clear to the reader that the study of form and position by coordinate systems is seriously damaged when restricted to Cartesian and polar models only. The dysmorphogeneses of transplantation cannot be interpreted if the interlacing of coordinate curves is not fully explored. Otherwise, in the absence of definitive morphogenetic assays, experimental data must be ambiguous.

Detection of Biological Coordinate Systems

To understand how data can be used to detect biological coordinate systems, let us look at the simplest case, analysis in a single dimension. For instance, what would be the appropriate coordinate system, Cartesian, polar, or otherwise, for a loop-shaped locus of tissue? We will ignore all aspects of its geometry except for the looping. That is, we will treat the item as a simple curve without width or thickness. In particular, the apparent "interior" of the loop is just an area on this paper, convenient for the sketching of the lines. To better understand the geometry we may distort it ad libitum, as it does not represent coordinated loci of actual tissue.

The Cartesian model assigns an ordinate to every point of the loop, an ordinate which runs on a vertical scale, from "up" to "down" and back again (Fig. 19). There is a highest point, A and a lowest point, B (or vice versa). According to the hypothesis behind the model, whenever any point x is relocated to a point y, the discontinuity of coordinate values which is created is filled in by intercalations on both sides. To draw the resulting configuration we may hold the coordinate curves level and bend the loop around appropriately, forming a level chart (Fig.20a). In this sketch the space between the intercalated peninsula and the original boundary is meaningless; only changes of sign of the coordinate gradient are shown. The reader may prefer instead to hold the loop fixed and split the coordinate curves, as in the coordination diagram (Fig.20b). Here contours leading to x separate the two loci of coordinate value y. Although we are not presently considering the interior of the loop, this figure suggests the existence of an interior point at which the locus for coordinate level y first becomes ambiguous. Either presentation indicates how relocating a tissue x should generate a small region symmetric about the new location of x. The reverse experiment, which relocates point y to location x, results in the same mirrored regeneration (Fig. 20c).

From this simple geometry we can draw certain formal deductions which the data must not contradict if the model is to apply. For

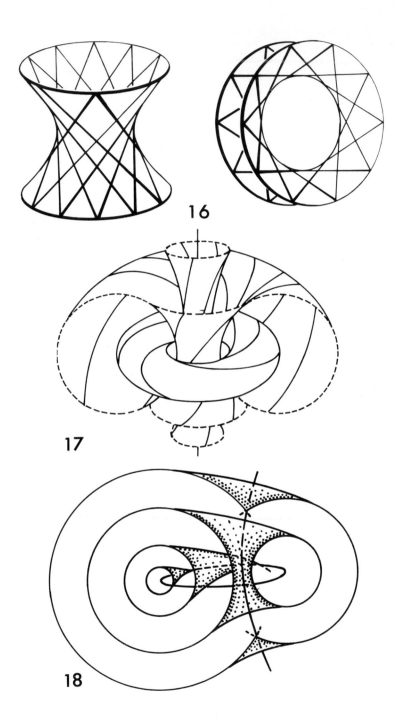

16

17

18

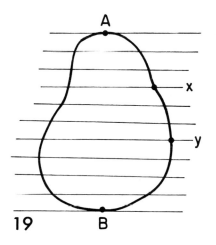

19

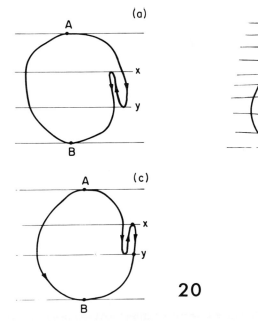

20

each point x that is not A or B there must be another point x', on
the other arc from A to B, that is <u>coordinated</u> with x according to
the literal meaning of that phrase suggested earlier.   Two such
pairs of coordinated equivalents, xx'   and yy', are shown in
Figure 21. Operationally speaking, points x and x' are
coordinated when the effect of transplanting x' to any locus y is
the same as the effect of transplanting x there.   The effect of
transplanting x to x', or vice versa, must be null. Points A and
B, highest and lowest, are uniquely characterized as the two
points to which no points can be coordinated in this sense.
Instead, if point A is transplanted to the position of point B, or
vice versa, there will result an intercalation which duplicates
the entire original loop of tissue (Fig. 22).

For any pair (x,x') of coordinated points, A is in between x
and x' on one arc of the loop and B is in between them on the
other   arc.   In geometrical language, the point-pair (A,B)
<u>separates</u> all pairs of coordinated points, but those pairs, like
(x,x')   and (y,y') in Figure 21, do not separate each other. Then
the special points A and B can never appear inside intercalated
regions, as neither is in between any other pair of coordinate
levels.

Other Cartesian loops can be sketched for which some of the
rules are violated in a systematic fashion. For instance, the
kidney-shaped level chart (Fig. 23a) corresponds to the
coordination diagram of Figure 23b. We see that some points have
a single coordinated point, like z or z', and others come in sets
of four, like the set y, y', y'', y'''. Finally, there is just
one set of three coordinated points x, x', x''. Of these three,
two, x' and x'', separate the points of the pairs, like z, from
the points of the quadruples, like y. Points A and A' are merely
a pair of coordinated points whose neighbors (y, y', y'', y''')
come in quadruples. The whole mirrored arc A-A' can be duplicated
experimentally by transplanting any x to the position of A or A'.
If we break the symmetry of A and A', as in Figure 24, the
resulting diagram is the same as Figure 20c, which came from a
general relocation within the simple system. The symmetric scheme
of Figure 23 arises from Figure 19 if the point x is transplanted
precisely to locus A.

In a quite different Cartesian scheme, Nature might have
duplicated B as well as A by imposing symmetry upon the cross-axis
of Figure 19 as well as the vertical axis. This provides
quadruples (x, x', x'', x''') of coordinate points except for A,
A', B, B', which are coordinated two by two. The resulting chart
(Fig. 25a) is clearer as the level chart of Figure 25b.   To
represent this loop on paper requires the illusion of three
dimensions.

All the Cartesian systems differ from the polar model in many
fundamentals.   In the basic polar scheme, or "clock model", there
are <u>no</u> corrdinated point pairs, but rather each point "tells a
different time". A suitable diagram replaces the level lines of
the Cartesian Figure 19 by radii from some formal center

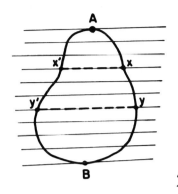

21

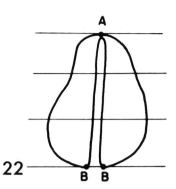

22

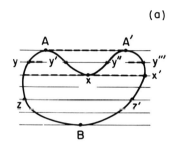

(a)

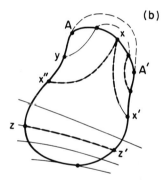

(b)

23

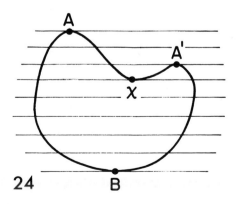

24

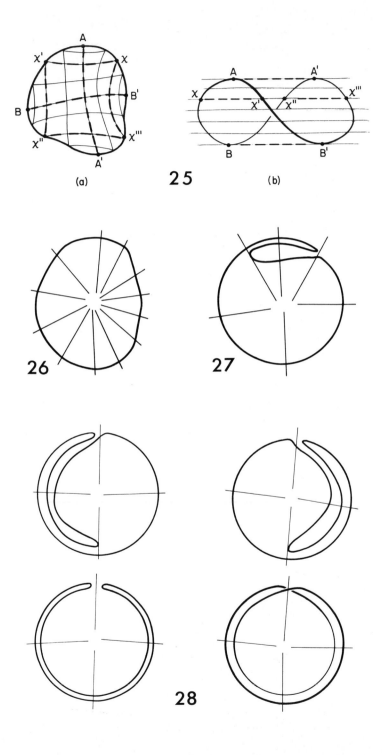

A

x'   x

B   B'

x''   x'''

A'

(a)

25

A   A'

x   x'   x''   x'''

B   B'

(b)

26

27

28

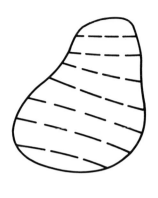

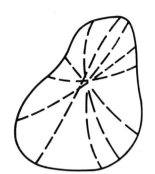

29

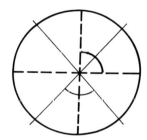
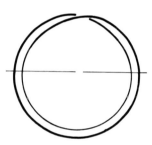

30

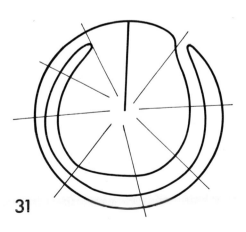

31

(Fig. 26). (This center is not to be presumed a point in the interior, which we are still proceeding without.) Nor are there, in this basic model, any special points on the circuit of the clock. The hypothesis behind the model demands, once again, that intercalation proceed via shortest paths (cf. Fig. 27). In this computation, any point may appear within the reduplicated segment.

There remains, nevertheless, a natural pairing of points of the loop, the pairing which is opposition: 12 o'clock versus 6, 3 o'clock versus 9, etc. These are point pairs for which the criterion of the shortest path is ambiguous. The organism cannot compute a reliable intercalation sequence, but will sometimes go clockwise, sometimes counterclockwise, more or less at random. The clock model demands that each point x of the clock have a single opposite point x' whose opposite, in turn, is x. While transplantation of the point x to most loci y will yield mirrored intercalations, as in the Cartesian case, transplantation of x to its opposite X+6 may result in any of the forms of Figure 28a-d. Two of these are mirrors, but two are full reduplications of the form--one clockwise (d), one counterclockwise (c).

I summarize these fundamental distinctions between the Cartesian and the polar models in terms of their natural pairing functions. Cartesian points are paired by the fact of coordination, equivalence under transplantation. Coordinate pairs (x, x'), (y, y') do not separate each other upon the loop of tissue, i.e. the interior lines of Figure 29a do not cross. Polar points are paired by the fact of opposition, ambiguity under transplantation. Each couple of pairs (x, x'), (y, y') separate each other upon the loop of tissue, i.e. the interior lines of Figure 29b all cross. The contrast between these models can thus be established "intrinsically", without recourse to any measurements or experiments upon the interior of the loop.

Like the Cartesian model, the polar scheme allows for systematic modifications. For instance, the "twenty-four hour clock" in Figure 30a, results in coordinated pairs (x, x') which are in opposition to other coordinated pairs (y, y'). In the figure coordination is shown by straight lines and opposition by 90 degree circular arcs. By analogy with Figure 28 we may draw out this same loop as a locus on the "true" cyclic coordinate as in Figure 30b. We saw this before (Fig. 28d) as one of the possibilities for intercalation between opposites. Another modification of the polar scheme introduces a fixed origin, 12 o'clock, which cannot be intercalated over. The "shortest path" is then reformulated to mean "the path omitting 12 o'clock" (Fig. 31; compare to Fig. 27).

These are the simplest cases of coordinate schemes, involving only a single spatial dimension. In this paper I have argued that the form of any empirical system can be properly established only by transplanting from each locus to every other locus, then submitting the findings to an exacting formal scrutiny. The appropriate methodology would have to include a probabilistic component reflecting experimental difficulties and the randomness of outcome intrinsic to biological computers.

Morphogenesis and Pattern Formation,
edited by T. G. Connelly et al.,
Raven Press, New York © 1981.

Discussion of Section V

STEINBERG: If neural folding is the consequence of this midline elongation as modeled by the stretched dental (rubber)dam, then removal of the notoplate-notochord complex ought to prevent neural folding.

JACOBSON: There is an experiment in which the embryo is cut into a half which has no notoplate or notochord in it. It does not elongate and it never closes itself into a tube, but it does roll up a little bit. The point is that I don't think that Nature works by dichotomies. I think it takes whatever it has available and uses a little bit of this and a little bit of that. What you are probably going to find is that there is some wedging and some elongation, rolling into a tube. Our job, and I think this is how the computer simulations really help, is to sort this out and see how much comes from one and how much comes from the other. That's what I hope we are leading to.

WOLPERT: This is an extremely impressive analysis. It's quite new to me that the elongation should lead to the closure of the tube. Am I right in thinking that the notochord is not playing a role in that elongation at that stage?

JACOBSON: The notochord is absolutely essential up to stage 15 and it's inseparable. There is no way that I can think of to separate it from the notoplate. We know that the notoplate is making those rearrangements so, in a formal sense, really it's the notoplate that's doing it; but the notochord is necessary for what it's doing. After stage 15, it is not necessary.

WOLPERT: That's when you begin to get the curling?

JACOBSON: Yes.

WOLPERT: I understand; so once again I wonder whether that analogy with the pigs was really a fair one because that was applying an extrinsic force to the system. Do you see my difficulty?

JACOBSON: I worried about that too, whether pulling on a sheet is the same as having a rod that expands in the midline. I asked our aerospace engineers, and they said: "That's totally secondary, you don't need to worry about that".

WOLPERT: So, it's the notoplate that is doing the elongation? I'm just trying to get a feel for what is causing that, because that in itself is very hard to understand.

JACOBSON: The relocation of those cells making more connections with the rest of the neural plate, so that it just attenuates along the line, requires a bias and a stabilization.

283

WOLPERT: What sort of program does one have to give the cells in order to make that rearrangement, and how cellular is this program (as opposed to extracellular)? You showed very beautifully that if you took a small fragment early on, it did its own thing. If you separate it into individual cells, so that they lose their coherence, do the individual cells do their own thing?

JACOBSON: Holtfreter and Burnside showed that you can isolate individual neural plate cells and they continue to elongate, but quantitatively, we don't know how much. That's difficult because they are curling.

WOLPERT: What sort of program do you have to give the cells in order to get that elongation?

JACOBSON: If it is indeed due to adhesive differences, you just have to have these two domains with adhesive differences in the range that allow for the Steinberg-type of mixing, and the constraint that those cells in the neural plate won't mix any more. Then perimeter elongation occurs.

BERNFIELD: I also wanted to ask you about the elongation of the notoplate. I think you have just answered it. You are hypothesizing that there is a difference in adhesion of the notoplate cells to the lateral plate cells.

JACOBSON: Yes, this is just one adhesive regime. There are probably others, but we haven't thought them all through yet.

BERNFIELD: Have you any idea what, in terms of their adhesive nature, would then be required for a change in adhesiveness from an early stage (stage 13) to the time when they become elongated?

JACOBSON: The working hypothesis that I presented doesn't require any change in adhesiveness to put it into that range; then the cells will work it out, given the bias and the stabilization in those early stages. Once a cell is a long rod it doesn't require so much stabilization. The problem is that it is an unstable boundary. It's like throwing alcohol in water.

BERNFIELD: Let me just ask you one more thing. Would the boundary between the two states of adhesion (notoplate versus the lateral plate) be the same regardless of where those cells are; whether they are elongated or placed in a more spherical shape?

JACOBSON: What you are asking is why don't we take some notoplate cells and some rest of the neural plate cells and disaggregate them. That's the kind of experiment we have to do, but we have just gotten to this point recently.

WAELSCH: Is there any correlation between the elongation of the cells and the state of determination in terms of nerve cell differentiation?

JACOBSON: This is still just a single cell thick neuroepithelium even as late as the brain-expansion stages. I don't know a thing about which cells are going to be glial cells or other cell types. All I know is that at the open neural plate stage these have the field characteristics of forebrain, midbrain and hindbrain as many people have shown. I don't think I'm answering your question.

WAELSCH: Haven't transplantation experiments been done at these different stages in order to ....

JACOBSON: The cells are all determined to be neural tissue by stage 13 and if you transplant a piece of beginning neural plate somewhere else it will make a host of neural derivatives.

MITTENTHAL: Let me ask a more specific version of Dr. Waelsch's question. Assume that you grafted the intubated brain region, which doesn't give the normal folding, into a normal embryo and then allowed it to continue to develop. If the normal ballooning out doesn't occur, do you think that the normal cell types will subsequently not differentiate? In other words, I'm asking you if you think it's possible that the determination of regions of the brain is a consequence of the ballooning which occurs previously?

JACOBSON: I know nothing about that, but I doubt it. I'm fairly certain that they're determined because since they are already in the neural plate, they must already be determined as far as being forebrain, midbrain and hindbrain.

MITTENTHAL: Isn't it possible that the direction of outgrowth of processes is influenced by the mechanical stresses that are set up by the ballooning?

JACOBSON: That's a whole new area that I haven't gotten into at all. Yes, I agree that it could very well have such an effect.

POOLE: Dr. Bookstein, I would like to make a comment and then ask a question. My comment is that I think that it's a little superficial to design coordinate systems according to the form. Form doesn't appear out of nowhere. It is generated by a bilateral system; it is generated through embryogenesis. There is a lot of classic information that says that there are coordinate systems in embryos and that they are graded along a particular axis. We live in a bilaterally symmetrical world. Doesn't that impose some restrictions on the types of coordinates that are significant for biological form-shaping systems? That's my comment.

My question is whether it might not be more important to look at the topological singularities the way Dave Stocum was suggesting and what Stu Newman was using in his model of chick limb outgrowth? Aren't the coordinate systems artificial. Perhaps the topological singularities in embryos might be important in specifying some degree of regulation.

BOOKSTEIN: I'll take the second question first. If your coordinate systems all have the same topology then, as in those analyses of van der Pol which all have the same underlying graph, then the information which is easiest to extract is certainly the parameteric information about the relation of the form to the topology and not the topology itself. For coordinate systems in embryos it may be that there is relatively little quantitative information and that the information is all topological. In that case, I would despair first of doing any kind of statistical analysis of populations, and second of doing any kind of analysis of variation. Rather, for the kinds of problems that will support intervention, I believe that the payoff for this, at least for quantitative morphometrics, has to be in areas which will support quantitation fairly straightforwardly. It is possible that the fundamental explanations of embryonic morphogenesis will involve topological universals; yet the study of their variations between species or over populations will involve quantitative measures within the same topology, so I'm not disagreeing with you.

On the point of bilateral symmetry, if I were studying what were bilaterally symmetrical in the projection I were using I would have to use a bilaterally symmetrical system, but these are all midsagittal, and so the question didn't arise in my analysis.

INKE: Did you observe any differences between the growth of the alveolar and the basal part of the mandible?

BOOKSTEIN: I was not able to do that because the data set which I was using for these outlines did not actually measure the alveolar part, but only connected it with a straight line where I could see it between the teeth. Thus, the data are insufficient. The next project is to do this, not on the basis of longitudinal data sets that happen to lie in archives, but to actually measure precisely what is required, probably on primates, and to analyze the part of growth of the parts of the mandible in greater detail. What you see is a holistic method and it is not powerful enough to make that distinction.

TREVOR: You discussed the problem of polar coordinates in which the point at the center is an awkward point. The angle at the very center of the coordinates is not defined. Polar coordinates have another problem as well. When you start at zero degrees and you go around the circle, the angle increases to 180 degrees, to 360 degrees and then right away it discontinuously jumps back to zero. That's no problem if you just want to use them as coordinates, but in Prof. Wolpert's work he says that coordinates represent a concentration of something or a phase-shift, something real that makes up these coordinates. I see a problem in this discontinuity and I wonder if you would comment on this?

BOOKSTEIN: That discontinuity can be removed simply by using the complex point on the circle as a coordinate. The angle is, in fact, a discontinuous representation of a continuously varying parameter. That isn't the problem I'm speaking of. The problem with polar coordinates is topological. There has to be a singularity inside the circle because it's gone around once and it has returned to its starting position, however it got there. It can go around the circle continuously. My main point was to bring these interpenetrating systems of polar coordinates to your attention because, as I say, they haven't been published in this century and no one but a few obscure archivists in math libraries know about them.

Morphogenesis and Pattern Formation,
edited by T. G. Connelly et al.,
Raven Press, New York © 1981.

Summary

Bruce M. Carlson

*Department of Anatomy and Division of Biological Sciences, University of Michigan, Ann
Arbor, Michigan 48109*

Instead of summarizing individual papers, I am going to try to construct a scheme of development that will highlight some of the major points of the meeting. As is always the case, this approach runs the risk of seeming to slight some ideas and to stress others.

Some of the most profound principles of morphogenesis are embodied in a morphologically simple phase of development which was not covered at this meeting. This is the transition from the single-celled zygote to the two-celled embryo. The zygote represents a potential individual and with time goes on to form a complete single individual. The two-cell stage also represents a single individual and normally develops as such. Yet, as has been shown in some of the oldest experiments in embryology, two individuals can be made to form merely by separating the blastomeres. In their original context, these experiments demonstrated the complete genetic and developmental potential of each blastomere. In the context of contemporary developmental biology, it could be very rewarding to devote more time to the problem of why, in normal development, the individuality inherent in each blastomere becomes subservient to the individuality of the organism as a whole. The essence of a number of the more complex regulative systems is probably embodied in the mechanisms controlling the integrity of the two-celled embryo.

There is increasing evidence (Wolpert) that early in development a coordinate system, probably superimposed upon the entire body, is established in the embryo. Nevertheless, there are still far more unknowns than facts. We do not know what kind of coordinate system or how early it is established. Embryologists are accustomed to thinking in terms of the Cartesian coordinate system, but are embryos? Bookstein showed us examples of many kinds of coordinate systems that could fit collected data. Perhaps one should design experiments so that the data could rule in or out certain of these systems. Regardless of the form of the coordinate system, if we are asked what we know about the physical basis for any coordinate system we can only honestly answer, virtually nothing.

Morphogenetic movements play a prominent role in many early developmental processes. Steinberg presented a number of amphibian systems in which cell sorting and migrations appear to be effected through differences in surface properties of cells in different germ layers or primordia. In recognition of the continuing discussions on the relative importance of direct cellular interactions versus matrix-mediated interactions in morphogenesis, it should be noted that extracellular matrix is very sparse in amphibian embryos, but it is plentiful in avian and mammalian embryos. The latter forms are the experimental objects commonly used in experiments involving the role of matrix, whereas amphibian embryos are favored by many investigators who work on cell-to-cell interactions.

After the germ layers have been laid down, the next major series of events is the formation of organ primordia (reviewed by Saxén). Almost every mechanism that has been proposed requires that groups of cells be able to receive signals or read cues and then respond to them. Regardless of one's bias regarding the nature of the signal there is some agreement about parameters of the system. (1) The process of receiving and responding is relatively slow, in the range of 10 or more hours. (2) The response of the receiving cells is different from what it would have been in the absence of the signal. (3) The nature of the response is appropriate to the genetic history of the cells. (4) The signal is usually general; the response is specific.

One of the first signal-response systems is the transformation of general ectoderm into the primordium of the nervous system, which was categorized by Saxén as a directive form of induction, probably mediated by diffusion. Even this classical, intensely studied system of induction was open to questions about the role of the matrix in the inductive process, and the possibility of transfer of positional values during induction.

As the primordia of most major organs are set up, there is a transfer from general to local developmental control. There is good evidence for positional effects during this phase. At this early phase of organogenesis, boundaries and organotypic characteristics are established, but fine control has not yet been exercised. Many organs begin to take shape as the result of continuous interactions between two tissue components. Usually one is dominant in controlling form and the other is permissive. In the dominant component the genetic message is becoming quite stable whereas it is less so in the permissive component. Once the dominant component is established, a firm memory is fixed in that tissue.

How might morphogenetic cell and tissue interactions be effected? One mechanism that has found particularly strong proponents among students of limb development (e.g. Wolpert) is by cells reading thresholds of diffusible substances along concentration gradients. Newman presented a specific model involving the diffusion of fibronectin in the limb bud.

Two specific models of cell-to-cell communication were proposed. On the basis of morphological evidence, Kelley stressed the potential importance of gap junctions as transfer sites of morphogenetic messages in limb mesenchyme. Steinberg presented new evidence of two varieties of aggregation factors on cells and suggested that this may be a potential basis for two-dimensional patterning, for example in retinotectal connections.

The importance of the matrix in communication between components of a system was often stressed during the symposium. Bernfield, using developing glands as his major example, presented considerable detail on the dynamics of cell surface and extracellular matrices and their relationship to branching morphogenesis. He cataloged four major cellular responses to the surrounding matrix: (1) proliferation, (2) change of cell shape, (3) cell adhesion, and (4) cell death. Kollar pointed out the many components in matrix and the large number of possible combinations of these components. He related specific cellular responses to specific alterations of the matrix and emphasized the potential informational content of the matrix.

In the development of external structures, where great precision of gross form is required, positional effects seem particularly important. There are, however, many models designed to explain how cells are assigned positional values. Some of the major options presented at the meeting were: (1) reading gradients of substances, (2) telling time, (3) cell-to-cell communication and (4) topological considerations involving the formation of peaks by factors such as squeezing. In the limb, cytodifferentiation is a late result of both matrix and positional effects. However specified, the mature cells in the limb retain a strong memory of their position. Positional memory is evident in regeneration experiments, particularly those involving displacement of components of the limb.

Morphogenesis of the nervous system is complex enough that it almost needs to be discussed in a separate category. Following primary induction, early development of the central nervous system involves a mix of proliferation, cell movement, changes in cell shape and mechanical factors. Enough has been learned about the two-dimensional behavior of amphibian neurulation for Jacobson and Gordon to construct useful computer models. Jacobson didn't dare speculate on how many years and how much more data would be required before modelling can be extended to a third dimension.

Caviness showed that pattern formation within the brain involves the radial migration of already specified cells along cellular guides (radial glial cells) into well-defined layers. These migrations require cells to pass through previously laid down layers of neurons. It is very difficult to attempt to analyze cortical layering by the traditional methodology of experimental embryology, but natural experiments in the form of genetic mutants with behavioral manifestations have helped greatly in understanding morphogenetic events in the brain.

The brain plays a prominent role in morphogenesis of the head. Both the brain and spinal cord, as well as the sense organs, induce protective coverings of hard tissue around themselves. Whereas the initial formation of the cranium depends upon inductive influences, the final shape of the skull is determined to a great extent upon forces generated by the brain and the pressure of the cerebrospinal fluid. Kollar has extended the morphogenetic role of the nervous system to the peripheral nerves by his hypothesis that nerves determine tooth pattern. The roles of growth and mechanical forces have received comparativeely little stress in most considerations of morphogenesis, but the presentations by both Smith and Bookstein graphically illustrated the importance of these factors when the overall formation of a structure is examined. This is particularly evident in the craniofacial region, but a number of the participants expressed a new-found awareness of the possible implications of these factors in early development.

There are innumerable varieties of abnormal development, which involve many types of mechanisms. Perrin stressed the importance of differentiating between the disturbance of normal developmental mechanisms and factors, such as destruction or pressure, which can lead to malformations. Gluecksohn-Waelsch demonstrated how through the study of mutants many aspects of development can be related to the genes. The number of effects that can be related to the malfunction of a single gene is often surprising. The possibility of relating some genetic syndromes to disturbances in regulatory genes was brought up.

Smith introduced the concept of deformation as opposed to malformation and the important role of mechanical factors in producing them. Equally important, he demonstrated means by which mechanical factors can be used in the correction of deformation in postnatal life. Variations in craniofacial growth and the ability to predict growth patterns both before and after corrective treatment are becoming increasingly prominent considerations in orthodontics and orofacial surgery. Bookstein showed the value of non-traditional means of taking measurements in this region and the extent to which the data can be dealt with mathematically.

The proceedings of this symposium demonstrated that there is still no central unifying theme underlying morphogenesis, although most of the research has settled along several major modes of thought. In some areas new or modified models await the acquisition of additional new data, and in other areas the data remain to be fit into potentially unifying models. The importance of interdisciplinary research looms ever larger, with biology and physics being combined in studies of cell aggregation, biology and chemistry in studies of the extracellular matrix and biology and mathematics in the modelling of morphogenetic processes. Will the field go full circle and like Driesch, again combine biology and philosophy?

Subject Index